Register Now for Online A Your Book!

SPRINGER PUBLISHING COMPANY
CONNECT™

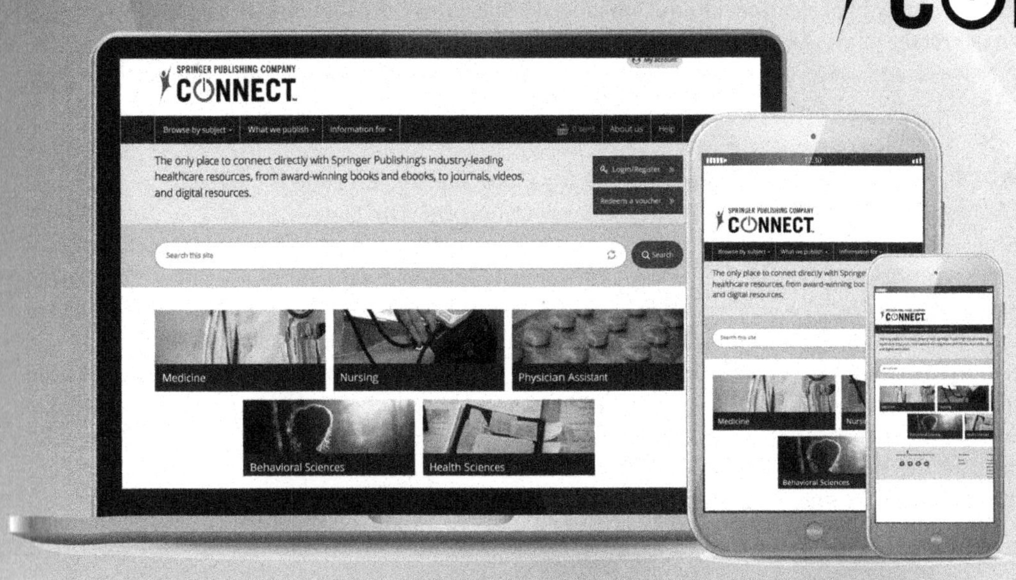

Your print purchase of *The DNP Project Workbook* **includes online access to the contents of your book**—increasing accessibility, portability, and searchability!

Access today at:

http://connect.springerpub.com/content/book/978-0-8261-7433-8 or scan the QR code at the right with your smartphone and enter the access code below.

8Y5CBG1K

Scan here for quick access.

If you are experiencing problems accessing the digital component of this product, please contact our customer service department at cs@springerpub.com

The online access with your print purchase is available at the publisher's discretion and may be removed at any time without notice.

Publisher's Note: New and used products purchased from third-party sellers are not guaranteed for quality, authenticity, or access to any included digital components.

Molly J. Bradshaw, DNP, APRN, FNP-BC, WHNP-BC, is an associate professor, DNP program coordinator, and faculty innovator at Eastern Kentucky University, Richmond, Kentucky. She completed her undergraduate nursing degrees at Eastern Kentucky University (1998, 2001); got her master's degree at the University of Kentucky (2005); and earned her doctor of nursing practice degree at Rutgers, The State University of New Jersey (2016). She is nationally board certified as both a family and a women's health nurse practitioner. She maintains an active clinical practice at First Choice Immediate Care, in Columbia, Kentucky. Her 21-year career in nursing includes diverse positions, including staff nurse (labor and delivery and the operating room), school nurse, nurse manager, nurse practitioner, and active service in the United States Navy Nurse Corps. Her academic scholarship is rooted in teaching innovation, use of infographics/social media, and the DNP Project. Her published works focus on clinical subjects such as prescribing habits of nurse practitioners and chronic disease management, including hypertension, chronic obstructive pulmonary disease, obesity, and multiple sclerosis. She currently serves as secretary of the American Association of Colleges of Nursing (AACN) Steering Committee for the Practice Leadership Network and as secretary for Pricilla's Cancer Foundation, operated by Dunnville First Baptist Church, Dunnville, Kentucky.

Tracy R. Vitale, DNP, RNC-OB, C-EFM, NE-BC, has been a nurse for more than 20 years and is currently an assistant professor and specialty director of DNP Projects/DNP Project courses at Rutgers, The State University of New Jersey School of Nursing, New Brunswick, New Jersey. She received her baccalaureate degree in nursing from The College of New Jersey (2000), her master's in nursing from the University of Phoenix (2006), and a doctor of nursing practice degree from Rutgers, The State University of New Jersey (2016). Prior to transitioning to academia in 2017, her nursing career included leadership positions in maternal–fetal medicine research, outpatient private maternal–fetal medicine and high-risk obstetrics practice, and labor and delivery/perinatal evaluation and treatment departments. Dr. Vitale sits on the board of directors for the Organization of Nurse Leaders of New Jersey and is actively involved with the mentorship committee for which she has spoken on a local, state, and national level about the mentorship of nurse leaders. She also serves on the advisory council for the New Jersey Collaborating Center for Nursing, which focuses on nursing workforce issues. Dr. Vitale also serves as a manuscript reviewer for select journals.

The DNP Project Workbook

A Step-by-Step Process for Success

Molly J. Bradshaw, DNP, APRN, FNP-BC, WHNP-BC

Tracy R. Vitale, DNP, RNC-OB, C-EFM, NE-BC

SPRINGER PUBLISHING COMPANY

Springer Publishing Company, LLC
11 West 42nd Street
New York, NY 10036
www.springerpub.com
http://connect.springerpub.com/home

Acquisitions Editor: Adrianne Brigido
Compositor: S4Carlisle Publishing Services

ISBN: 978-0-8261-7432-1
ebook ISBN: 978-0-8261-7433-8
Instructor's PowerPoints ISBN: 978-0-8261-7434-5
Chapter/Lesson Mapping to DNP Essentials ISBN: 978-0-8261-7435-2
Rutgers DNP Project ISBN: 978-0-8261-7431-4
Supplementary Editable Activities ISBN: 978-0-8261-7437-6

DOI: 10.1891/9780826174338

Qualified instructors may request supplements by emailing textbook@springerpub.com
An editable activities supplement with materials for Chapters 1, 3, 4, and 7 is available from www.springerpub.com/dpw

Supplemental DNP Project documents for Chapter 10 are available at connect.springerpub.com/content/book/978-0-8261-7433-8/ch10

21 22 23 / 5 4

Printed in the United States of America by Gasch Printing.

For my grandparents and my family, who have always supported me in life, school, work, and faith. For numerous others who seem to show up at just the right times in my life. For my faithful K-9 companion, Macho, the Yorkie. For a special person who encouraged me to believe in my dreams. What would I have done without you?

MOLLY J. BRADSHAW

This text is dedicated to those who have always supported my efforts, encouraged me, and told me I could accomplish anything I put my mind to, especially my parents, Joseph and JoAnne; my husband, Joe; and my children, Joseph and Sophia. I would also like to acknowledge the support of my colleagues, including Lydia, Molly, Sue, and Sharon, for their continued guidance and support. You all have allowed me to achieve more than I could have ever imagined. I hope to inspire others as much as you have done for me. I'd also like to acknowledge those who have literally been by my side throughout this entire nursing journey, including Jack, Harvey, and Darius.

TRACY R. VITALE

Contents

Faculty Contributors and Reviewers

Maureen Anderson, DNP, APN, CRNA
Assistant Professor, Director of Simulation
Division of Advanced Nursing Practice
Rutgers School of Nursing
Rutgers, The State University of New Jersey
New Brunswick, New Jersey

Tracy Arnold, DNP, RN
Assistant Professor
Associate Dean for Hunt School of Nursing
Gardner Webb University

Irina Benenson, DNP, FNP-C, CEN
Assistant Professor
Division of Advanced Nursing Practice
Rutgers School of Nursing
Rutgers, The State University of New Jersey
New Brunswick, New Jersey

Debra Bingham, DrPH, RN, FAAN
Associate Professor
University of Maryland
Baltimore, Maryland

Molly J. Bradshaw, DNP, APRN, FNP-BC, WHNP-BC
Associate Professor, DNP Program Coordinator
Department of Baccalaureate and Graduate Nursing
Eastern Kentucky University
Richmond, Kentucky

David G. Campbell-O'Dell, DNP, APRN, FNP-BC, FAANP
President
Doctors of Nursing Practice, Inc.
Key West, Florida

Thomas Christenbery, PhD, RN, CNE
Professor and Director of Program Evaluation
Vanderbilt University
Nashville, Tennessee

Jill Cornelison, DNP, RN
Associate Professor
Department of Baccalaureate and Graduate Nursing
Eastern Kentucky University
Richmond, Kentucky

Mary DiGuilio, DNP, APN, FAANP
Assistant Professor
Specialty Director for the Adult-Gerontology Nurse Practitioner Program
Rutgers, The State University of New Jersey

Margaret Dreker, MPA, MLS
Information and Education Librarian
Rutgers, The State University of New Jersey
New Brunswick, New Jersey

Mercedes Echevarria, DNP, APN-C
Associate Professor and Assistant Dean for the Doctor of Nursing Practice Program
George Washington University
Washington, District of Columbia

David Anthony Forrester, PhD, RN, ANEF, FAAN
Professor
Division of Nursing Science
Rutgers School of Nursing
Rutgers, The State University of New Jersey
New Brunswick, New Jersey

Karen Gilbert, MLS, MPH
Associate University Librarian
Library Liaison to the Health Sciences
Eastern Kentucky University
Richmond, Kentucky

Patricia Hindin, PhD, CNM, RYT 200
Associate Professor, Fellow
Division of Advanced Nursing Practice
Rutgers School of Nursing
Rutgers, The State University of New Jersey
New Brunswick, New Jersey

Sharon Lock, PhD, APRN, FNAP, FAANP
Professor and Assistant Dean of Faculty Practice
Director of the Wilmore Faculty Practice
University of Kentucky
Lexington, Kentucky

Rachel Mack, PhD, DNP, APRN, C-FNP, CNE
Associate Dean of Academic Affairs
Frontier University
Hyden, Kentucky

Marilyn Oermann, PhD, RN, ANEF, FAAN
Thelma M. Ingles Professor of Nursing
Director of Evaluation and Educational Research
Duke University
Durham, North Carolina

Nancy Owens, DNP, APRN, FNP-C
Associate Professor
Department of Baccalaureate and Graduate Nursing
Eastern Kentucky University
Richmond, Kentucky

Sallie Porter, DNP, PhD, APN, RN-BC, CPNP
Associate Professor
Division of Advanced Nursing Practice
Rutgers School of Nursing
Rutgers, The State University of New Jersey
New Brunswick, New Jersey

Gina Purdue, DNP, RN, CNE
Associate Professor
Department of Baccalaureate and Graduate Nursing
Eastern Kentucky University
Richmond, Kentucky

Lori Smith, DNP, APRN, FNP-C
Assistant Professor
Director of the Graduate Nursing Program
Henderson State University

Grace H. Sun, DNP, APRN, FNP-BC
Assistant Professor
Texas Tech University Health Sciences Center

Tracy R. Vitale, DNP, RNC-OB, C-EFM, NE-BC
Assistant Professor
Division of Advanced Nursing Practice
Rutgers School of Nursing
Rutgers, The State University of New Jersey
New Brunswick, New Jersey

Student Contributors and Reviewers

Brenda Caudill, DNP, APRN

Angela Clark, DNP, RNC-OB

Martha De Crisce, DNP, APN, FNP-C

Christine Leithead, DNP, APRN, FNP-C

Tarnia Newton, DNP, MSN, FNP-C

Aleksandra Novik, BBA, DNP, APN-C

Michelle Santoro, DNP, APN, FNP-C

Angela Wood, DNP, APRN, FNP-C, PPCNP-BC

Margaret Zoellers, DNP, APRN, FNP-BC

Foreword

It is a great honor and privilege to have been asked to introduce this valuable book, *The DNP Project Workbook: A Step-by-Step Process for Success*, a book that offers a most welcome guide to those of you who aspire to earn your DNP degree and lead nursing, healthcare, and society now and into the future.

The DNP degree is a leadership credential in problem-solving. As a DNP-prepared nurse, you will be expected to lead nursing, health policy, and healthcare. In fact, a key tenet of the Institute of Medicine's (IOM's) report, *The Future of Nursing: Leading Change, Advancing Health* (IOM, 2011), is that "Nurses should be full partners, with physicians, and other health professionals, in redesigning health care in the United States" (p. 8). This means that as a DNP-prepared nurse, you will be expected to lead interprofessional partnerships and collaborate with stakeholders at every level of the current and future healthcare system, including among nurse generalists, APRNs, and other healthcare providers and policy makers.

According to the American Association of Colleges of Nursing (AACN; 2015), the purpose of designing and implementing a scholarly, evidence-based DNP Project is that it should be an academic experience that allows you to demonstrate competency of the DNP Essentials. Achieving these Essentials requires you to engage in leadership behaviors and utilize evidence to solve complex problems. The DNP Project experience should help prepare you to lead changes at the highest levels of clinical practice and policy, and ultimately improve the overall quality of healthcare (AACN, 2015).

Our new healthcare environment is rapidly changing and demanding better care for individuals, improved health outcomes for populations, and lower costs for consumers. In this new environment of rapid change and increasing complexity, DNP-prepared nurses are being challenged to lead healthcare systems that offer universal accessibility, coordination across all points of care, and the delivery of high-quality, safe care—and all this at an affordable price. This environment challenges DNP-prepared nurses to understand and embrace collaboration, team-based care, and partnerships, and to focus on providing excellence for healthcare consumers in achieving optimal health outcomes (Salmond & Forrester, 2016).

Informed by the historical underpinnings of nursing and advanced practice nursing, this workbook provides DNP students with the strategies to engage in evidence-based practice change and leadership opportunities in which to apply these strategies to the realities of advanced practice nursing. It offers DNP students a clear focus on professional practice, clinical leadership, and policy making. Here, leadership is conceptualized as being concerned with the APRN's ability to influence others by building highly productive teams and identifying and working with stakeholders to reach specific goals in order to achieve excellence in nursing and healthcare.

This book offers a wealth of strategies that will be tremendously helpful to DNP students in achieving excellence by developing, implementing, evaluating, and disseminating high-quality DNP Projects. Real-world examples and useful exercises are provided. DNP students are challenged to think critically, plan ahead, and be strategic in their decision-making in choosing meaningful, feasible project designs and methods. Students are invited to look ahead to the future and ponder the possibilities of a desired future for nursing and healthcare.

This much-needed book is an excellent resource for guiding the next generation of DNP-prepared nurses who strive to lead and improve patient-related outcomes. It is my hope that *The DNP Project Workbook: A Step-by-Step Process for Success* will educate, inspire, and empower its readers to lead nursing, health, healthcare, and society into a better, healthier future.

Please enjoy your journey as you proceed with your DNP program of study and carry out your DNP Project.

David Anthony Forrester, PhD, RN, ANEF, FAAN
Professor, Division of Nursing Science, Rutgers University School of Nursing
Clinical Professor, Rutgers University Robert Wood Johnson Medical School
New Brunswick, New Jersey

REFERENCES

American Association of Colleges of Nursing. (2015). The doctor of nursing practice: Current issues and clarifying recommendations. Retrieved from https://www.aacnnursing.org/Portals/42/News/White-Papers/DNP-Implementation-TF-Report-8-15.pdf

Institute of Medicine. (2011). *The future of nursing: Leading change, advancing health.* Washington, DC: National Academies Press. Retrieved from http://www.nationalacademies.org/hmd/Reports/2010/The-Future-of-Nursing-Leading-Change-Advancing-Health.aspx

Salmond, S. W., & Forrester, D. A. (2016). Nurses leading change: The time is now! In D. A. Forrester (Ed.), *Nursing's greatest leaders: A history of activism* (pp. 269–286). New York, NY: Springer Publishing Company.

Preface

WHY YOU NEED THIS WORKBOOK

Your choice to pursue the DNP degree requires the completion of a DNP Project. For most students, the thought of this academic requirement is overwhelming at first. The most difficult part is the beginning. You need a place to start. You need a process to follow that creates momentum toward success. We are here to help! Let us be your guide. The purpose of this workbook is to deliver a step-by-step process toward finishing your DNP Project. The lessons engage you in active learning, give you real-world context, and support you with practical tips and advice. The workbook helps you avoid stalemate, minimizes your frustration, and encourages you to think like an innovative problem-solver. Our goal is to help you and your team make meaningful changes in practice that can improve health outcomes for the patients and populations we serve.

THE VISION AND INSPIRATION FOR THIS WORK

The vision for this workbook started with my own DNP experience. I know now that my experience was typical. I struggled in the beginning. I changed my topic around and couldn't seem to find that perfect question to ask. Faculty used words and phrases that contradicted. For example, one would say "Your research project," and then another would say "No, you are not doing research," which confused me terribly. I could not sort out what was good to know in class versus what I needed to know for creating the project. I felt like certain classmates were ahead of me, that their ideas were so great, and that I was falling behind. It was all overwhelming, to the point of tears. I didn't know how to break down the process of creating the project.

My classmate Tracy R. Vitale also had reservations at the beginning of the process. "Making the decision to even return for a DNP was not easy. Maybe it was the 5-year-old twins, two dogs, and the husband I had at home or trying to figure out how I would balance working full time with returning to school full time. I came to the program having a general idea of the topic I wanted my DNP Project to be about ... even though I didn't quite know exactly what the actual project would be." The good news is that we all made it. We all graduated. But having a workbook to break down the steps would have been tremendously helpful.

Frustration with the DNP Project process became my motivator. Being a nurse educator in a sprawling BSN–DNP program, I committed to finding out for myself everything to be known about the DNP Project. I was going to make myself an expert and learn to teach the components of project development in a systematic way. My timing coincided with an opportunity to become the Director of DNP Projects at my school. What followed next became the basis of what we teach you in this workbook.

First, I created key documents for our department. These documents outlined the minimum requirements for the DNP Project as described by the American Association of Colleges of Nursing (AACN). I made a chart comparing the differences between the DNP and PhD degrees. I rewrote the DNP tool kit for our school and pitched it to the faculty for approval. These revised documents and quick references helped create a more common language to use when discussing the DNP Project. (We are going to share similar documents with you in this workbook.)

Then, with these faculty-approved documents in hand, I started hosting "DNP Project workshops." The workshops were offered outside of classroom time, and ahead of courses in which the DNP Project proposal would be written. It gave students an opportunity to learn about the specifics of the project, do exercises to develop their ideas, and get feedback in a group context. Students commented:

- "I have a better understanding and foundation of what the DNP Project is and what I need to complete. Having taken this workshop, I no longer feel like a 'deer in headlights.' Despite still feeling apprehensive and anxious about the process, I have a stronger feeling that I can complete this within the time frame allotted."
- "Just the fact that we got an insight on what the project is about and what the steps will be in completing it. I knew nothing about this project and was terrified of it, but after coming to this workshop I feel a bit more comfortable knowing what is expected."

I tracked the attendees over the course of their DNP Projects and found that those who attended the workshops experienced less anxiety and made better overall project progress compared to their peers. As a final step, I began a basic audit of the DNP Projects completed by the graduating class. I used the DNP Essentials and the minimum DNP Project requirements outlined by AACN (2015) as a starting point. This process gave me better clarity on what elements need improvement in our program.

Ultimately, the inspiration for this work centers first on you—my student, my colleague. Students in DNP programs are registered nurses. Therefore, we are already colleagues. As a faculty member or mentor, you are hiring me, engaging me, to help guide you to a higher level of practice. Our commitment to you in return is to make things as simple, manageable, and feasible as possible. If you work hard with us, you will finish strong. But our real driver has to be our patients. They face complex problems and need our help. The DNP degree is about giving you a new skill set to assist your patients. The DNP Project is an opportunity to practice those skills in a real-world context, with the help and guidance of your DNP faculty.

WHAT TO EXPECT FROM THE WORKBOOK

The DNP Project Workbook: A Step-by-Step Process for Success is a collection of individual lessons spanning 10 chapters. Overall, the workbook starts with fundamental, knowledge-based information regarding the DNP Project. It then moves through the development of the DNP team, the feasibility of project ideas, and later through the elements of developing, implementing, evaluating, disseminating, and sustaining the project. Real-world projects are explored in Chapter 10, Finishing Strong: Project Profiles and Empowerment, and tips, advice, and expert commentary are offered throughout.

The lessons are designed to be completed in short intervals. In our experience, DNP students are better able to complete shorter lessons over a given time span. This makes it easier to manage with full-time work, families, and so on. Each lesson gives you some brief background information and then leads you through an active learning exercise. At the end of each lesson, we offer advice for next steps, remind you of key milestones, and recommend additional references and resources. The lessons build on one another as the chapter progresses.

The workbook is designed with usability and flexibility in mind. Open, white space is available in each lesson if you prefer to write directly in the workbook. Electronic versions are offered as well; these can be filled out electronically if you need to send a copy to a faculty member. You might need a fresh clean copy to begin a lesson again. There are forms that will help you better document and organize ideas, communicate with stakeholders, and track your progress. Also, we understand that there is variation across DNP programs in terms of the order in which content is taught. Having the lessons broken down individually allows you to complete them in the order that best correlates with the requirements at your school. In addition, the workbook includes useful instructor resources so that the process can be easily implemented into courses—there are PowerPoint slides that summarize content and chapters and lessons are mapped to the AACN DNP Essentials.

This is a unique product because it is a workbook, not a "textbook" in the traditional sense. It is a platform intended to generate momentum. Our tone and language are purposely nonacademic, conversational, and slightly raw. We want you to feel that we are guiding you and teaching you as mentors. We recognize that this information is not always comprehensive. Rather, it is a place to start. To supplement the context of activities, we refer to outside sources, like the Institute for Healthcare Improvement (IHI). We draw inspiration from outside, nonhealthcare business concepts. We also correlate the content of the lessons with more detailed reading available in the Springer DNP library. If you find that you need more information, we point out target chapters, specific content, and additional resources that you can further explore.

A LIVING PROCESS

I often refer to the DNP Project process as a "living process." It is organic, growing, and always under development. Why? Because it a practice-focused doctorate. Practice changes. Practice evolves. As the healthcare system evolves, as patients/populations evolve, as evidence evolves, so must the DNP Project process. The DNP Projects of today should look nothing like the DNP Projects of the future. We must change to meet the needs of the patients and the discipline.

The constant here is the approach we take to solving problems. What is the problem? What has been done so far to address the problem? What resources and evidence do we have to inform solutions? Can we implement a change in practice and measure its impact? Should we continue that practice or abandon it and make new changes? It is the approach to problem-solving that helps us set a standard for "minimum expectations" of a DNP Project. The key milestones lead to addressing a problem in practice.

This is a critical conversation because as a student you will hear faculty talking about "rigor" in the DNP Project process. We talk about this more in the workbook, but for now, embrace the idea of quality. We want you to do quality work that meets a minimum set of expectations based on national standards and the requirements at your school. The minimum expectations ensure a degree of equity among DNP Projects.

"But I want to do a 'good' project," you say? Of course, we want that for you, too. But remember that you are entering a living process. As you complete this work, we ask that you and your faculty be open to new ideas. A "good" project is a completed project that engaged a student in a meaningful learning experience while meeting national and program expectations. There is no such thing as a "perfect" project, unless unicorns also exist.

FINAL THOUGHTS

Together, our experience offers a variety of perspectives as both faculty and former DNP students. We are both still engaged in clinical practice—I am a nurse practitioner and Tracy, my coauthor, is a nurse executive. We represent a DNP spectrum: (a) a large, research-based school of nursing in an urban setting; and (b) a smaller regional, online program, catering to rural populations. In this workbook we present to you a united front of DNP content to serve you so that you can impact your communities, our nation, and the world.

Regardless of the size of your institution, DNP core courses are based on the DNP Essentials. The core courses of a DNP curriculum offer opportunities for you to gain new knowledge and skills. This allows you to examine a complex problem through multiple lenses. Each course offers something that can contribute to the DNP Project. The DNP Project will morph as you complete these courses. Do not expect your first ideas to be your final ideas or you will likely be disappointed. Sit back, keep an open mind, and learn something new.

The common thread of problem-solving runs through the fibers of nursing and at our core is a constant in our profession. We are problem solvers. That is truly what the DNP degree is all about. Keep in mind that this is hard work; it should be, you will graduate with a doctoral degree. We want to help you through this process step-by-step. Hang with us. Just start here, let's work hard, and you will finish strong!

Molly J. Bradshaw

Introduction

The DNP degree is a terminal degree in nursing that requires a high level of professionalism. Before you begin, we have organized a series of tasks that you should complete to be fully prepared for the DNP Project process. These tasks include suggested activities for self-assessment, tips for getting organized, and recommendations for basic skill sets that are necessary, yet not typically included in coursework.

WRITING A PROFESSIONAL BIO

Having a professional bio is perhaps one of the most important pieces you can write about yourself. Consider it to be the first impression of who you are, what you have done, and highlight your areas of interest. It is often difficult to write because, by nature, most of us are not very good about boasting or self-promotion. Keep in mind that professional bios can appear in a variety of formats, including an organization's website spotlighting employees, a personal website, or even on social media platforms like LinkedIn, Facebook, or Twitter. Bios are used as speaker introductions during professional presentations and even in online courses to introduce yourself to other students. Regardless of the forum, a personal bio allows you to highlight your interests, expertise, and the work you have done in a succinct format.

Helpful Hints:

- Keep it to an appropriate length. Aim for about 10 sentences. However, recognize this may need to be adjusted based on what the bio is for: Twitter/Instagram bios will be short due to space limitations; website bios can be longer; speaker bios will also be relatively short (about 10 sentences).
- Use the correct tense. Write your bio in the third person.
- Remember that this is a living document. The biography will change as your accomplishments and career evolve. Edit and revise your personal bio often to keep it current.
- Showcase your accomplishments. Include at least one professional accomplishment.
- Tell us about you, the person. Consider a statement about your life outside of your work, like maybe something about your hometown, family, or a hobby/interest.

PROFESSIONAL PICTURES

We have already discussed establishing yourself through your professional identity. Now you should have a picture to go along with it. We are not talking about a picture of you relaxing on the beach or having a good time at your favorite sporting event. We are talking about a professional headshot … not far from what we all did in kindergarten when we showcased our pearly-white smiles. Remember, this is your time to make a first impression—make yourself look the part both online and in person.

Helpful Hints:

- Look the part. Look like the professional you are presenting yourself to be.
- The photo does not need to cost a fortune. Look to see whether your current employer or school offers the option of professional photos. If not, consider a local photography studio.
- Wear something you feel confident in. Avoid patterns, seasonal outfits, or clothes you would wear to a party. Remember, this is a picture intended to reflect you as a professional.
- Use your photo on any platform you can. Since you invested the time and effort in getting a professional headshot, use it as your visual identity for those social media accounts and websites.

WRITING A CURRICULUM VITAE

Once you make the decision to look for that dream job, you need to be prepared to reach out to potential stakeholders, organizations, and potential employers. Having a curriculum vitae (CV) that is written well provides you the opportunity to showcase why you are a good fit for the organization. Understand that résumés are summative and generally shorter, no longer than one page. CVs, on the other hand, are longer and provide a more thorough, comprehensive summary of all you have accomplished.

Helpful Hints:

- Keep it simple. Avoid a cute, creative font. Choose one that is simple and easy to read. Consider using Times New Roman, Arial, Calibri, or Cambria for example.
- Use an appropriate font size: Keep the text at 11 or 12 points. Your name and section headers can be slightly larger at 14 or 16 points.
- Consistency is critical. If you are underlining section titles, do so for all of them.
- Formatting is important. White space is a good thing. Keep margins consistent (1 inch on all sides is standard).
- Add a summary statement/CV objective: Include a short paragraph explaining why you are the person best qualified for the position.
- Include all necessary sections. Include contact information (including email, website, phone number, etc.); education; work experience; presentations/publications; research experience; licensure/certifications; awards; and additional training/skills, including additional languages spoken.

BUSINESS CARDS

In the age of technology does it even make sense to have a business card? Some tech experts even argue that business cards are obsolete in today's technological world. True, but consider the fact that there are still "old school" professionals who find the business card much more tangible than a text that may get lost or forgotten about in a smartphone. Business cards are also not subject to a bad Wi-Fi connection or dead spots. Consider the business card to be an extension of your online identity.

Business cards allow for a quick, immediate exchange of information in a variety of settings like conferences, guest lectures, and presentations. Imagine this scenario: You are presenting your DNP Project (or other research) at a conference and decide to check out the other posters. If someone is interested in speaking with you but your poster is unattended, leaving a bunch of business cards will allow the person to grab one and have your information so they can reach out to you at a later time.

Helpful Hints:

- Create a card specific to you as a professional. Depending on the nature of your DNP Project, you may or may not want to use the same cards given to you by an employer. Distinguish/appreciate the student role versus the employee role.
- Include the appropriate email. Again, consider the best approach for people to contact you. If you are not planning on staying with your employer, it may be better to use a personal professional account.

- List your name and email address at minimum. We recommend you use your full name, credentials, and preferred email address at minimum.
- Keep the look professional. Be sensitive to color, logos, and so forth. Do not use logos without permission.

LEARNING STYLE

Understanding your learning style facilitates success. This workbook is designed to work for students of various learning styles through clear direction, action, and reflection. Although there are many assessments available to determine one's learning style, we recommend simply starting with the VARK Learning Inventory (http://vark-learn.com/the-vark-questionnaire).

LEADERSHIP STYLE

Just as learning style varies, so does leadership style. No way is the "right" way, but certainly some methods are more effective than others at different points of time. It is important to recognize the different types of leadership and how these impact those being led. In the following, we outline different types of leadership styles and historical figures past and present who have been identified with a specific leadership style.

- Authoritarian: Needs individual control of all decisions. "What I say goes." Minimal to no input from others. *Examples:* Steve Jobs (Apple), Bill Gates (Microsoft)
- Laissez-Faire: A hands-off approach to leadership in which others are the decision makers. Can surround themselves with experts who can get the job done. Conversely, sometimes this leadership style can have the opposite result and productivity is very low. *Examples:* Andrew Mellon (industrialist/philanthropist), Ronald Reagan (U.S. president)
- Democratic: Leader works together with others during the decision-making process. *Example:* George Washington (U.S. president)
- Bureaucratic: Leadership follows a strict hierarchy with clear rules and positions of power. *Examples:* Winston Churchill (British prime minister), Colin Powell (former U.S. secretary of state)
- Charismatic: Relies on charm and charisma to influence people using the art of persuasion. These leaders use their conviction and commitment as their motivation. *Examples:* Mother Teresa (missionary), Lee Iacocca (Crysler Motors)
- Transformational: Leader and team work together toward a common goal and "big picture." *Examples:* Martin Luther King, Jr. (American minister), Walt Disney (Disney)

Helpful Hints:

- Be inspired. Think about what is important to you and what inspires you. Use this as motivation and create goals. Use that motivation to lead your team.
- Appeal to your team: Your goals must align with the goals of those you hope will follow.
- Reward and recognize achievement: Whether the victories are small or big, celebrate and reward accomplishments.
- Develop and demand: Develop your team with the skills members need and demand quality work.
- Keep going: Don't ever give up. Setbacks will happen, but a true leader will persevere.
- Know your leadership style: What type of leader are you? Consider taking an online leadership self-assessment to see.

BASIC TECHNOLOGY SKILLS

Basic technology skills are a requirement for the DNP Project. The skills identified here are not necessarily always skills that are taught as part of the program, but rather ones you need to learn/refine on your own. It is also not uncommon for students to come without the skill set, yet we expect it. It behooves you to become familiar with these computer programs as early in your DNP program as possible. Although it will take some time on the front end to learn, this investment will pay off 10-fold on the back end when the programs can work for you and make life much easier. Talk to your DNP faculty about preferences for technology. Some software may be offered free of charge through your school. Resources may also be available through the libraries that teach you how to use key software programs.

Helpful Hints:

- Familiarize yourself with Word-processing programs: Microsoft Word, Google Docs, etc.
    - Key skills:
        - Creating a table of contents using levels of headings
        - Formatting/inserting tables and figures
        - Creating hanging indents for reference pages (for those required to use APA)
        - Proper use of page and section breaks
        - Integrating EndNote/RefWorks into Word
- Familiarize yourself with data-management systems: Microsoft Excel, SPSS, etc.
    - Key skills:
        - Data entry
        - Creating graphs and tables from data sets
        - Use of basic formulas for data analysis
- Familiarize yourself with presentation software: Microsoft PowerPoint, Google Slides, Prezi, etc.
    - Key skills:
        - Professional presentation design; proper use of images, art
        - Use of notes section
        - Use of presenter mode (for schools with projection abilities)
        - How to embed videos
- Familiarize yourself with citation management software: EndNote, RefWorks, Zotero, etc.
    - Key skills:
        - How to import/export citations
        - Use of EndNote/RefWorks in Word to "cite as you write"
        - How to change formatting for different reference styles

TIME-MANAGEMENT STRATEGIES

We all recognize that life is happening at the same time as your DNP Project. Careers, children, spouses, and even parents and grandchildren are all vying for your attention. It's hard to say no, but recognizing the need to find balance is important.

Helpful Hints:

- Be committed: Once you sit down to work, commit to staying with it for the time you set aside. Avoid distractions during this time—do not check emails, take phone calls, or check social media. If this is time set aside for school work, then keep it that way.
- Keep a schedule: Planning out a timeline and sticking to it help create some accountability.
- Schedule time to think: You will not be innovative if you are exhausted.
- Use your calendar: It is another way to stay organized; set deadlines and block off time as designated to complete your tasks.
- First things first: Prioritize your work. The work that rises to the top of the to-do list should be done first.

- Say no. You do not need a reason to say no. Sometimes saying no is the best way to ensure your work gets completed. Avoid overcommitment. Saying yes to something is time taken away from writing your DNP Project proposal/final project.
- Plan ahead: Plan your weeks ahead of time. Start on Sunday and figure out what needs to be accomplished. This allows you to focus and set goals for the week's activities.
- Schedule breaks: Planning for a break periodically helps you avoid burnout.
- Stay organized: This includes keeping your workspace organized as well as your mind.
- Take care of yourself: This means both physically and mentally. Physical activity like exercise or yoga is helpful. Also important is to make sure you get enough sleep. This also includes setting aside some relaxation time.
- Delegate: If there are tasks that can be delegated, do so!

CREATING GOOD WRITING HABITS

The DNP Project and other doctoral work require high-level scholarly writing. If academic writing is not a strong skill for you, seek help early and often. Many schools provide assistance with writing for graduate students. However, we observe that students fail to take advantage of these services, or seek outside services, in a timely manner. Writing requires practice and time. It is imperative to establish good writing habits as a doctoral student.

Helpful Hints:

- Workspace: Establish a designated workspace where you will go when you are ready to write.
- Make it a date: Set writing goals on your calendar.
- No way; today's the day: List daily nonnegotiable responsibilities.
- Make it a date: Write 5 out of 7 days for 50 minutes at a time (use a timer).
- Just write it: Sit in your chair and write anything on a blank page.
- Stay on schedule: When the timer goes off, get up and move. As scheduled, go back for another round.
- Keep track: Track your writing time when you are done.
- Keep a buddy: Have an accountability buddy who you can check in with; text them when you've finished writing and tell them how long you worked.
- Proofread: Despite feeling like you know your paper inside and out, proofread it. In fact, have someone else read it. The challenge is that we know what it is supposed to say, but that doesn't mean that is what it actually says.
- Know your limitations: Although it is a large investment, consider the possibility of using your college/university's writing center or even hiring an editor.
- Have a backup of your files: Save your documents to a flash drive or a cloud account, email them to yourself, and so on. Consider the situation of a friend whose car was broken into: Not only was her laptop (with her project on it) stolen, but so was the flash drive containing the only other version of the project.
- Name your files appropriately: Include your last name, date, and keyword/phrase in the file name. If you just save files by course or week of the assignment, you may not be able to find things later.

COMMUNICATION

As the project evolves, it is imperative to keep a record of your communications with your DNP team, stakeholders, and others.

Helpful Hints:

- Keep a communication log: Document dates when you communicated, topics discussed, and next steps. Keeping this log allows you to establish clear goals and timelines in order to keep you on track.
- Consider timing: If you are asking someone to read your paper and provide constructive feedback, recognize that it is unrealistic to expect a return of your paper within 24 to 48 hours. Faculty, editors, writing centers, among others, are busy. Although your work is certainly important, reading your paper is not their only obligation. If you are looking for feedback prior to submitting for a grade or the next phase of your project, plan accordingly to give the reader an appropriate time frame to review the material—usually about a week or 2.
- Follow-up: If you send an email, generally, a response within 48 to 72 hours is customary. Plan ahead with your faculty and understand the process for communicating emergencies. Lack of planning does not constitute an emergency.

In summary, an introduction to common elements of professional behavior, basic technology skills, and self-assessment accelerate your success in the DNP Project process. Moving forward, we recommend and caution you that you should fully discuss DNP program requirements with your faculty. We are now ready to begin the work of the DNP Project.

RESOURCES

The *DNP Project Workbook* includes a robust ancillary package. Qualified instructors may obtain access by emailing textbook@springerpub.com. Available instructor resources:

- Chapter-Based PowerPoint Presentations
- Chapter/Lesson Mapping to DNP Essentials

Purchasers of this book may access the following resources via http://connect.springerpub.com/content/book/978-0-8261-7433-8:

- Supplementary Editable Activities
- Supplemental Sample DNP Projects

1

Understanding the DNP Degree and DNP Project

Molly J. Bradshaw, Tracy R. Vitale, Rachel Mack, and Sallie Porter

Lessons

OBJECTIVES

The purpose of this chapter is to introduce fundamental concepts of the DNP degree and the DNP Project. The student will complete a series of lessons designed to introduce basic information that is necessary to start the process of DNP Project planning.

By the end of this chapter, you will be able to:

- Compare and contrast the DNP and PhD terminal degrees in the context of nursing roles.
- Analyze the minimum requirements of a DNP Project.
- Critique DNP Projects to examine content.

INTRODUCTION

The first step of the DNP Project process is to establish a solid foundation. In this chapter, we present some of the fundamental documents on which the DNP degree and DNP Project are based. It is very important that you read these documents and complete the activities presented in the lessons in order. They build on one another. Each lesson is broken down so that you can do the work in manageable segments. Some lessons will take longer than others, but you will be able to pick up easily where you left off. You may feel that you are reading some phrases over and over again. That's okay, repetition is a teaching technique used to reinforce key information. We talk to you in the first person, just as if we are sitting together in a classroom. We speak frankly, honestly, and in plain language. Our goal is to be your guide.

As a professional nurse, I despise things that waste my time. In this process, we will not waste your time either! We guarantee that the information we are about to share with you is 100% applicable to the degree and the project. We know the information is not comprehensive. But it's a great start. Our goal is to partner with you and your faculty. We want to share with you what we have learned to save you time and streamline your effort. We know that you will be more productive as a student if you have some foundations in place. Fine-tuning comes later. You have to start somewhere. To finish this DNP Project you have to understand the game.

Why is it even necessary to get a terminal degree in nursing? Why do you want this degree for yourself and your nursing career? In the first lessons, we are going to think that through. The DNP is a degree; it's not a role in nursing. So it's important that you know why you are here and that you have a vision for what you want to get out of this learning experience.

You will also have to be able to explain what a DNP degree is and how it is different than a PhD. This is the #1 question you are going to get from everyone you know, "What is a DNP?" Then they will say "Oh, like a PhD?" or "Oh, like a medical doctor?"—No. The DNP is a practice-focused terminal degree in nursing (American Association of Colleges of Nursing [AACN], 2006). You may feel like a parrot because you will have to explain this over and over. Be patient and respond with the heart of a teacher. The DNP degree is a relatively new degree in the grand scheme of academics. We have to patiently educate our colleagues and the public. That starts with understanding this yourself.

We need nurses with the ability to problem solve at high levels. That's what this degree is about, the highest level of nursing practice. The DNP Project at its core is a supervised, high-level problem-solving process. The DNP student must identify problems; assess the situation; and use evidence to develop, implement, and evaluate outcomes and process. Our solutions must be sustainable and designed to impact the patients we serve. Ours is not a one-and-done experience. It is an experience that you need some help with the first time around so that later you can lead a project to make practice changes and improve health. It's more like a see one, do one, teach one career experience. It is rooted in concepts of evidence-based practice and quality improvement.

In a DNP program, you will *not* be doing "research" in the traditional sense of the word. Just to make sure we are clear, we are including an entire lesson about what the word "research" technically means and how to use it properly at the doctoral level. The DNP Project is about taking research that already exists, evaluating it, and then finding ways to translate, implement, and utilize it in the practice setting. Did you know that it takes 17 years to translate research into practice (Morris, Wooding, & Grant, 2011)? Our colleagues take the lead of generating nursing research. They are the experts of nursing science. We, the DNPs, with PhDs take the lead by deciding how to translate, utilize, and evaluate the impact of that research on patients because we are the experts of nursing practice (AACN, 2015).

At the conclusion of the chapter, we dive into the development of a DNP Project. We guide you through the expectations for DNP Projects, as outlined by the AACN. We help you prepare questions for faculty as you review the project expectations at your school. Most important, we review some projects together. The chapter ends with some suggestions and clarification on group DNP Projects.

Start here and work hard, so that you can finish strong. Let's begin.

REFERENCES AND RESOURCES

American Association of Colleges of Nursing. (2006). *The essentials of doctoral education for advanced nursing practice.* Retrieved from https://www.aacnnursing.org/Portals/42/Publications/DNPEssentials.pdf

American Association of Colleges of Nursing. (2015). *The doctor of nursing practice: Current issues and clarifying recommendations* [White paper]. Retrieved from https://www.aacnnursing.org/Portals/42/News/White-Papers/DNP-Implementation-TF-Report-8-15.pdf

Morris, Z. S., Wooding, S., & Grant, J. (2011). The answer is 17 years, what is the question: understanding time lags in translational research. *Journal of the Royal Society of Medicine, 104*(12), 510–520.

MY GOALS FOR UNDERSTANDING THE DNP DEGREE AND DNP PROJECT ARE TO:

Lesson 1.1

WHY GET A TERMINAL DEGREE?

BACKGROUND

The Institute of Medicine's (IOM; 2011a) report, *The Future of Nursing* continues to offer a vision for the evolution of nursing practice. This critical document points out a need for nurses prepared at the doctoral level and calls specifically for an increase in nurses with the DNP degree (IOM, 2011a). The DNP is a terminal nursing *practice* degree (American Association of Colleges of Nursing [AACN], 2004). To better understand the vision of *The Future of Nursing* (IOM, 2011a), it is critical to understand what the DNP degree is and what it is not. It is even more important to understand why this degree is necessary. Why do you want this degree? What skills will it add to your nursing practice? Nursing skill sets evolve over time. Nurses need new skills to navigate and solve problems in complex healthcare environments. Nurses need to lead and *practice* at the highest levels.

LEARNING OBJECTIVES

- Distinguish the DNP degree from other terminal degrees.
- Articulate why the DNP degree is necessary for nursing's future and your future.

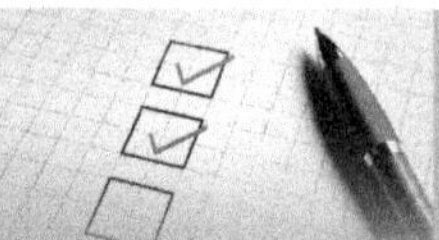

Activities

Read the IOM (2011b), *Future of Nursing* report brief and the AACN's (2004) position statement on DNP education. Use the information in these documents to list the key points of these documents. Talk to colleagues and faculty members to clarify concepts and engage in further discussion.

The Future of Nursing report brief describes four key messages. Write the key messages in the spaces provided.

1. ______________________________

2. ______________________________

3. ______________________________

4. ______________________________

Other Notes From *The Future of Nursing* Report

The AACN (2004) Position Statement on the Practice Doctorate in Nursing describe the climate of the practice doctorate at the time of its writing. It provides context to better understand the evolution of the DNP degree. A series of recommendations are made. Review the document and recommendations, and then write your answers to the following prompts and questions.

The idea of "practice" is defined in the context of three major categories. List them.

1. ______________________________

2. ______________________________

3. ______________________________

According to the AACN (2004) document under review, what are some key distinctions of the "practice-focused" DNP degree compared to the "research-focused" PhD degree? Complete the chart and take notes. The first one is done for you.

DNP: "PRACTICE-FOCUSED" DEGREE	NOTES
Less emphasis on theory and metatheory	PhD places more focus on nursing theories

At the time of publication of this document (2004), how was the need for the DNP degree perceived? Describe why it was important to the future of nursing practice.

List three reasons the DNP degree is necessary for you and your nursing practice.

1. ______________________________

2. ______________________________

3. ______________________________

SUMMARY

The DNP degree is practice focused. The DNP degree is not research focused. The DNP-prepared nurse is influential in leading change. The DNP-prepared nurse is an expert in their clinical field who can identify problems, develop evidence-based solutions, and evaluate the impact of the solution on health-related outcomes. The DNP degree offers a skill set to ensure that nurses meet the expectations of *The Future of Nursing* report (IOM, 2011a). Next steps:

- Discuss this activity with colleagues and faculty.
- Visit the "Campaign for Action" website (https://campaignforaction.org/about), which includes goals stemming from *The Future of Nursing* (IOM, 2011a) report.
- Read more about the IOM's, Future of Nursing Report on Education.

REFERENCES AND RESOURCES

American Association of Colleges of Nursing. (2004). *AACN position statement on the practice doctorate in nursing.* Retrieved from https://www.aacnnursing.org/Portals/42/News/Position-Statements/DNP.pdf

Institute of Medicine. (2011a). *The future of nursing: Leading change, advancing health.* Washington, DC: National Academies Press. Retrieved from https://www.nap.edu/read/12956/chapter/1

Institute of Medicine. (2011b). *Report brief: The future of nursing: Leading change, advancing health.* Retrieved from http://nationalacademies.org/hmd/%7E/media/Files/Report%20Files/2010/The-Future-of-Nursing/Future%20of%20Nursing%202010%20Report%20Brief.pdf

RELATED TEXTBOOK

Dreher, H., & Glasgow, M. (2017). *DNP role development for doctoral advanced nursing practice.* New York, NY: Springer Publishing Company.

Chapter 1: The Historical and Political Path of Doctoral Nursing Education to the Doctor of Nursing Practice Degree

Lesson 1.2

NURSING DEGREE VERSUS NURSING ROLE

BACKGROUND

There is a difference between your nursing degree and your nursing role. The Institute of Medicine's (IOM; 2011) report, *The Future of Nursing: Leading Change, Advancing Health* recommends that nurses transition seamlessly through a career of lifelong learning. After completing the baccalaureate degree in nursing (BSN), nurses should consider what their role in nursing will be—staff nurse, nurse manager, executive, or advanced practice nurse, for example. These roles will require additional education and training beyond the BSN.

Getting the DNP degree may or may not change your role in nursing. Depending on the your nursing role, the degree options may vary. At each degree level there are certain essential skills outlined by the American Association of Colleges of Nursing (AACN) that are expected of all nurses with the given degree, BSN, MSN, or DNP. In addition, universities and institutions may have additional degree requirements that extend beyond the requirements for nursing practice. The DNP degree prepares the nurse to engage in the highest levels of nursing practice (AACN, 2006).

LEARNING OBJECTIVES

- Consider the options for nursing roles beyond the BSN.
- Describe the Consensus Model for Advanced Practice Nursing.
- Trace the options for completion of the DNP degree.

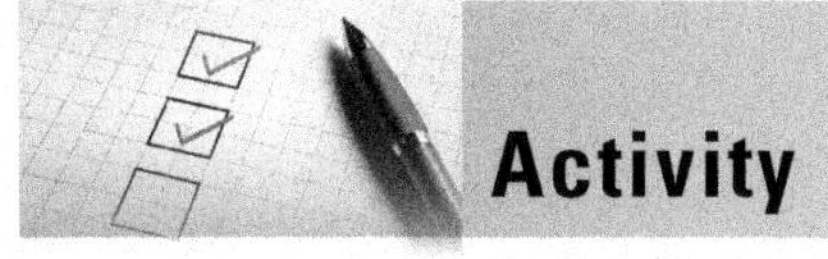

Activity

Examine the options for nursing roles beyond the BSN. List your current role. Select your future role. Are they the same? Or will your role change?

Hint

For this exercise, do not state that you are a nurse educator in your current role or indicate that nurse educator will be a future role. Consider *only* your nursing practice role. There are two reasons for this. First, to be a nurse educator, you must be an expert in an area of nursing practice. Second, all nurses need additional training to achieve the competencies required of a nurse educator (National League for Nursing, 2012). The focus of the DNP degree is to make you an expert in your area of practice. The nurse educator role is a separate and distinctive role (more on this later).

My current nursing role: ____________________

My future nursing role: ____________________

For nurses who are considering roles in advanced practice nursing, it is imperative to be aware of what is commonly known as the "Consensus Model." The National Council of State Boards of Nursing (NCSBN) published a model to better illustrate the various advanced practice roles in nursing. The goal of this model is to provide some unity, standardization, and regulation of these roles across the country. Published in 2008, one of the key features of the model is the process for choosing the advanced nursing role.

Review the information on the Consensus Model (www.ncsbn.org/aprn-consensus.htm).

Step 1: Choose your advanced practice nursing role.

Step 2: If applicable, choose your population of focus and complete the required training.

Step 3: Obtain licensure in your state.

Step 4: Specialize further within your role, population, and training via additional education.

Now, fill out your information:

____

Advanced Practice Training/Specialization

____

Licensure

____

Population of Focus

____

Your Role

Now with your future nursing role in mind, highlight your current highest nursing degree. Then trace the options for completing the DNP degree (Figure 1.1).

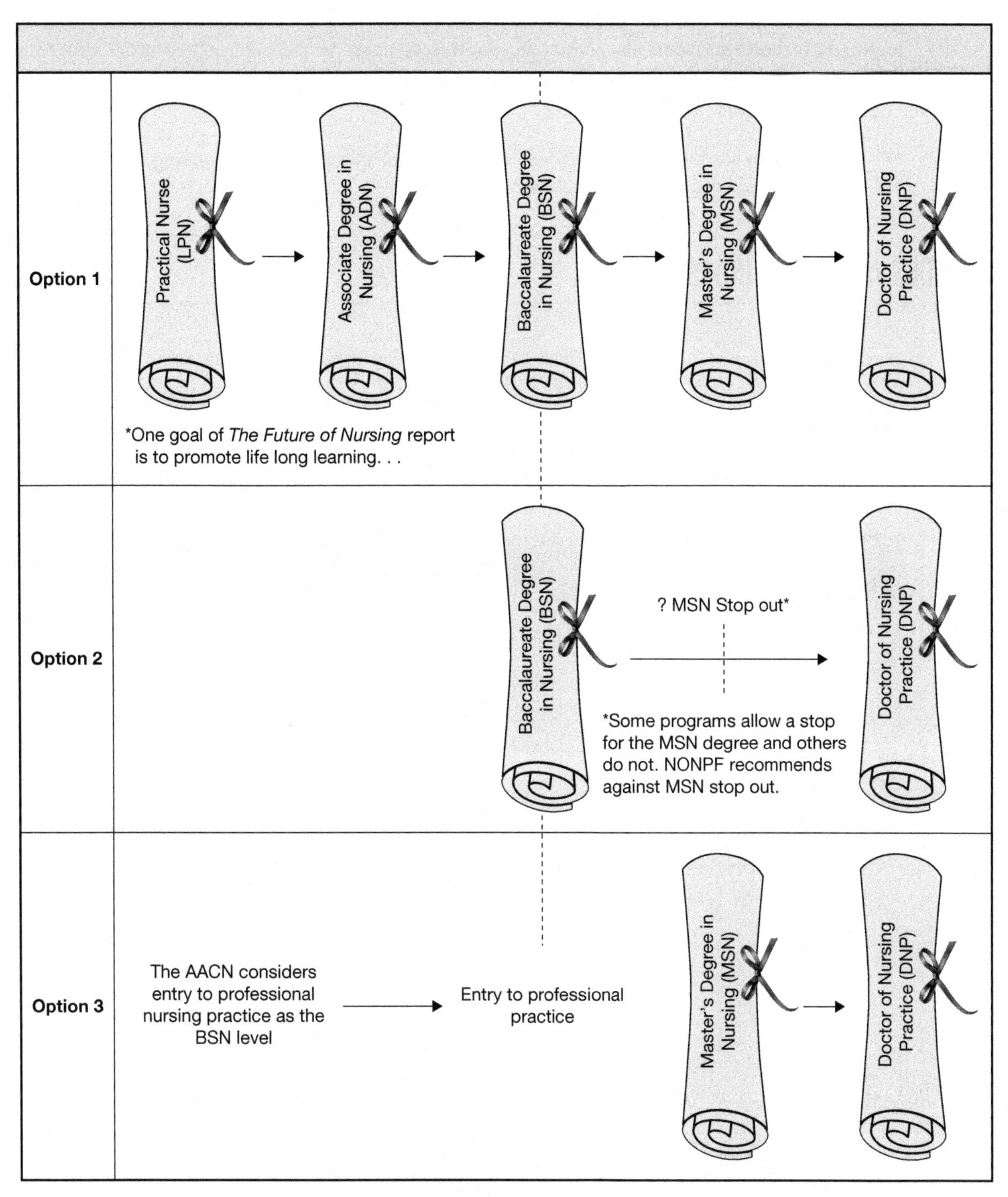

Figure1.1 Three common pathways to a DNP degree. AACN, American Association of Colleges of Nursing; NONPF, National Organization of Nurse Practitioner Faculties.

SUMMARY

After completing the BSN, select your role in nursing. If it is in advanced practice, understand what is required to achieve licensure. Depending on your role, you may have the option to practice with a range of degrees—BSN, MSN, DNP, or an other terminal degree. The DNP degree ensures that a nurse has basic, essential skills to practice at the highest levels of nursing. Next steps:

- Make a list of questions for your faculty regarding your nursing role and nursing degree.
- Ensure that you are clear on expectations.

REFERENCES AND RESOURCES

American Association of Colleges of Nursing. (2006). *Doctor of nursing practice essentials*. Retrieved from https://www.aacnnursing.org/Portals/42/Publications/DNPEssentials.pdf

Institute of Medicine. (2011). *The future of nursing: Leading change, advancing health*. Washington, DC: National Academies Press.

National League for Nursing. (2012). *Nurse educator core competency*. Retrieved from http://www.nln.org/professional-development-programs/competencies-for-nursing-education/nurse-educator-core-competency

RELATED TEXTBOOK

Dreher, H., & Glasgow, M. (2017). *DNP role development for doctoral advanced nursing practice*. New York, NY: Springer Publishing Company.

Chapter 2: Role Theory and the Evolution of Professional Roles in Nursing
Chapter 3: The Evolution of Advanced Practice Nursing Roles
Chapter 4: How Doctoral-Level Advanced Practice Roles Differ From Master's Level
Chapter 5: The Role of the Practitioner
Chapter 6: The Role of the Clinical Executive
Chapter 7: The Role of the Educator
Chapter 8: The Role of the DNP in Quality Improvement and Patient Care Initiatives
Chapter 9: The Clinical Scholar Role in Doctoral Advanced Nursing Practice

Lesson 1.3

"RESEARCH": WHAT DOES THE WORD MEAN?

BACKGROUND

Do you know what the word "research" means? According to Merriam-Webster, the word "research" means:

- Careful or diligent search
- Collecting of information on a given subject
- Investigation or experimentation aimed at discovery or interpretation of facts

The use of the word "research" can cause confusion when discussing the DNP Project or when discussing scholarly activity. Sometimes the person using the word "research" in a sentence does not give it the same meaning as the person reading or listening to the sentence does. This may be a potential source of frustration, confusion, and disconnection on the key differences between the DNP and PhD. Sounds crazy? Let me give you an example.

"I am going to do some research **on diabetes." (Nurse)**

WHAT DOES THIS MEAN? WRITE THE POSSIBLE EXPLANATIONS

Most likely, this nurse simply meant that she was going to look up some information about diabetes. The word was used as a general verb, about a high-level, precise, execution of the scientific method. Because we are all at different levels, with different experiences, we could easily misunderstand each other. We must use terminology with a clear understanding of meaning. The purpose of this lesson is to retrace what you have learned about the term "research" during your education to date and ensure that you understand the intent of the word when used in the future.

LEARNING OBJECTIVES

- Define the term "research."
- Utilize the term "research" in an appropriate context.

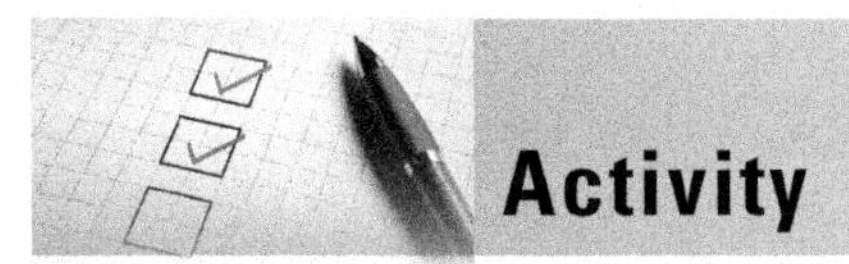

Activity

Let's break this down by discussing what you learned about science and research in elementary school. First, you probably had a poster in your classroom describing the scientific method: Question, hypothesize, experiment, observe and record, analyze, and share results. Do you recall learning this?

What was the point of learning this in elementary school? At first, it is to give you a basic knowledge of the scientific method and process. As people advance in their education, their use of the scientific method may become more refined. In high school, the use of this method probably applied to chemistry experiments. At higher levels, you engage more in the scientific process.

Let's look at another example. In undergraduate courses, you may have participated in a microbiology experiment. Your project may have sounded like this:

1. Question: Which surface has more germs, a student desk or the bathroom sink?
2. Hypothesis: I predict the bathroom sink has more germs.
3. Experiment: Swab the surface of (a) a desk and (b) a bathroom sink. Incubate for 24 hours.
4. Observe and Record: Document colony counts.
5. Analyze: Which surface grew more germs? The sink grew more germs than the desk. Is the hypothesis accepted or rejected? Accepted.
6. Share results: Based on our experiment, the bathroom sink has more microbes than the desk. We recommend the staff clean the surface of the sink twice daily.

Would you consider this type of work research? Who designed this experiment? The teacher. Who was the leader of this experiment? The teacher. But you were there, engaged, and applying knowledge at a higher level.

APPLICATION

At the doctoral level, you are at the highest levels of nursing practice and nursing science. Nursing scientists all use the same scientific method to answer questions. They are using very precise and exact methods which that can be reproduced. They are taking careful measurements, using validated instruments on properly sampled populations. They intend for the results of their experiment to be used in practice. When the term "research" is used in doctoral conversation, it is generally intended to mean high-level nursing research.

The PhD-prepared nurse is the driver and leader of nursing science. Other nurses, with varying degrees, may assist the PhD-prepared nurse in the research process. However, these nurses are participating in the scientific process; they are not leading or designing the actual experiment.

In a later lesson, we talk more about qualitative versus quantitative data, about the role of the DNP-prepared nurse, and so on. The point here is to ensure that we understand the meaning of the word "research" and to give caution on both its use and intended meaning in doctoral conversation. This applies to faculty and students—choose your words carefully!

If your intended meaning of "research" is to search or gather information on a subject, try to use some of these synonyms: Investigate, inquire, explore, probe, or fact-finding. Next steps:

- Consider reading a completed PhD dissertation.
- Discuss the term "research" with your faculty; how will it be used in communication?

RELATED TEXTBOOK

Christenbery, T. (Ed.). (2018). *Evidence-based practice in nursing.* New York, NY: Springer Publishing Company.

Chapter 1: Nursing's Commitment to Best Clinical Decisions

Figure 1.2 Representations of the Scientific Method

Table 1.2 Distinguishing Characteristics of EBP, Research, and QI

Lesson 1.4

UNDERSTANDING THE DNP ESSENTIALS

BACKGROUND

The American Association of Colleges of Nursing (AACN) is a national organization focused on academic nursing. Collectively, the organization is composed of 814 schools of nursing, over 45,000 faculty members, and 513,000 students from both public and private universities. The AACN, in collaboration with partnering organizations, recommends a set of essential skills for nurses at each degree level—the BSN, the MSN, and the DNP. In other words, these are skills that all nurses should have at that degree level regardless of their role in nursing. These Essentials are used to establish expectations of graduates and ensure the quality of nursing education programs (AACN, 2018).

The current DNP Essentials were published in 2006 and are the cornerstone of the DNP curriculum. At the time of this writing, they are under revision. The DNP Essentials outline fundamental content and competencies that are required to achieve the DNP degree. Academic DNP programs seeking accreditation from the Commission on Collegiate Nursing Education (CCNE) must demonstrate that the Essentials are addressed in the DNP program (AACN, 2006).

The DNP Essentials are also closely related to the DNP Project. The DNP Project is an opportunity to operationalize the concepts with faculty input and supervision. The project is one way to demonstrate competency of the Essentials. The project itself does not have to include all the Essentials, but it will include many or most of them (AACN, 2015). Mastery of the DNP Essentials may also occur during didactic activities that take place as a part of DNP coursework. They may also be incorporated into the DNP practice experience required for the DNP degree (AACN, 2015). The DNP practice experience itself will be discussed in detail in a later activity.

It is critically important that you understand the DNP Essentials. This will not happen immediately. In fact, you will complete entire courses to fully master the concepts. In this lesson, we introduce the DNP Essentials. The goal is to ensure that you have enough information to begin thinking about how the DNP Essentials will impact the DNP Project. It may be helpful to return to this lesson later as you progress through your DNP program.

LEARNING OBJECTIVES

- Read the DNP Essentials.
- Define each Essential.
- Prepare questions for coursework and use of the DNP Essentials in the DNP Project.

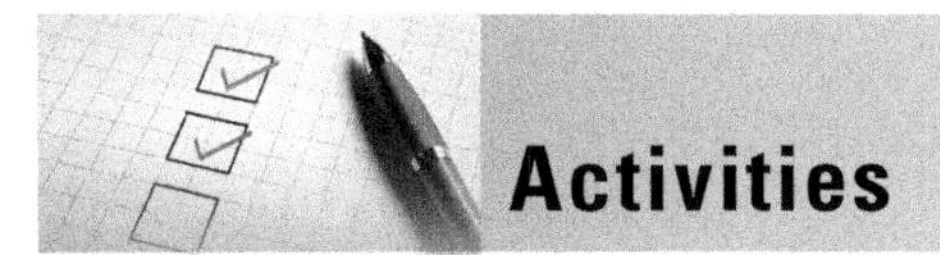

Activities

Read the AACN DNP Essentials (2006) document. As you read about each Essential, write a basic definition of each using your own words. Write down any questions you have for your faculty.

Essential I: Scientific Underpinnings for Practice

Definition:

Question(s):

Essential II: Organizational/Systems Leadership for Quality Improvement and Systems Thinking

Definition:

Question(s):

Essential III: Clinical Scholarship and Analytical Methods for Evidence-Based Practice

Definition:

Question(s):

Essential IV: Information Systems/Technology and Patient Care Technology for the Improvement and Transformation of Healthcare

Definition:

Question(s):

Essential V: Healthcare Policy for Advocacy in Healthcare

Definition:

Question(s):

Essential VI: Interprofessional Collaboration for Improving Patient/Population Health Outcomes

Definition:

Question(s):

Essential VII: Clinical Prevention and Population Health for Improving the Nation's Health

Definition:

Question(s):

Essential VIII: Advanced Nursing Practice

Definition:

Question(s):

SUMMARY

If you review the MSN Essentials and compare them to the DNP Essentials, you might argue that they are very similar. The key difference is the level at which these skills are executed. For example, an MSN-prepared nurse might participate in a team to develop a change in the practice environment. But the DNP-prepared nurse is equipped and prepared to be the leader of the team. Again, the DNP degree is designed to equip nurses for the highest levels of practice and leadership, to drive change, and improve health outcomes (AACN, 2004). Next steps:

- Continue work toward mastery of the DNP Essentials.
- Consider the DNP Essentials as you develop the DNP Project.

REFERENCES AND RESOURCES

American Association of Colleges of Nursing. (2004). *AACN position statement on the practice doctorate in nursing.* Retrieved from https://www.aacnnursing.org/Portals/42/News/Position-Statements/DNP.pdf

American Association of Colleges of Nursing. (2006). DNP Essentials. Retrieved from https://www.aacnnursing.org/DNP/DNP-Essentials

American Association of Colleges of Nursing. (2015). *The doctor of nursing practice: Current issues and clarifying recommendations*. Retrieved from https://www.aacnnursing.org/Portals/42/News/White-Papers/DNP-Implementation-TF-Report-8-15.pdf

American Association of Colleges of Nursing. (2018). Who we are. Retrieved from https://www.aacnnursing.org/About-AACN

RELATED TEXTBOOK

Christenbery, T. (Ed.). (2018). *Evidence-based practice in nursing*. New York, NY: Springer Publishing Company.

Preface: Goals of This Book

Chapter 19: EBP: The Sequential Layering of BSN, MSN, and DNP Competencies and Opportunities

Table 19.1 AACN EBP Essentials Crosswalk

Lesson 1.5

COMPARING THE DNP AND PhD

BACKGROUND

The DNP is an option for a terminal practice degree in nursing. The curriculum for the DNP degree is based on the American Association of Colleges of Nursing (AACN, 2006) DNP Essentials. The DNP degree is different than other terminal degree options. Again, it is a practice-focused degree, not a research-focused degree (AACN, 2006). The DNP degree itself does not determine one's nursing role. It ensures that nurses have a skill set to engage in practice at the highest levels of nursing (AACN, 2006). Ideally, DNP- and PhD-prepared nurses should collaborate to maximize health-related outcomes.

In this lesson, the DNP degree is compared to other terminal-degree options in nursing, specifically, the PhD. Being clear on this concept will add clarity to the DNP Project. A word of warning: This has historically been one of the most challenging concepts to explain since the inception of the DNP degree. Students are often unable to articulate the differences even as they applied for their degree program. For many students, the, "ah-ha!" moment does not come until later in their program of study. We want you to feel clear from the beginning so that you can be more successful.

LEARNING OBJECTIVES

- Outline the components of the DNP degree and PhD degree.
- Compare and contrast the elements of the degrees.

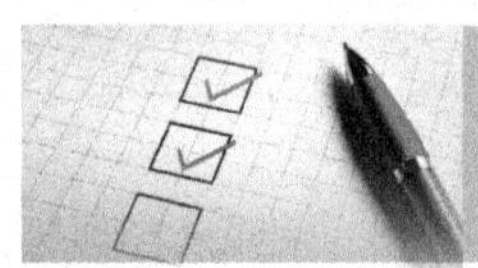

Activities

At the most fundamental level, the AACN defines the DNP as a practice-focused degree and the PhD as a research-focused degree. Practice is broadly defined as "any form of nursing intervention that influences healthcare outcomes for individuals or populations" (AACN, 2004, p. 2). The DNP Essentials go on to discuss research focus as "knowledge-generating" (AACN, 2006, p. 3) and more intently focused on concepts of theory, methodology, and statistical precision (AACN, 2006).

Concepts related to the degrees are broken down in the following tables by category: DNP or PhD. Information from the AACN has been translated into each box for you. Use additional resources to add information to each concept. Suggested material can be found under "References and Resources" in this section. Make sure to write down questions for discussion with your faculty member.

CONCEPT	DNP (PRACTICE FOCUSED)	PhD (RESEARCH FOCUSED)
Purpose of degree	Prepare nurses at the highest level of nursing *practice*: • Generate new knowledge via practice innovation or evidence-based QI* • Translate research into practice†	Prepare nurses at the highest level of nursing *science*: • Generate new knowledge via application of rigorous scientific methods • Conduct research to advance nursing science
Students	Committed to a career in practice	Committed to a career in research
Program outcomes	Healthcare improvement by: • Practice contributions • Practice scholarship • Policy changes • Leadership in practice	Healthcare improvement by: • Scientific contributions • Scientific scholarship • Scientific inquiry • Leadership in research
Notes:		

*QI, quality improvement. Remember that these are nursing degrees, and they are not nursing roles.
†All nurses will complete additional training to prepare them for their nursing roles.
Source: Data from the American Association of Colleges of Nursing. (2006). DNP Essentials. Retrieved from https://www.aacnnursing.org/DNP/DNP-Essentials; American Association of Colleges of Nursing. (2015). *The doctor of nursing practice: Current issues and clarifying recommendations* [White paper]. Retrieved from https://www.aacnnursing.org/Portals/42/News/White-Papers/DNP-Implementation-TF-Report-8-15.pdf

CONCEPT	DNP (PRACTICE FOCUSED)	PhD (RESEARCH FOCUSED)
Final academic product	DNP scholarly project	Dissertation
Faculty/experts advising the student	DNP Team	Committee
Intention	The DNP Project is a learning experience. The DNP Project is meant to improve outcomes in a local context/population: • Transferrable outcomes • One project cycle /degree	The PhD dissertation is a learning experience. The PhD dissertation is meant to provide information that can be generalized to a larger context/population: • Generalizable outcomes • Multiple experiments/degree

CONCEPT	DNP (PRACTICE FOCUSED)	PhD (RESEARCH FOCUSED)
Approach	Implement change and evaluate: • Identify problems • Gather/critique research • Determine best practice • Implement solutions • Evaluate outcomes/process • Adopt/abandon practice • Repeat.	Scientific research methods: • Formulate a question • State hypothesis • Conduct an experiment • Record/interpret findings • State the results • Share outcomes for potential use in practice • Repeat.

Source: Data from the American Association of Colleges of Nursing. (2006). DNP Essentials. Retrieved from https://www.aacnnursing.org/DNP/DNP-Essentials; American Association of Colleges of Nursing. (2015). *The doctor of nursing practice: Current issues and clarifying recommendations* [White paper]. Retrieved from https://www.aacnnursing.org/Portals/42/News/ White-Papers/DNP-Implementation-TF-Report-8-15.pdf; White, K. M., Dudley-Brown, S., & Terhaar, M. F. (Eds.). (2020). *Translation of evidence into nursing and healthcare* (3rd ed.). New York, NY: Springer Publishing Company.

In reviewing this information, write down at least two thoughts or questions you have for your faculty.

1.

2.

Why DNP and PhD? Rachel Mack, PhD, DNP, APRN, C-FNP, CNE

Students, colleagues, and friends have asked me repeatedly why I have two doctoral degrees. My answer is twofold, and my response is always the same. I completed my DNP degree first, as I felt it was important for me to complete a terminal degree that was clinically focused. I am a practicing family nurse practitioner. However, I work not only as a family nurse practitioner but also as a nurse educator in academia. So I felt it was equally important for me to complete my PhD in nursing education.

I learned so much wonderful information in both programs, but they were very different. The DNP program track that I completed was specifically designed for advanced practice nurses who already hold a master's degree in nursing and national certification as an advanced practice nurse. The program was not focused on gaining content that would allow me to specialize in a specific nursing role, but to provide coursework that assisted me in growing as a clinical leader and aided in developing the skills that I needed to effect positive change in the healthcare system. The DNP program helped me improve my critical thinking skills, evaluate evidence-based research, and to translate my knowledge into practice.

I enjoyed my DNP program immensely. But I wanted to develop my competency in research, so I applied for the PhD in the nursing education program. I felt strongly that I needed to complete this degree to be an expert in the field of nursing education. I was also acutely aware of the nurse faculty shortage that we are facing in the United States. My PhD program prepared me to be an expert nurse educator and researcher, which assists me in helping to advance nursing science. This program helped me develop skills in curriculum development, course evaluation, curriculum design, backward design, information technology, research, and theory development. This type of work is not the focus of a DNP program.

In my opinion, completing both degrees has been very beneficial in advancing my knowledge in research, clinical practice, and nursing education. Nurses with a DNP degree can be hired as faculty since it is a terminal degree. However, additional education-specific knowledge is needed beyond the DNP degree. I encourage you always to continue to learn and grow in your area of specialty. We can make positive changes in our healthcare systems by increasing our knowledge and understanding through furthering our education.

DNP or PhD? DNP and PhD! Sallie Porter, DNP, PhD, APN, RN-BC, CPNP

DNP students occasionally ask me why I chose to obtain both a DNP degree and a PhD degree. The answer is relatively simple: As a clinician, I wanted to hold the highest clinical practice degree available to me—the doctor of nursing practice. I usually add that if the DNP degree had come along a bit sooner, that might have been my truly terminal terminal degree.

However, what I learned as a PhD student (I got that degree first) certainly supported my learning as a DNP student. The PhD degree provided me with multiple research method courses, much more than I received in my DNP program, and also a deeper understanding of data analysis (although I am still learning). My PhD gave me the time to develop my content expertise in a narrow area and gave me the flexibility to participate in three different fellowships during my time as a student. The opportunity to interact outside of your institution and learn with other professions provided a sound basis for much of what I do and value today. It also gave me plenty of opportunities to write—pretty much every assignment was to write a research-based paper or a research project. And to read—the required reading load was tremendous, especially for a person like me who worked full time. Overall, the PhD program really did help me learn to think differently and better.

My DNP degree program was more fast paced and was presented in a 3-day weekend model that met once a month. The model was designed to move you relatively quickly through the still-evolving DNP degree content. I already had my master's degree and post-master's pediatric nurse practitioner certification, so the content was strictly DNP degree content and not the role content that many students are trying to master as well in a BSN-to-DNP degree program. I cannot emphasize enough what a challenge it can be to learn a new role as part of a doctoral degree. New things I learned in the DNP degree program included a systematic review as a method, that many PhD nurses did not truly understand the DNP degree, the struggles of group work, and how important understanding your stakeholders and setting are to implementing change. Overall, the DNP degree provided me with the information needed to take knowledge and implement it in a way to improve health outcomes.

As evidenced by the sheer numbers of nurses working to obtain their DNP degree and the plethora of new and planned DNP programs, I would say that nurses have voted with their feet and the DNP degree won! Of course, we still do need nurse scientists. We need DNP-educated nurses to further assume leadership positions in healthcare institutions, professional associations, schools of nursing, and governmental and health policy agencies. We also need to ensure that DNP-educated nurses determine what the degree encapsulates and how best to process learners to that end point. The DNP may be a terminal degree, but for nurses, patients, and healthcare, it is just the beginning of a wonderful journey that I believe will ultimately change healthcare for the better.

SUMMARY

The DNP is a practice-focused degree with an emphasis on implementing and evaluating changes in the healthcare setting. The PhD is a research-focused degree centered on more traditional concepts of science. In the next lesson, we will further explore the elements of the DNP Project. Next steps:

- Continue to explore the distinguishing features of both the DNP and the PhD to promote future collaboration by reading the article by Murphy, Staffileno, and Carlson (2015) referenced here.
- Talk to your faculty if you have questions.

REFERENCES AND RESOURCES

American Association of Colleges of Nursing. (2006). DNP Essentials. Retrieved from https://www.aacnnursing.org/DNP/DNP-Essentials

Murphy, M., Staffileno, B., & Carlson, E. (2015). Collaboration among DNP- and PhD-prepared nurses. *Journal of Professional Nursing, 31*(5), 388–394. doi: 10.1016/j.profnurs.2015.03.001

White, K. M., Dudley-Brown, S., & Terhaar, M. F. (Eds.). (2020). *Translation of evidence into nursing and healthcare* (3rd ed.). New York, NY: Springer Publishing Company.

RELATED TEXTBOOK

White, K. M., Dudley-Brown, S., & Terhaar, M. F. (Eds.). (2020). *Translation of evidence into nursing and healthcare* (3rd ed.). New York, NY: Springer Publishing Company.

Lesson 1.6

EVIDENCE-BASED PRACTICE AND QUALITY IMPROVEMENT

BACKGROUND

All nurses should be committed to the idea of using the best information available to make the best decisions they can for their patients. The term "evidence-based practice (EBP)" is defined as "the conscientious, explicit, and judicious use of the integration of current best evidence, clinical expertise, and patient values into the decision-making process for patient care" (Christenbery, 2018, p. 5). Although good in theory, use of evidence in clinical practice can be difficult. There is certainly a tendency to continue behaviors because "that's the way we have always done it" in nursing. But with this mind-set, we are not delivering the best possible care to our patients.

The Institute for Healthcare Improvement (IHI) states that the goal should be to improve the health of our patient populations by providing access to quality care at affordable costs (IHI, 2018). This has been coined "The Triple Aim." If we include the self-care of the healthcare team, this is referred to as "The Quadruple Aim" (Figure 1.2).

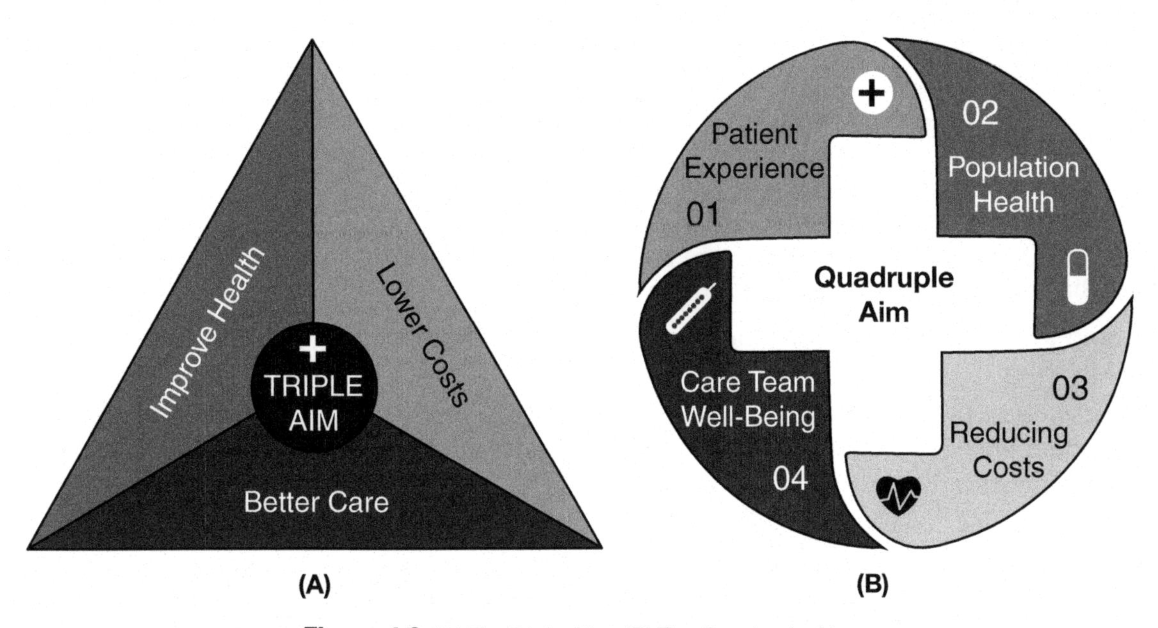

Figure 1.2 (A) The Triple Aim. (B) The Quadruple Aim.

Even Florence Nightingale used evidence to improve the quality of nursing care. The modern momentum to improve quality in healthcare is well articulated in a series of documents published by the Institute of Medicine (IOM), *To Err Is Human* in 1999 and *Crossing the Quality Chasm* in 2001. *The Future of Nursing* report (IOM, 2011) is a key document that every DNP student needs to read and review in detail. The links to the document summaries are provided here:

- 1999: *To Err Is Human* (https://www.nap.edu/read/9728/chapter/1)
- 2001: *Crossing the Quality Chasm* (https://www.nap.edu/catalog/10027/crossing-the-quality-chasm-a-new-health-system-for-the)
- 2011: *The Future of Nursing: Leading Change, Advancing Health* (https://www.nap.edu/read/12956/chapter/1)

These documents point out that the current healthcare system is flawed. The system itself is not safe. People are harmed by preventable errors when they enter the healthcare system. There is variation in cost and quality of care (IOM, 1999, 2001).

Healthcare professionals were also not receiving the knowledge and skills they needed to improve the situation. In 2003, the IOM released *Health Professions Education*, which states that health professional education programs should include competencies in five areas: (a) patient-centered care, (b) quality improvement, (c) interprofessional collaborative practice; (d) health information technology, and (e) EBP (IOM, 2003). When you align the publication of these documents with the origins of the DNP degree in the early 2000s, it is clear to see a relationship. Nurses with a practice focus need a higher level of skill and education to be change agents in the modern healthcare environment. Specifically, they need to improve their knowledge of EBP and engage in quality improvement and quality assurance.

LEARNING OBJECTIVES

- Examine the IOM documents *To Err Is Human* and *Crossing the Quality Chasm*.
- Define the qualities of "good" healthcare.
- Compare and discuss the features of three process models:
  - The steps of the EBP process
  - IHI: Model for Improvement
  - The scientific method

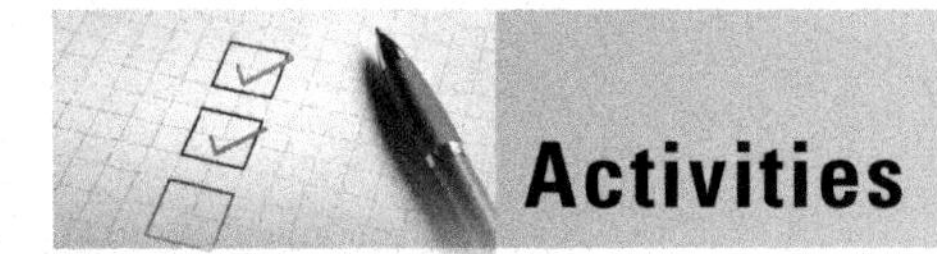

Activities

Use the summary of the IOM (1999) report, *To Err Is Human,* to extract these key points:

At least 44,000 people die annually from a medical error that could have been prevented (IOM, 1999). What are some of the types of errors that occur?

According to the report, errors are not really caused by "bad apples" but are more commonly caused by what?

The goal set was to reduce preventable errors by 50% or more. To achieve this goal a strategy for improvement was described, using a four-tiered approach. What are those four tiers?

1. ______________________________

2. ______________________________

3. ______________________________

4. ______________________________

Read the summary of the IOM (2001) report, *Crossing the Quality Chasm.* This document outlines six specific attributes of "good" or "quality" healthcare. Use the document to describe the intended meaning:

Safe:

Effective:

Patient centered:

Timely:

Efficient:

Equitable:

If the healthcare system were to be redesigned, what are some general principles to use? There are 10 rules for redesign listed in the IOM (2001) report, *Crossing the Quality Chasm*.

Based on your clinical practice today, do you think quality is being achieved? Is there room for improvement?

There are many models and frameworks for making changes and improving the quality of healthcare. Remember that both a DNP- and a PhD-prepared nurse can make improvements in healthcare. But they use different approaches. The DNP-prepared nurse is more likely to use models and frameworks rooted in EBP and quality improvement (QI). The PhD-prepared nurse will use the scientific method. Look at each model (Figures 1.3–1.5) and read the supplemental materials. How do these frameworks compare and how do they contrast?

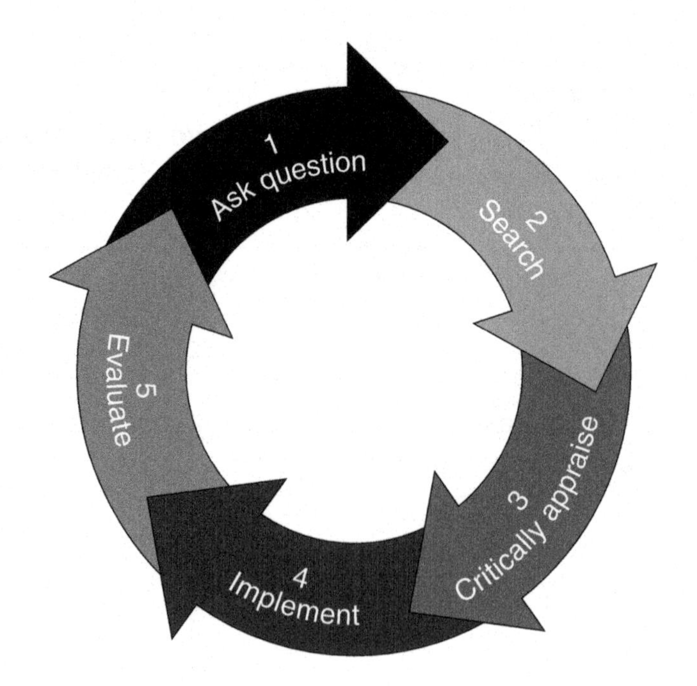

Figure 1.3 The steps of the EBP process. EBP, evidence-based practice.

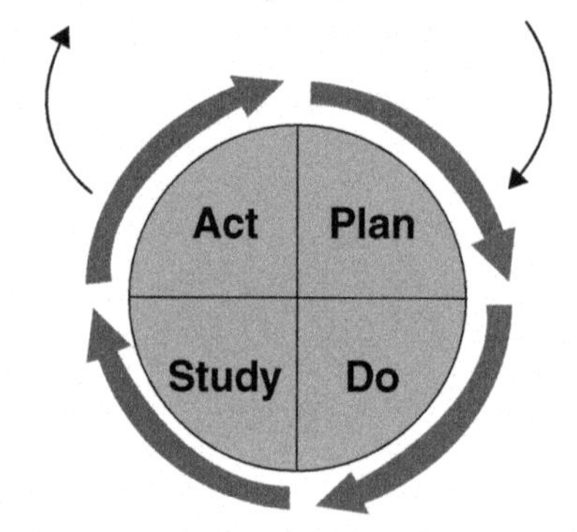

Figure 1.4 Model for Improvement.

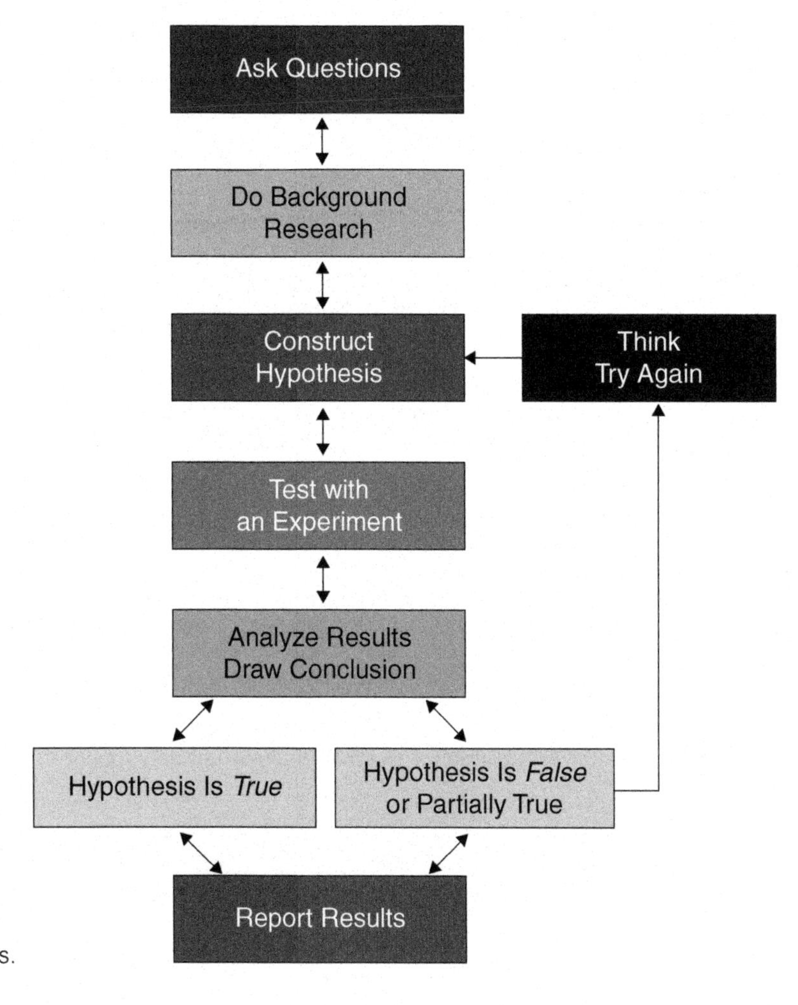

Figure 1.5 Scientific method.
Source: Reproduced with permission from Langley, G. J., Moen, R. D., Nolan, K. M., Nolan, T. W., Norman, C. L., & Provost, L. P. (2009). *The improvement guide: A practical approach to enhancing organizational performance*. San Francisco, CA: Jossey-Bass.

SUMMARY

The DNP Project is an academic experience designed to help prepare nurses to lead changes at the highest level in the practice setting, which will improve the quality of healthcare (American Association of Colleges of Nursing, 2006, 2015). The DNP Project is rooted in concepts of EBP and QI. It borrows concepts and terminology from science and research but does not fully embrace the precise rigor of the scientific method because it has a different purpose. Next steps:

- Explore more about the EBP process at https://fuld.nursing.osu.edu/offerings-overview
- Explore more about the IHI Model for Improvement at www.ihi.org/resources/Pages/HowtoImprove/default.aspx
- Consider enrolling in the free IHI Open School courses available at www.ihi.org/education/IHIOpenSchool/Pages/default.aspx
- NOTE: You can earn a FREE Certificate in Basic Quality from IHI. Read the details: www.ihi.org/education/IHIOpenSchool/Courses/Pages/OpenSchoolCertificates.aspx

REFERENCES AND RESOURCES

Agency for Healthcare Research and Quality. (2008). Six domains of quality in healthcare. Retrieved from https://www.ahrq.gov/talkingquality/measures/six-domains.html

American Association of Colleges of Nursing. (2006). *The essentials of doctoral education for advanced nursing practice.* Retrieved from https://www.aacnnursing.org/Portals/42/Publications/DNPEssentials.pdf

American Association of Colleges of Nursing. (2015). *The doctor of nursing practice: Current issues and clarifying recommendations* [White paper]. Retrieved from https://www.aacnnursing.org/Portals/42/News/White-Papers/DNP-Implementation-TF-Report-8-15.pdf

Berwick, D., & Whittington, J. (2008). The Triple Aim: Care, health, and cost. *Health Affairs, 27*(3), 759–769. doi: 10.1377/hlthaff.27.3.759

Institute for Healthcare Improvement. (2018). Science of improvement. Retrieved from http://www.ihi.org/about/Pages/ScienceofImprovement.aspx

Institute of Medicine. (1999). To err is human: Building a safer healthcare system, summary. Retrieved from http://www.nationalacademies.org/hmd/~/media/Files/Report%20Files/1999/To-Err-is-Human/To%20Err%20is%20Human%201999%20%20report%20brief.pdf

Institute of Medicine. (2001). Crossing the quality chasm, summary. Retrieved from http://www.nationalacademies.org/hmd/~/media/Files/Report%20Files/2001/Crossing-the-Quality-Chasm/Quality%20Chasm%202001%20%20report%20brief.pdf

Institute of Medicine. (2003). *Health professions education: A bridge to quality*. Washington, DC: National Academies Press. Retrieved from http://www.nationalacademies.org/hmd/Reports/2003/Health-Professions-Education-A-Bridge-to-Quality.aspx

Institute of Medicine. (2011). *The future of nursing: Leading change, advancing health*. Washington, DC: National Academies Press.

Langley, G. J., Moen, R. D., Nolan, K. M., Nolan, T. W., Norman, C. L., & Provost, L. P. (2009). *The improvement guide: A practical approach to enhancing organizational performance*. San Francisco, CA: Jossey-Bass.

RELATED TEXTBOOKS

Christenbery, T. (Ed.). (2018). *Evidence-based practice in nursing*. New York, NY: Springer Publishing Company.

Hickey, J. V., & Brosnan, C. A. (Eds.). (2017). *Evaluation of health care quality for DNPs* (2nd ed.). New York, NY: Springer Publishing Company.

Lesson 1.7

WHAT IS A DNP PROJECT?

BACKGROUND

To provide high-quality healthcare, *The Future of Nursing* report (Institute of Medicine, 2011) envisions a workforce with a skill set to lead change, utilize evidence, and ensure optimal patient outcomes. The DNP degree is a terminal practice-focused degree intended to prepare nurses for this endeavor. The curriculum for the DNP degree is based on the American Association of Colleges of Nursing (AACN, 2006) DNP Essentials. The final academic product of the DNP degree is called a "DNP Project" (AACN, 2015).

The DNP Project is meant to be a learning experience. It is an opportunity to apply skills learned in didactic courses in a real-world context (AACN, 2015). The nature of DNP Projects has evolved and continues to evolve. This is logical as the problems of nursing practice are dynamic and unlikely to remain the same over time. Thus, the goal is to equip nurses with high-level problem-solving skills so that they can continue to lead and engage in projects beyond graduation.

The DNP Project is also highly controversial. The requirements and elements of the project vary based on the nurse's role, partnering agency, university requirements, and other variables. When the DNP Project was conceptualized, there was no agreement on what it should entail. At some universities, the DNP Project was first modeled after the dissertation completed by PhD candidates. Some schools initially used a portfolio model in which students collected work from different courses to complete a final product. Some schools permitted group projects and others did not. There were schools that permitted integrative or systematic reviews as a final project. In short, the DNP Project did not have clear expectations. The debate over the DNP Project continues, but there has been some recent clarification.

In 2015, the AACN published a white paper titled, "The Doctor of Nursing Practice: Current Issues and Clarifying Recommendations." The document attempted to set a minimum expectation for all DNP Projects. Regarding the project, the AACN states, "It is important that the translation of knowledge into the practice setting by way of a final scholarly project be clarified to ensure consistency of learning" (p. 3). In other words, when someone graduates with a DNP degree, we want to be assured that the student projects are at least equitable. The contents of the document are only recommendations from the AACN Task Force. Some schools broadly interpret the recommendations. However, it is our opinion that this document represents very reasonable expectations and should be utilized throughout the DNP curriculum until updated or revised.

In this lesson, we will dissect this document to establish a baseline for your DNP Project. In later lessons, we incorporate expectations from your university and guide you through other project considerations.

LEARNING OBJECTIVES

- Read the AACN's (2015), "The Doctor of Nursing Practice: Current Issues and Clarifying Recommendations."
- Dissect elements of the document to inform your DNP Project.

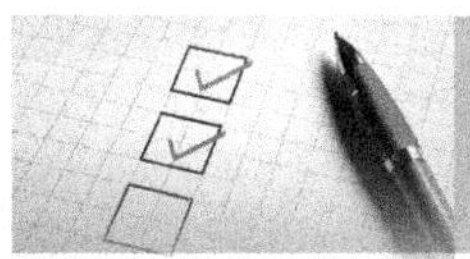

Activities

Use the AACN (2015) document to extract and outline key information. We help you dissect the meaning of the sections as you work.

Section II. The DNP Project, p. 3. Complete this sentence.

Title: "The final scholarly project should be called ____________________________."

Learning Point: Do not call it a "capstone project." The word"capstone" is confusing because it is used in other levels of nursing (BSN) and even in other professions. Do not call it "research" or a "dissertation" because these are the academic products of the PhD degree. Even faculty may use these words incorrectly. We should say "DNP Project." Encourage everyone to refer to this clarification.

Section II. The DNP Project, p. 4. Complete these sentences.

Scholarly Product: "the elements of the DNP Project should be the same for all students and include planning, implementation, and evaluation components. ... All DNP Projects should:

a. "Focus on a change ______________________________."

b. "Have a system or ______________________________."

c. "Demonstrate ______________________________."

d. "Include a plan for ______________________________."

e. "Include an evaluation of ______________________________."

f. "Provide a foundation for ______________________________."

Learning Point: These are minimum expectations. Some projects may be more robust on one element compared to the others. Remember that we have to start somewhere in establishing equity and standards of quality for DNP Projects.

Section II. The DNP Project, p. 5. Complete this sentence.

"Dissemination of the DNP Project should include ______________________________."

Learning Point: It is important to share what you learn from your DNP Project with others. Colleagues may want to implement something similar in their work setting. The public may benefit from some part of the information. Remember at the highest levels of practice and scholarship, it is often necessary to share information in different ways depending on the audience. You should disseminate the project findings in multiple ways. We believe for this body of scholarship you should have a final academic paper, a final presentation to stakeholders, and a final poster (or other product that is easily shared at a conference, online, etc.). Review the Appendix for additional suggestions. Later we review the requirements for your university.

Section II. The DNP Project, p. 5. Take notice and investigate.

The AACN recommends the use of a digital repository to catalog and share DNP Projects. Many schools and universities have these available and require all doctoral students to use them. Independent repositories are also available. Be careful to follow organizational policies on their use and comply with requirements for de-identification of sensitive project information. Here are the links to some repositories for you to explore:

- The Virginia Henderson Library: www.nursingrepository.org/
- The Doctors of Nursing Practice Organization: www.doctorsofnursingpractice.org/doctoral-project-repository/
- Eastern Kentucky University: https://encompass.eku.edu/dnpcapstones/
- University of San Francisco: https://repository.usfca.edu/dnp/
- University of Massachusetts Amherst: https://scholarworks.umass.edu/nursing_dnp_capstone/
- University of Texas at San Antonio: http://library.uthscsa.edu/2011/09/etd/

Section II. The DNP Project, p. 5. Answer the following question.

DNP Project team: Why should the term "DNP Project team" be used instead of "committee"?

Answer: ____

Learning Point: The DNP Project process needs to be differentiated from the PhD dissertation process. Again, many faculty may not use this term appropriately. Please refer them to this clarifying point.

SUMMARY

Now you have started reading about the minimum expectations of a DNP Project as outlined by the AACN. In the next lesson, we explore the requirements at your university. As the chapter concludes, we return to the AACN document to help clarify other project-related concepts such as the type of project, considerations for group projects, the DNP practice experience, and the DNP practice hours. Next steps:

- Access the DNP Project requirements at your university.
- Read them and reflect on how they relate to what you have learned in this lesson.

REFERENCES AND RESOURCES

American Association of Colleges of Nursing. (2006). *The essentials of doctoral education for advanced nursing practice.* Retrieved from https://www.aacnnursing.org/Portals/42/Publications/DNPEssentials.pdf

American Association of Colleges of Nursing. (2015). *The doctor of nursing practice: Current issues and clarifying recommendations.* Retrieved from https://www.aacnnursing.org/Portals/42/DNP/DNP-Implementation.pdf

Institute of Medicine. (2011). *The future of nursing: Leading change, advancing health.* Washington, DC: National Academies Press.

RELATED TEXTBOOK

Christenbery, T. (Ed.). (2018). *Evidence-based practice in nursing.* New York, NY: Springer Publishing Company.

Unit II: Designing and Implementing Evidence-Based Practice Projects

Lesson 1.8

DNP PROJECT REQUIREMENTS AT YOUR SCHOOL

BACKGROUND

The minimum expectations for DNP Projects are informed by the DNP Essentials and further clarified by the American Association of Colleges of Nursing (AACN) report, "The Doctor of Nursing Practice: Current Issues and Clarifying Recommendations" (AACN, 2015). The individual school or university further outlines its expectations for DNP Projects.

LEARNING OBJECTIVES

- Outline the DNP Project requirements at your school.
- Compare the content to what you have learned so far.
- List questions to clarify with faculty.

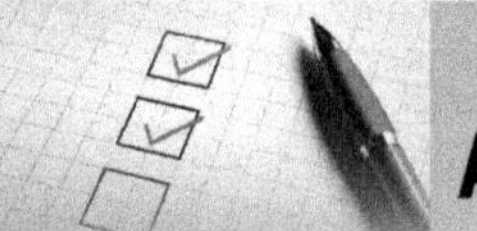

Activities

It is the student's responsibility to ensure that they have read the DNP Project requirements at their school. A list of questions follows to help you extract key information and organize it. Compare the information gleaned to what you have learned. Make a list of questions to further clarify with your faculty.

What is the date or version of your DNP Project requirements? ______________________________

Who is your academic advisor? ______________________________

His or her contact information: ______________________________

____

____

What type of DNP degree program are you enrolled in? ______________________________

What is your anticipated date of graduation? ______________________________

Take some notes. In reviewing this information, how does the DNP Project process work at your school? Here are some points to consider.

- How is the topic for the DNP Project chosen?
- At what point in your curriculum do you need to have the topic solidified?
- Who determines where, or in what context, the DNP Project will be implemented?
- What is the process for creating the DNP team?
- What are the requirements for the DNP team members?
- What types of DNP Projects are permitted or have been completed at your school?
- Does the school permit group projects? If so, how does that process work?
- How is the DNP Project proposal written? Is there a dedicated course for this or is it completed outside of coursework?
- What is the process for proposal approval?
- How does the student and school partner with agencies and other project stakeholders involved in the project?
- Is there support available to the student for project-related writing and statistics?
- What are the final steps of writing, presenting, and disseminating the project?
- Does the school provide a checklist for you to follow?

Questions for Faculty

SUMMARY

There will be more questions as you go along. Keep a list of your questions for faculty. Please do not feel overwhelmed at this point. In this lesson, you are simply being introduced to project information at your school so that you can plan. If you know what to expect, it is much easier to complete the process. In the next lesson, we review some actual DNP Projects. By seeing some final products, you can get a sense of what you are trying to accomplish. Next steps:

- Access two completed DNP Projects from your school and read them for the next activity.
- If your access is limited, utilize the online repositories listed previously to select projects to review. Your faculty may also assign projects for the class to review for later discussion.

REFERENCES AND RESOURCES

American Association of Colleges of Nursing. (2015). *The doctor of nursing practice: Current issues and clarifying recommendations*. Retrieved from https://www.aacnnursing.org/Portals/42/DNP/DNP-Implementation.pdf

These are some examples of DNP Project requirements from various universities:

Chamberlain University. (2018). *Doctor of nursing practice (DNP) project & practicum handbook*. Downers Grove, IL: Author. Retrieved from https://www.chamberlain.edu/docs/default-source/current-students/dnp-project-practicum-handbook.pdf?sfvrsn=30

Purdue University. (2016). *Doctor of nursing practice: Practice inquiry project guidelines and checklist*. West Lafayette, IN: Author. Retrieved from https://www.purdue.edu/hhs/nur/students/graduate/documents/policies/dnp-project-guidelines.pdf

Rutgers School of Nursing. (n.d.). DNP toolkit. Retrieved from http://nursing.rutgers.edu/students/DNP-Toolkit

Lesson 1.9

REVIEW OF COMPLETED DNP PROJECTS

BACKGROUND

During the first course of my program, the faculty recommended reading a completed DNP Project. "How in the world can you accomplish a goal if you have no idea of what you are trying to achieve?" said Dr. Sabrina Chase. I regret to tell you that it took me almost four semesters to take this advice. When I finally did, it was much easier to see the path to the end. I want you to be better than me—read some projects now! In fact, we will review a few together.

In this lesson, I would like you to select two complete projects from your school to review if possible. Then, I will select some projects to review with you. Our goal is to see how DNP Projects are developed based on what we have learned. We will use the minimum expectations published by the American Association of Colleges of Nursing (AACN, 2015) to guide our discussion.

I need to make a disclaimer before we begin. I am not here to categorize the projects in this review as "good projects" or as "bad projects." The projects I have selected have something to offer to spark conversation and promote learning. I purposely selected projects that can be freely accessed, in full, online. I tried to select topics that most nurses could relate to in some clinical way. Just to ensure respect and transparency, I am including a link to my own DNP Project along with my review of my project in hindsight.

I have yet to read a "perfect" DNP Project, including my own. I have yet to read a DNP Project and not think, "Maybe they could have done this?" or, "Maybe that would have worked better?" The reality is that DNP Projects exist in the real world. DNP Projects are practice based, like the degree. Practice is messy! It's dirty, it's hands-on, and it does not exist in a test tube. The final write-up of a DNP Project rarely sheds full light on the challenges, obstacles, or politics of the process. The DNP Project offers a learning experience. If you get through the process once with the help of your faculty, the idea is that you will do after you graduate. In the final academic write-up, we are sharing what we learned—the good, the bad, and the ugly.

LEARNING OBJECTIVES

- Inventory select elements of completed DNP Projects.
- Summarize observations and discuss them with classmates and faculty.

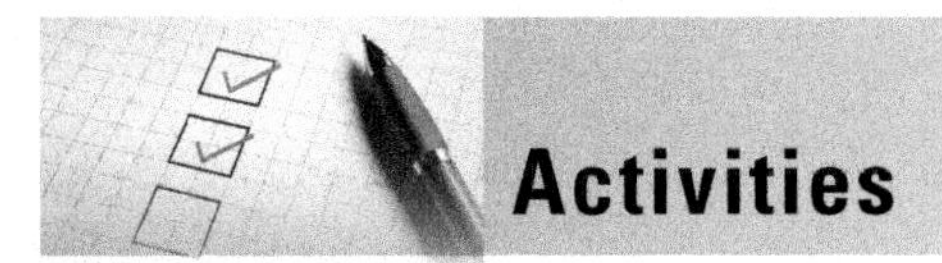

Activities

Read the following completed DNP Projects. Take notes as you identify the DNP Project expectations described by AACN (2015). (Editable versions of these activities may be accessed in a supplemental forms document available at springerpub.com/dpw. This supplement is also available at connect.springerpub.com/content/book/978-0-8261-7433-8.)

DNP Project Review I

Project Title: "The 5A's Model for Smoking Cessation: Engaging Health Care Providers and Overcoming Barriers to Change." Retrieved from https://sigma.nursingrepository.org/handle/10755/620614

AACN PROJECT ELEMENTS	REVIEW NOTES
What was "changed" in practice and how did it impact healthcare outcomes?	
Was there a focus on a population or system? Explain.	
How did the project demonstrate implementation? What was done?	
What outcomes or processes were evaluated?	
How was practice or policy impacted by the project?	
How will the project be sustained?	
Were plans for future scholarship discussed?	

DNP Project Review II

Project Title: "Standardizing Smoking Cessation Intervention for Patients in an Acute Care Setting" (see Supplement 1.1, available at connect.springerpub.com/content/book/978-0-8261-7433-8/ch01).

AACN PROJECT ELEMENTS	REVIEW NOTES
What was "changed" in practice and how did it impact healthcare outcomes?	
Was there a focus on a population or system? Explain.	
How did the project demonstrate implementation? What was done?	
What outcomes or processes were evaluated?	
How was practice or policy impacted by the project?	
How will the project be sustained?	
Were plans for future scholarship discussed?	

How are the two projects similar and how are they different?

DNP Project Review III

Project Title: "Improving Communication in the Clinical Environment Through Bedside Shift Report: A Quality Improvement Project." Retrieved from https://sigma.nursingrepository.org/handle/10755/621114

AACN PROJECT ELEMENTS	REVIEW NOTES
What was "changed" in practice and how did it impact healthcare outcomes?	
Was there a focus on a population or system? Explain.	
How did the project demonstrate implementation? What was done?	
What outcomes or processes were evaluated?	
How was practice or policy impacted by the project?	

AACN PROJECT ELEMENTS	REVIEW NOTES
How will the project be sustained?	
Were plans for future scholarship discussed?	

Based on these three reviews, what have you learned about DNP Projects?

1.

2.

3.

What questions do you still have?

1.

2.

3.

SUMMARY

I will make one final remark. It may seem off-topic. It may seem inappropriate. Unfortunately, you will get its meaning as you read more and more completed DNP Projects. *Writing well is important.* You are completing a *doctorate* after all, the highest level of practice and scholarship. As you read completed DNP Projects, you might observe poor sentence structure, improper punctuation, poor grammar, lack of American Psychological Association (APA) style, and a whole series of other deficiencies. *This is not okay!* If you struggle with academic writing, please get help early and often. Get or hire someone to proofread your work. Your ability to communicate in writing reflects on the professionalism of our nursing community. Please give your writing or writing development the attention it deserves. Next steps:

- Continue to read and review DNP Projects, especially those related to your topic.
- Investigate writing support.
- Review the author's evaluation of her own DNP Project, available at http://npmollyb.wixsite.com/who4nprx/dnp-project-critique

REFERENCES AND RESOURCES

American Association of Colleges of Nursing. (2015). *The doctor of nursing practice: Current issues and clarifying recommendations* [White paper]. Retrieved from https://www.aacnnursing.org/Portals/42/News/White-Papers/DNP-Implementation-TF-Report-8-15.pdf

Dols, J., Hernandez, C., & Miles, H. (2017). The DNP Project: Quandaries for nursing scholars. *Nursing Outlook, 65*(1), 84–93. doi: 10.1016/j.outlook.2016.07.009

Rousch, K., & Tesoro, M. (2018). An examination of the rigor and value of the final scholarly projects completed by DNP nursing students. *Journal of Professional Nursing, 34*(6), 437–443. doi: 10.1016/j.profnurs.2018.03.003

Waldrop, J., Carusol, D., Fuchs, M., & Hypes, K. (2014). EC as PIE: Five criteria for executing a successful DNP final project. *Journal of Professional Nursing, 30*(4), 300–306. doi: 10.1016/j.profnurs.2014.01.003

RELATED TEXTBOOK

Bonnel, W., & Smith, K. (2018). *Proposal writing for clinical nursing and DNP Projects.* New York, NY: Springer Publishing Company.

Lesson 1.10

THE DNP PRACTICE EXPERIENCE AND PRACTICE HOURS

BACKGROUND

When nurses hear the words "clinical" or "clinical practice," they immediately envision nursing school and nursing activities related to direct patient care. That experience was necessary to train you as a general nurse and perhaps as an advanced practice nurse. But for the most part, the traditional sense of the clinical experience for nurses has to do with preparing you for your role in nursing.

As you recall, the DNP is a degree and is not a role in nursing. However, there are certain skills and competencies, called the "DNP Essentials," that are expected of all nurses who hold a DNP degree, regardless of role. To become an expert on the DNP Essentials, you will need to have a learning experience to ensure that you are prepared at the highest levels of practice. The "DNP practice experience" occurs as part of your DNP academic program and is designed to immerse you in opportunities to operationalize the DNP Essentials. The DNP Project is a significant part of this "DNP practice experience." However, some DNP Essentials may also be learned as part of certain coursework depending on the design of your curriculum. Be clear that the DNP practice experience is not necessarily the same as you imagine "clinical" to be in other parts of nursing.

The American Association of Colleges of Nursing (AACN, 2006) states that to be expert in the DNP Essentials, 1,000 hours of practice beyond the BSN are needed. When you enter your DNP program, the faculty will determine the number of hours needed to meet this requirement based on your nursing education upon enrollment and intended program of study. For example, if you are a new BSN graduate going into a DNP program, you may complete 1,000 (or even more) practice hours to meet the requirements for both your new nursing role (advanced practice) and the DNP Essentials. If you are a nurse with a master's degree in nursing, you may receive some credit of supervised practice hours for work completed during that degree. Your work experience does NOT count toward the DNP degree. The AACN is very clear that the 1,000 hours must be completed in the context of a supervised academic program (AACN, 2006).

The DNP practice experience should be diverse and not purely focused on direct patient care. Students can be placed in nontraditional environments to expand their knowledge of health-related issues. As a faculty member, I have place students with social workers, attorneys, chief financial officers, pharmaceutical/insurance companies, the military, and other entities involved in healthcare. Be open-minded. Be clear on how the experience is helping to advance competency of the DNP Essentials and/or the agenda of the DNP Project.

LEARNING OBJECTIVES

- Review the AACN clarification of the DNP practice experience.
- Discuss expectations for the DNP practice experience.
- Clarify the number of hours you needed to meet the 1,000-hour requirement.

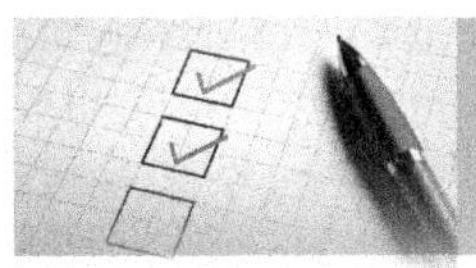

Activities

Read "The Doctor of Nursing Practice: Current Issues and Clarifying Recommendations, section IV on Practice Experience, Practice Hours, and Collaborative Partnerships" (AACN, 2015). Schedule a meeting with your faculty advisor and discuss the following:

- How many hours do you need to meet the 1,000-hour requirement?
- How do you track the completion of your hours?
- How is the DNP practice experience executed at your school?
- Who is responsible for "approving" the activities of the DNP practice experience?

SUMMARY

In Chapter 9, The DNP Experience, we will discuss the DNP practice experience further and give an exam of potential activities. Be sure to clarify any questions you have as you begin the DNP Project process. As a sidenote, we recommend that you keep a log of everything you do related to the DNP Project process. A form to assist you with this is provided in the Appendix of the workbook. Write things down as you go and later you can discuss what counts or does not count with your faculty. Don't stress about the idea of 1,000 hours because it will go by very quickly as you engage in this process. Next steps:

- Finish reading the "The Doctor of Nursing Practice: Current Issues and Clarifying Recommendations" (AACN, 2015).
- Review your university policy on group DNP Projects before beginning the next activity.

REFERENCES AND RESOURCES

American Association of Colleges of Nursing. (2006). *Doctor of nursing practice Essentials.* Retrieved from http://www.nationalacademies.org/hmd/Reports/2010/The-Future-of-Nursing-Leading-Change-Advancing-Health/Report-Brief.aspx

American Association of Colleges of Nursing. (2015). *The doctor of nursing practice: Current issues and clarifying recommendations.* Retrieved from https://www.aacnnursing.org/Portals/42/News/White-Papers/DNP-Implementation-TF-Report-8-15.pdf

Lesson 1.11

GROUP DNP PROJECTS

BACKGROUND

According to the American Association of Colleges of Nursing (AACN, 2015), group DNP Projects are acceptable when they are appropriate to the program and practice area. Like all group projects, it is difficult to determine the exact contributions of each group member without good planning, clear expectations, and a sound process for evaluation. In this lesson, we will examine the pros and cons of group DNP Projects.

In favor of group DNP Projects are those who assert that the technique promotes teamwork and collaboration. Faculty might argue that in some cases group DNP Projects are necessary because of faculty shortages, lack of collaborative partnerships, or clinical/political limitations. These are valid points. In contrast, others argue that as the DNP is a terminal degree, an individual project is only natural. How else can one demonstrate clear competency of DNP Essentials? After all, there is really no such thing as a group PhD dissertation. Again, these are valid points.

The AACN (2015) is not against the idea of group DNP Projects as long as certain standards are met. Specifically, they state, "each DNP student must have a leadership role in at least one component of the project and be held accountable for a deliverable" (p. 4). AACN also states that guidelines for the project and a rubric for individual student evaluation must be established at the beginning of the DNP Project process. Examples are provided to support these positions.

LEARNING OBJECTIVES

- Size up the pros and cons of a group DNP Project.
- Decide whether your DNP Project will be an individual or group project.
- Cultivate expectations for planning and evaluation if a group project is selected.

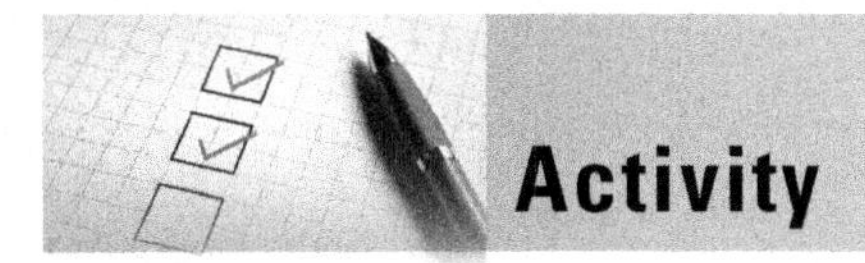

Activity

Review the requirements for DNP Projects at your school to determine whether a group project is even a possibility. If your school does not permit group projects, you can proceed to the chapter summary. If the school does permit group projects, start by reviewing a completed group DNP Project from your school if available. Then answer the questions that follow. When you are finished, we suggest scheduling a meeting with the appropriate faculty member to discuss the group project further. Questions to consider:

- How many students can work in a group?
- How are the groups determined?
- How is each student graded and evaluated as an individual?
- Have group projects been successful in the past?
- Is there a project-planning form the school recommends to use to get organized?
- What happens if one of the students is not able to finish the project?
- What happens if one student is completing the work successfully and other members are not?

My Opinion of Group Projects Molly J. Bradshaw

As a DNP program director, I have mentored both individual and group DNP Projects. I feel compelled to share my personal views and experiences with you on this topic. First, I firmly believe that the majority of DNP students should be completing individual DNP Projects. Because the DNP represents the highest level of practice and is a terminal degree, I feel that it is imperative that there is clear evidence that is a student demonstrates competency in all aspects of the degree program. This is very difficult to evaluate fairly as a faculty member unless the exact individual evaluation is used on all students. If students must be individually evaluated, it personally does not save me time as a faculty member to allow group projects.

I have also witnessed tragedy happen in the context of group projects. In one case the spouse of a student developed terminal cancer and the student had to stop participating in the program. As a result, the other student could not finish the project and started over on a new, individual project. In other cases, especially in the BSN–DNP tracks, some students were not academically successful in courses, which prohibited their progress on the DNP Project. My advice to you is to be very, very clear about what happens to your progress if there are difficult circumstances. If the group project is optional, are you willing to risk a delay of graduation for the sake of your partner?

I also live in a world of other realities. For example, nursing is desperate for clinical sites and clinical placements. In certified registered nurse anesthetist (CRNA) programs, it is not reasonable to allow students to do individual projects in the same, few, precious clinical sites that we have available. Midwifery faces the same limitation. It would burn out our clinical partners. Thus, group projects may be a program requirement in such cases.

The bottom line is that I worked hard for my DNP degree. Personally, I do not want to see us handing out DNP degrees without clear evidence that high standards were met. Therefore, faculty should insist on compliance with the AACN (2015) recommendations for group projects and agree on the number of students per project in advance. To assist you, a planning form to use for group projects is included in the Appendix.

NEXT STEPS

- If you are going to be doing a group DNP Project, complete the planning form.
- Schedule a meeting to discuss your plans with your faculty.

REFERENCES AND RESOURCES

Forehand, J., Leigh, K., Farrell, R., & Spurlock, A. (2016). Social dynamics in group work. *Teaching and Learning in Nursing, 11*(2), 62–66. doi: 10.1016/j.teln.2015.12.007

American Association of Colleges of Nursing. (2015). *The doctor of nursing practice: Current issues and clarifying recommendations.* Retrieved from https://www.aacnnursing.org/Portals/42/News/White-Papers/DNP-Implementation-TF-Report-8-15.pdf

CHAPTER SUMMARY

Now you have a basic understanding of the DNP degree and DNP Project. We have gone through some of the fundamental information. We compared the terminal nursing degrees of DNP versus PhD. We examined requirements and read completed DNP Projects. Take a moment to reflect on what you have learned:

After completing the lessons, I learned:

I still have questions about:

I am going to take this knowledge and put it into action. Two specific things I need to do are:

1.

2.

2

Assembling the DNP Team and Becoming a Leader

Tracy R. Vitale, Molly J. Bradshaw, and David Anthony Forrester

Lessons

OBJECTIVES

The purpose of this chapter is to provide an understanding of the roles played by various stakeholders in the DNP Project and help students position themselves as the project lead. By the end of this chapter, you will be able to:

- Identify key stakeholders playing a role in the DNP Project.
- Distinguish the various roles each stakeholder has in the development, implementation, and evaluation of the DNP Project.
- Develop a plan for creating the DNP team.
- Utilize nursing history to frame leadership of the DNP Project.

INTRODUCTION

Successful completion of a DNP Project requires the support of a team. There are some things that you need to understand as you build the team that will support you during this experience. Good leadership starts with good self-awareness, so remember to complete the suggested leadership evaluation tools.

The American Association of Colleges of Nursing (AACN) recommends that the group involved with the DNP Project at the academic level be called "DNP team" and not "committee." The team is usually composed of the DNP student, a main faculty member, and at least one additional member. Often, a team includes a contact person at the organization or agency where the project will take place. Sometimes students have an influence in determining the members making up the DNP team. At other schools, the members are assigned. Likewise, the agency representative may not be optional. Before completing this chapter, it is a good idea to have your school requirements accessible as you work.

Remember the primary goal of the DNP team is to support you through this process. The DNP team assists the student in planning, data analysis, dissemination, and other critical project milestones. The expectation is that upon graduation, you will be skilled, experienced, and able to lead a change initiative independently. The final evaluation of the student is always the responsibility of the faculty (AACN, 2015). Again, refer to your school's requirements.

Based on our experience, we recommend that you keep the DNP team to as few members as possible. You can seek assistance and input from a multitude of sources. But it is not always necessary for the contributors to be an official part of the DNP team. The fast-paced realities of DNP Projects may not accommodate such a large team. Please ensure that you speak to your DNP chair first before officially seeking or inviting members to the team. This person will help you decide whether the contributor should officially be on the team or not.

Students often feel conflicted about input they get from faculty teaching a course versus feedback from their DNP team. Who has the final say in green-lighting your project idea? Usually, the main faculty member assisting with your DNP Project, who is called the *DNP chair*. The DNP chair may not be the faculty member teaching your project-related courses. In other words, you may be taking a class called "Project Planning" with a faculty member who is grading you on proposal development, but the actual approval of the proposal is made by the DNP chair and DNP team. It is important to know how the academic organizational structure works. How will your DNP chair be selected/appointed? How are grievances handled?

The DNP student must also be a leader in the healthcare setting, not simply a manager (Forrester, 2016). What is the difference? Nursing leadership involves visionary, long-term thinking, behavior modeling, trust, and other qualities (Forrester, 2016). Nursing management takes a short-term and task-oriented view that maintains a status quo often by following rules and guidelines (Forrester, 2016).

Nursing has a rich history of leadership. You will be joining its ranks. Take time to indulge in reading and learning about the plight of other nursing leaders. How does their work apply to the problem you are facing? We are working hard in order to finish strong! Let's begin.

REFERENCES

American Association of Colleges of Nursing. (2015). *The doctor of nursing practice: Current issues and clarifying recommendations* [White paper]. Retrieved from https://www.aacnnursing.org/News-Information/Positions-White-Papers/DNP-Implementation-TF-Report-8-15.pdf

Forrester, D. A. (2016). *Nursing's greatest leaders: A history of activism*. New York, NY: Springer Publishing Company.

MY GOALS FOR ASSEMBLING THE DNP TEAM AND BECOMING A LEADER ARE TO:

Lesson 2.1

WHY TEAM VERSUS COMMITTEE?

BACKGROUND

The American Association of Colleges of Nursing (AACN, 2015) recommended the term *committee* be replaced with the term *DNP Project team* in order to further differentiate the team that oversees the DNP Project from those assisting PhD students. Clear expectations are outlined by the AACN that the DNP Project team is made up of the student (or group of students), a doctorally prepared faculty member, as well as a practice-focused mentor and/or agency representative. Additional personnel (e.g., experts, mentors) may also contribute to the project as needed in a formal or informal capacity (e.g., medical expert, librarian). Although this may seem like semantics, consider how the two terms really do differ from one another. Merriam-Webster (2019a, 2019b) definitions:

Committee: "a person to whom a charge or trust is committed or a body of persons delegated to consider, investigate, take action on, or report on some matter."

Team: "a number of persons associated together in work or activity."

It is important to recognize that DNPs are expected to change practice through interprofessional collaboration. DNP Essential VI focuses on interprofessional communication for improving patient and population health outcomes. This is realized through the collaborative efforts required to work through the DNP Project. Depending on the nature of your project, you will work with various professionals such as physicians, advanced practice nurses, registered nurses, administrators, staff, and possibly interdisciplinary personnel, including pharmacists, politicians, and others. Everyone brings a different perspective and area of expertise to the table, yet all can provide insight to the project. A distinguishing feature of the DNP- versus MSN-prepared nurse is that the DNP nurse is not just a contributor, but a leader in this capacity.

LEARNING OBJECTIVES

- Outline the differences between committees and teams.
- Identify benefits of DNP teams over DNP committees.

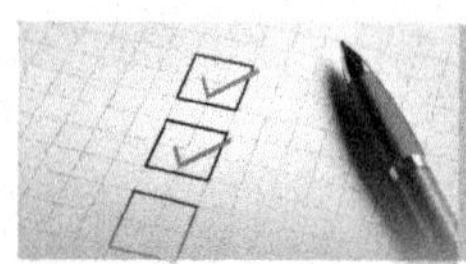

Activities

Consider how the roles and responsibilities of an interprofessional team for a community hospital vary from a rewards/recognition committee for a community hospital. Reflect on your experience with both teams and committees and identify the differences between the two.

____

____

____

Write down at least two thoughts or questions you have for your faculty.

1. ____________________

2. ____________________

SUMMARY

Teams are different from committees. They include people who are all working toward a common goal and are much more inclusive. Start to hardwire your brain to refer to those who assist you with your project as your *DNP team members*. Next steps:

- During project planning consider the nature of team dynamics.
- Be mindful and alert, looking for colleagues and faculty with interests similar to yours.

REFERENCES AND RESOURCES

American Association of Colleges of Nursing. (2015). *The doctor of nursing practice: Current issues and clarifying recommendations* [White paper]. Retrieved from https://www.aacnnursing.org/News-Information/Positions-White-Papers/DNP-Implementation-TF-Report-8-15.pdf

Committee. (2019a). In *Merriam-Webster's online dictionary*. Retrieved from https://www.merriam-webster.com/dictionary/committee

Team. (2019b). In *Merriam-Webster's online dictionary*. Retrieved from https://www.merriam-webster.com/dictionary/team

RELATED TEXTBOOK

Marshall, E. S., & Broome, M. E. (2016). *Transformational leadership in nursing.* New York, NY: Springer Publishing Company.

Chapter 10: Building Cohesive and Effective Teams

Lesson 2.2

ROLE OF THE STUDENT

BACKGROUND

As a DNP student, you will experience a shift in your practice, leadership responsibilities, and expectations. As a doctoral student, you are held to a higher standard and expected to produce outcomes on a much higher level. The bar is justifiably raised and you are expected to meet, if not exceed, those expectations. But to start? Some students will have leadership experience. Others may be newly graduated from a

BSN program. We are starting with your leadership role on the DNP team. Later, the skills that you learn can be translated to accomplish high-order practice.

LEARNING OBJECTIVES

- List key roles of DNP team members in the DNP Project.
- Develop a plan for creating the DNP team.
- Prepare for successful leadership of the DNP team.

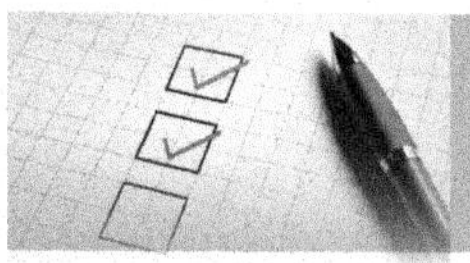

Activities

Refer to the DNP Project requirements at your school and answer the following questions:

1. What are your responsibilities as a student according to the requirements at your school?

2. Who is your primary DNP Project faculty member (i.e., your *chair*)? Or how is the primary faculty member chosen?

Primary Faculty (DNP Chair) Name:

Email/Phone Number:

3. How are additional DNP team members selected or chosen at your school? At what point in the curriculum is this decision made? As a discussion point with your faculty, you may preidentify potential team members. Make a list and discuss with your primary faculty member.

Name:

Email/Phone Number:

Organization:

Why this person would make a good DNP team member:

Name:

Email/Phone Number:

Organization:

Why this person would make a good DNP team member:

Name:

Email/Phone Number:

Organization:

Why this person would make a good DNP team member:

In reviewing this information, write down at least two thoughts or questions you have for your faculty.

1. ______________________________

2. ______________________________

When the team is assembled, students are expected to keep records of communication with team members. The DNP Team Member Communication Form included in the Appendix will help you. What other strategies can help you maintain consistent and effective communication with your DNP team for each step of your project? Make a list.

1.

2.

3.

4.

5.

SUMMARY

The student is the leader of the DNP team and is supported by a primary faculty member and additional team member(s). Sometimes additional people will contribute to the project in formal or informal ways. You have the responsibility to lead the project from concept through implementation and dissemination. Next steps:

- Continue to explore strategies to help you in the role of the leader of the DNP Project.

RELATED TEXTBOOKS

Forrester, D. A. (2016). *Nursing's greatest leaders: A history of activism.* New York, NY: Springer Publishing Company.

Part 2: Modeling the Way

Part 3: Inspiring a Shared Vision

Part 4: Challenging the Process

Marshall, E. S., & Broome, M. E. (2016). *Transformational leadership in nursing.* New York, NY: Springer Publishing Company.

Chapter 8: Personal Perspectives on Role Integration

Chapter 9: Leadership Skill Set for the Advanced Practice Nurse

Chapter 10: Developing the Skill Set for the Executive Nurse Leader

Lesson 2.3

ROLE OF THE FACULTY AND ACADEMIC TEAM MEMBERS

BACKGROUND

Recalling the recommendations of the American Association of Colleges of Nursing (AACN, 2015), the DNP Project should include a team that includes a doctorally prepared faculty member who can not only serve as a mentor but also be responsible for the evaluation of the final DNP Project. Recognizing that at times there may be many hands in the pot, it is important to be able to differentiate everyone's roles and responsibilities, which may vary by school and program.

Traditionally, the role of course faculty is to provide you with the skill set related to the DNP Essentials. For example, course faculty may guide a student through a literature review or provide the logistics of writing the academic papers related to the project. If course faculty are different from your DNP Project team, it becomes even more important to recognize the relationships and determine their impact on the project.

LEARNING OBJECTIVES

- Identify the roles/responsibilities of the primary faculty/academic team members who have a role in the DNP Project.

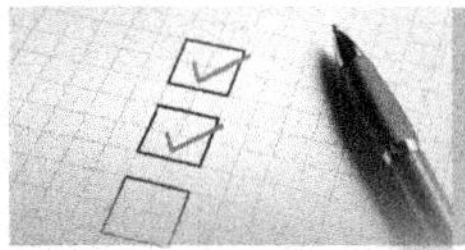

Activities

Review any school content that outlines the responsibilities of the DNP faculty and DNP team members so that you know how they can support you through your project. Often, this information is located in the DNP Project requirements for your school. List their primary roles/responsibilities as related to the DNP Project:

1.

2.

3.

4.

5.

In reviewing this information, write down at least two thoughts or questions you have for your faculty.

1. ______________________________

2. ______________________________

SUMMARY

The faculty are available to support you in a number of ways. It is your responsibility as the team leader to ensure effective coordination with both your DNP Project course faculty and those associated with your specific DNP Project. Be prepared to use this knowledge when you create a communication plan for the development and writing of your DNP Project.

REFERENCE AND RESOURCE

American Association of Colleges of Nursing. (2015). *The doctor of nursing practice: Current issues and clarifying recommendations* [White paper]. Retrieved from https://www.aacnnursing.org/Portals/42/News/White-Papers/DNP-Implementation-TF-Report-8-15.pdf

RELATED TEXTBOOK

Forrester, D. A. (2016). *Nursing's greatest leaders: A history of activism.* New York, NY: Springer Publishing Company.

Part 2: Modeling the Way

Part 3: Inspiring a Shared Vision

Part 4: Challenging the Process

Lesson 2.4

ROLE OF THE DNP PRECEPTOR AND ORGANIZATION REPRESENTATIVE

BACKGROUND

DNP preceptors and organization representative have roles in your DNP education and DNP Project. Under most circumstances, the DNP team will include the DNP preceptor or another representative of the partnering organization. This team member is the expert on practice and/or organizational context.

The role of the DNP preceptor includes being able to lead, teach, consult, coach, supervise, support research, manage, facilitate, and be a resource to the student. The role of the preceptor is not only to provide direct supervision in the DNP Project experience hours but also to guide your development in a clinical environment in order to promote both critical thinking and self-awareness. Regardless of your type of DNP program, your preceptors and organization required leaders will provide you with the support for you to develop the skills necessary to be a DNP.

Organizational and systems leadership is the focus of DNP Essential II. It is expected that you will not only be able to direct patient care but also that of the greater community. Your DNP skill set will include the ability to conceptualize care delivery models that are feasible within the current context of not only the organization but also the political, cultural, and economic state (American Association of Colleges of Nursing [AACN], 2006). AACN Essential VIII focuses on advanced nursing practice. Although the preceptor may have a responsibility to the DNP student in the clinical setting, it is possible that skills learned may be of help as you navigate the DNP Project.

LEARNING OBJECTIVES

- List potential skills and/or project contributions from DNP preceptor(s), organization representative, and champions.

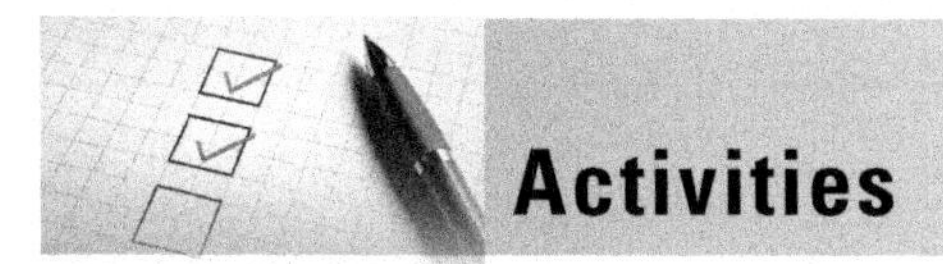

Activities

Next to each DNP Essential, list a potential skill that you can learn from the preceptor. Note how that skill contributes to your DNP Project.

DNP ESSENTIAL	SKILL TO LEARN/PROJECT CONTRIBUTIONS
I. Scientific Underpinnings for Practice	
II. Organizational and Systems Leadership for Quality Improvement and Systems Thinking	
III. Clinical Scholarship and Analytical Methods for Evidence-Based Practice	
IV. Information Systems/Technology and Patient Care Technology for the Improvement and Transformation of Healthcare	
V. Healthcare Policy for Advocacy in Healthcare	
VI. Interprofessional Collaboration for Improving Patient and Population Health Outcomes	

DNP ESSENTIAL	SKILL TO LEARN/PROJECT CONTRIBUTIONS
VII. Clinical Prevention and Population Health for Improving the Nation's Health	
VIII. Advanced Nursing Practice	

SUMMARY

Project champions are discussed in a later section, but basically these are formal or informal organization leaders with the ability to influence change. You can read more about historical nursing champions in *Nursing's Greatest Leaders: A History of Activism* (2016) by D. Forrester.

REFERENCES AND RESOURCES

American Association of Colleges of Nursing. (2006). *The essentials of doctoral education for advanced nursing practice* [White paper]. Retrieved from https://www.aacnnursing.org/Portals/42/Publications/DNPEssentials.pdf

Forrester, D. A. (2016). *Nursing's greatest leaders: A history of activism*. New York, NY: Springer Publishing Company.

RELATED TEXTBOOK

Forrester, D. A. (2016). *Nursing's greatest leaders: A history of activism*. New York, NY: Springer Publishing Company.

Part 2: Modeling the Way

Part 3: Inspiring a Shared Vision

Part 4: Challenging the Process

Lesson 2.5

THINKING THROUGH THE PROS AND CONS OF ADDITIONAL TEAM MEMBERS

BACKGROUND

The American Association of Colleges of Nursing (AACN, 2015) indicates that it may be necessary for additional personnel to assist with the DNP Project throughout the project stages. However, having multiple team members may create a situation in which there are competing motives. At this point, we have explored the roles and responsibilities of the student, primary faculty, and DNP preceptor/organization representative. Do you need additional contributions to your project? There are pros and cons to having more people involved in the intricacies of the project.

LEARNING OBJECTIVES

- Identify the pros and cons of adding additional team members to the project.

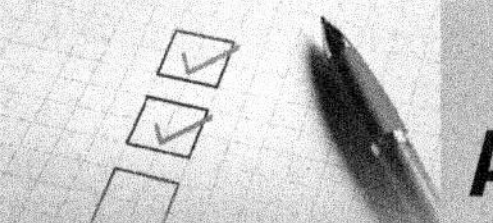

Activities

Consider the following examples in which additional team members may benefit or hinder the DNP Project process. Reflect on how you would best handle the situation and whether you would add the third person as a team member.

Example 1: A student is developing a quality-improvement (QI) project focused on improving exclusive breastfeeding rates in the neonatal ICU. The student's team currently includes a faculty member who provides expertise in DNP Project writing/navigating institutional processes and a team member who provides clinical expertise as a doctorally prepared neonatal nurse practitioner. The student suggests adding a lactation consultant who is assigned to the neonatal ICU as a team member due to this person's expertise and likely investment in seeing this project succeed.

Example 2: A student is conducting a QI project to develop a code sepsis protocol for the emergency room of an acute care setting. Knowing there is a tremendous amount of literature and standards of care to review for both the background and the significance and formal review of the literature, the student is looking to include the librarian as a third team member.

Determine additional stakeholders who are potential team members; consider the pros and cons of adding them as official team members.

STAKEHOLDER	PROS/CONS	DISCUSSION POINTS
1.		
2.		
3		
4.		

In reviewing this information, write down at least two thoughts or questions you have for your faculty.

1. ______________________________

2. ______________________________

SUMMARY

Various people may be able to provide guidance and assistance in the development and implementation of the DNP Project, but not all should be a part of the team. To move forward, it is important to understand the difference between potential contribution versus role responsibility. Consider the need for a formal role on the DNP team versus acknowledging their contributions in the final DNP Project. As a next step, discuss any potential team members with your DNP chair or primary faculty.

REFERENCE AND RESOURCE

American Association of Colleges of Nursing. (2015). *The doctor of nursing practice: Current issues and clarifying recommendations* [White paper]. Retrieved from https://www.aacnnursing.org/Portals/42/News/White-Papers/DNP-Implementation-TF-Report-8-15.pdf

RELATED TEXTBOOK

Forrester, D. A. (2016). *Nursing's greatest leaders: A history of activism.* New York, NY: Springer Publishing Company.

Part 2: Modeling the Way

Part 3: Inspiring a Shared Vision

Part 4: Challenging the Process

Lesson 2.6

CREATING YOUR DNP TEAM

BACKGROUND

The DNP Project is led by the DNP student. The DNP student is supported by the DNP team. The majority of DNP teams are made up of the student (or group of students), a doctorally prepared faculty member (chair), as well as a practice-focused mentor, organizational leader, interdisciplinary leader related to the project, and so on (AACN, 2015). Additional personnel (e.g., experts, mentors) may also contribute to the project in a formal or informal capacity with varying levels of support.

LEARNING OBJECTIVES

- Review institutional requirements for DNP team members.
- Identify potential DNP team members.
- Select DNP team members.

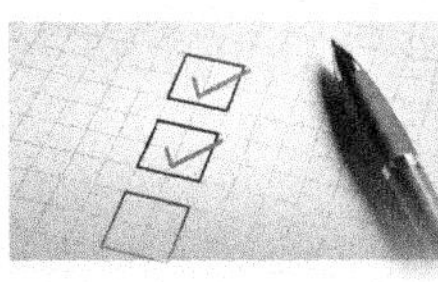

Activities

Identify at least one faculty member and one practice-focused expert who could potentially be members of your team. Include rationales for why you have selected specific personnel. You may return to this activity depending on the project progression rules at your school.

POTENTIAL ROLE	POTENTIAL TEAM MEMBERS	PROJECT CONTRIBUTION
1. DNP Project Chair		
2. Practice Expert		
3. Organization Representative		
4. Other Member		

SUMMARY

The team that you create will drive the project. Surrounding yourself with a team that can provide you with the guidance, support, and expertise you need will help you at the most critical times of the process. Discuss with your faculty/DNP chair the process for formally inviting members to the team.

REFERENCE AND RESOURCE

American Association of Colleges of Nursing. (2015). *The doctor of nursing practice: Current issues and clarifying recommendations* [White paper]. Retrieved from https://www.aacnnursing.org/Portals/42/News/White-Papers/DNP-Implementation-TF-Report-8-15.pdf

RELATED TEXTBOOK

Forrester, D. A. (2016). *Nursing's greatest leaders: A history of activism.* New York, NY: Springer Publishing Company.

Part 2: Modeling the Way
Part 3: Inspiring a Shared Vision
Part 4: Challenging the Process
Part 5: Enabling Others to Act

Lesson 2.7

HISTORIC NURSING LEADERSHIP TO FRAME YOUR LEADERSHIP ROLE

BACKGROUND

At the time I began studying for my DNP degree, I had been an RN for 15 years. I regret to report that I had never found the time to read Florence Nightingale's (1859) *Notes on Nursing*. Could I call myself an expert leader and know really nothing about the iconic nursing leaders?

During my doctoral education, I made a commitment to improve my knowledge of historical nursing leadership. They say history repeats itself. Could we appreciate historic nursing leadership to prepare us for new leadership roles in nursing? I think so. These leaders identified problems and found ways to make a change in practice and address the problems to improve outcomes for their patients. The process of problem-solving and concepts of leadership are not new. If they can lead, so can I, and so can you.

LEARNING OBJECTIVES

- Examine historic nursing leadership to inform future practice.

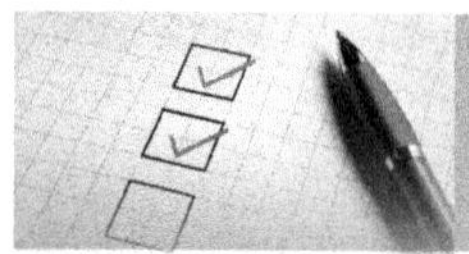

Activities

Identify five leaders of interest to you; here is a list of suggestions. Investigate and read about them. Next to each nursing leader, list the major health problem(s) these leaders challenged and the strategies they used to change nursing practice.

- Mother Mary Aikenhead (Irish; 1787–1858): Arguably the first visiting nurse in the world
- Dorothea Lynde Dix (American; 1802–1887): Widely known as a pioneer crusader for the mentally ill

- Florence Nightingale (British; 1820–1910): Acclaimed to be the founder of "modern nursing"
- Clara Barton (American; 1821–1912): Humanitarian and founder of the American Red Cross
- Edith Louisa Cavell (British; 1865–1915): World War I nurse heroine who faced a firing squad
- Lillian D. Wald (American; 1867–1940): Founded the Henry Street Settlement, which evolved into the Visiting Nurse Service of New York
- Clara Louise Maass (American; 1876–1901): Sacrificed her life in the fight against yellow fever
- Margaret Higgins Sanger (American; 1879–1966): Birth-control activist and sex educator who opened the first birth-control clinic in the United States and established Planned Parenthood
- Elizabeth Kenny (Australian; 1880–1952): Challenged conventional wisdom and promoted a controversial new treatment approach for poliomyelitis
- Mary Breckinridge (American; 1881–1965): Established the Frontier Nursing Service (FNS) to provide healthcare in the Appalachian Mountains of Eastern Kentucky
- Luther Christman (American; 1915–2011): Advocate for race and gender equality in nursing
- Mary Elizabeth Carnegie (American; 1916–2008): Fought for racial equality

SELECTED LEADER	PROBLEMS THEY FACED	STRATEGIES TO CHANGE PRACTICE

Are any of the problems or strategies relevant in the practice of nursing today?

Do their leadership strategies apply to your leadership of this project? List three useful points.

1.

2.

3.

DNPs and Nursing's Distinguished History of Leadership: D.A. Forrester

One of the key messages of the Institute of Medicine's report on *The Future of Nursing: Leading Change, Advancing Health* (Institute of Medicine [IOM], 2011) is that "Nurses should be full partners, with physicians, and other health professionals, in redesigning health care in the United States" (pp. 1–11). DNP-prepared nurses are expected to take on frontline leadership roles in evidence-based nursing practice, administration, education, research, and health policy-making. DNP nurse leaders are needed to transform the healthcare system, and therefore advance the health of society. In the health policy arena, DNPs must recognize their role in leading policy making. They must be a visible and vocal presence on high-performing teams, advisory committees, commissions, and boards. Only then will DNPs and all nurses be full partners in advancing the nation's health systems and improving patient care (IOM, 2011).

DNPs must participate in leading the nursing profession and society into the future. Studying nursing leadership and nursing history through the stories of some of the nursing discipline's most prominent leaders fills an educational gap for many nursing students and nurses regarding nursing, nursing leadership, nursing history, and nursing's impact on society (Forrester, 2016). Historic nurse leaders exemplify courage, bravery, fearlessness, open-mindedness, and innovation.

Nursing's history is replete with the life stories of many great nurse leaders. Ours is a distinguished history of nursing leadership, activism, and impact. Over the centuries, nursing leaders have modeled vision, intelligence, resourcefulness, and political awareness. Nursing's leaders have demonstrated a continuing commitment to advancing the discipline and meeting the increasingly complex needs of society.

Although the fascinating life stories of so many historic nurse leaders were lived out long ago and far away, they are just as relevant today as when they occurred. These nurses' stories tell of the evolution of nursing and society over the centuries and around the world. Their stories facilitate an exploration of the very nature of leadership.

In the aggregate, nursing offers a compelling history, not only of events and people within the context of their times, but of the contributions of so many visionary women who had the sheer courage, tenacity, and passion to move the nursing profession into the future—to the betterment of society around the world.

The domain of leaders is the future (Kouzes & Posner, 2017). DNP nurse leaders must lead nursing, health, healthcare, and society into a better future. "*Exemplary nursing leadership* is active, future-oriented, and produces change" (Forrester, 2016, p. 5). The life stories of nursing history's greatest leaders inspire DNP-prepared nurse leaders to become activist agents of change striving for a better future for nursing, health, healthcare, and society.

NEXT STEPS

- Continue to improve your knowledge of historic and current nursing leaders.
- Who are the current nursing leaders in your discipline? What do you know about them?

REFERENCES AND RESOURCES

Forrester, D. A. (2016). *Nursing's greatest leaders: A history of activism.* New York, NY: Springer Publishing Company.

Institute of Medicine. (2011). *The future of nursing: Leading change, advancing health.* Washington, DC: National Academies Press.

Kouzes, J. M., & Posner, B. Z. (2017). *The leadership challenge* (6th ed.). San Francisco, CA: Jossey-Bass.

Nightingale, F. (1859). *Notes on nursing: What it is and what it is not.* London, UK: Harrison.

RELATED TEXTBOOK

Forrester, D. A. (2016). *Nursing's greatest leaders: A history of activism.* New York, NY: Springer Publishing Company.

Part 6: Encouraging the Heart

Part 7: The Future

CHAPTER SUMMARY

Chapter 2, Assembling the DNP Team and Becoming a Leader, builds on leadership concepts and focuses on the logistics of assembling the DNP team. You will have to lead this team, but the other members provide support. Your leadership skills must translate to the practice setting to create change and improve health outcomes. Use inspiration from other nurse leaders, past and present, to guide you.

Reflection

List two things that you have learned about the DNP Project team:

1.

2.

What points do you need clarification about?

1.

2.

NOTES

3

Identifying Problems and Project Topics

Molly J. Bradshaw, Tracy R. Vitale, Mercedes Echevarria,
Patricia Hindin, Jill Cornelison, Sharon Lock,
and Maureen Anderson

Lessons

OBJECTIVES

DNP students struggle to identify problems that would make suitable topics for their DNP Projects. In this chapter, the student will complete a series of exercises to help them think through and brainstorm ideas for the project. Students who have already identified a topic will still benefit by completing the lessons to ensure that they have fully examined their ideas. The goal is to identify a problem of interest and draft a problem statement. By the end of this chapter, you will be able to:

- Inventory potential DNP Project topics at the global, national, and local levels.
- Examine health-related problems within the context of systems, technology, and policy.
- Explain the impact of health problems on populations.
- Select an appropriate problem as the topic of the DNP Project.
- Draft a problem statement.

INTRODUCTION

In 1953, Alex Faickney Osborn wrote a book titled *Applied Imagination*. In the book, he coined the term *brainstorming*. *Brainstorming* refers to the process of creating ideas and writing them down without critiquing them. We will use guided brainstorming as a way to collect ideas and write them down to inspire the topic of your DNP Project. Later, you will critique them and present the outcome to your faculty.

Ideas for DNP Projects are based on problems. When I ask DNP students about their project topics, I will *always* begin by asking them this question, "What is the *problem* that you have identified?" I follow up by saying next, "How does that impact patients?" It will be helpful for you to adopt this strategy. If you talk about your project, start by stating the problem. Follow up by explaining how it impacts patients or a population. At this point, you should refrain from talking about the intervention of the project. Don't let your mind be distracted or jump ahead in the process. "I am going to educate ..." or "I am going to do a chart audit..." —no, stop! These ideas are premature for now. Keep them written down, but off to the side. The intervention is not informed until you can fully understand what the problem is and what issues impact the problem.

In my experience, post-master's DNP students tend to have an easier time identifying the problem they want to address because they are already working in a nursing role. These students tend to struggle more later in the process when the intervention turns out to be different from what they have envisioned. They take feedback with hesitation and sometimes reluctance, or at least I did. As we move through the lessons in this chapter, I ask that you keep an open mind. Your project problem, intervention, and evaluation plan will evolve as you go through the process. Even if you already have a project topic, problem, or practice gap in mind, you need to complete the work of this chapter to ensure that you have thoroughly brainstormed and considered the problem from every angle.

In contrast, students who are in BSN–DNP programs struggle in a different way. There is enormous pressure because they are completing the DNP degree and training for a new nursing role at the same time. In my experience, these students sometimes feel indifferent to the DNP Project because they are more focused on finishing the requirements for advanced practice or a new nursing role. If BSN-DNP students are asked to identify problems, they will most likely identify problems that they have experienced or observed as a registered nurse. They are also more likely to describe problems at their current place of employment, which often changes after they graduate. Likely, the BSN-DNP student may not be working at all as they go through school that heightens their anxiety as they hear classmates talking about projects in their place of employment.

I would like to just offer some friendly advice to BSN–DNP students. First, you have to consider what you want your doctoral expertise to be related to. What will advance your career more? Doing a project related to your current role/situation? Doing a project related to the role you are transitioning to? Second, you do not have to be employed by an organization to do a project there. Consider partnering with the organization you want to work for in the future. This same advice might apply to the post-master's DNP student looking to change her or his career trajectory or organizations in the future. It is simply food for thought. Please consult your faculty to discuss this further.

Problems are also experienced in the context of organizations. This brings us to our next point. The topic of your DNP Project will have to be a problem that both you and your stakeholders identify as a priority. Often, problems are broad, and there may be flexibility as it translates to a DNP Project. In other circumstances, an organization may be very specific about the problem they need help with. You will need to have detailed discussions with your faculty and organizational representatives to sort out the exact context of the problem. Eventually, you will need to do more investigation or root-cause analysis once the priority is identified. Your task now is simply to find problems.

Most importantly, problems in the healthcare setting are experienced by patients, families, and populations. We want you to think about the problem from every possible angle. What is experience of those we serve with this problem? Find inspiration from your population and then consider where this population exists in daily life. Healthcare does not always occur in the four walls of a building, hospital, or clinic.

In summary, remember that these lessons are intended to spark a massive, yet organized brainstorm. Our goal is to ensure that you have fully explored potential problems that could translate to your project topic. In the end, you need to make a final selection and discuss it with your faculty. We will draft a problem statement and you will be able to revise it in in the first lesson of Chapter 4, Developing the DNP Project Background and Context. You may need to revisit this chapter multiple times to reach this goal. Let's begin.

REFERENCE

Osborn, A. F. (1953). *Applied imagination*. Oxford, UK: Scribner's.

MY GOALS FOR IDENTIFYING PROBLEMS AND PROJECT TOPICS ARE TO:

Lesson 3.1

YOUR INITIAL IDEAS

BACKGROUND

Upon admission to DNP programs, students are often asked about a topic for their DNP Project. Some students have well-developed ideas, and this chapter helps enrich those thoughts. Others students are not sure where to start. Start here. Our goal is to help you identify the problem you will work on for your DNP Project. Keep an open mind. Remember that brainstorming is meant for exploring ideas, not critiquing ideas (Stausmire & Ulrich, 2015). The purpose of this lesson is to document initial thoughts, ideas, and experiences as potential topics for the DNP Project. It is the first in a series of brainstorming sessions. The activity is broken down into three parts: your initial thoughts, your favorite clinical subject, and your experiences.

LEARNING OBJECTIVES

- Document, in detail, what you have been thinking about related to the project.
- List your favorite clinical subjects, topics, and diagnosis.
- Reflect on your own experiences.
- Catalog your top three ideas.

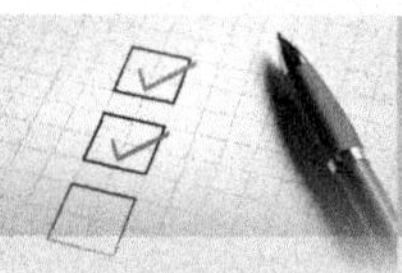

Activities

This is a brainstorming session. The goal is to document your ideas. Respond to each prompt. Set a timer allowing 5 minutes for each prompt. Write whatever comes to mind—sentences, phrases, or words. Avoid trying to edit, analyze, or get it just right. We help you with that later. (Editable versions of these activities may be accessed in a supplemental forms document available at springerpub.com/dpw. This supplement is also available at connect.springerpub.com/content/book/978-0-8261-7433-8.)

Brainstorming Prompt 1: Your Initial Thoughts About the DNP Project

When you started the DNP program, what were you considering for your project? Why?

Brainstorming Prompt 2: Your Favorite Clinical Subject

Make a list of your favorite clinical subjects, topics, or diagnoses; and explain why you like them.

CLINICAL SUBJECT	WHY I LIKE THIS SUBJECT
Example, Diabetes	Interesting, I have a family hx, relevant to family nurse practitioners (FNPs)

Brainstorming Prompt 3: Your Experiences

In your experience (personal or professional), what are the healthcare problems that frustrate you the most? Why? Think of this in terms of patients, families, populations, healthcare organizations/systems, policies, technology, colleagues, and so on.

NEXT STEPS

Now, take a highlighter and review what you have read. Highlight the three ideas that you like the most. Write those ideas below using only two to three words. At the end of the chapter, we will come back to these three concepts.

Example: Distress in diabetics

1. ______________________________

2. ______________________________

3. ______________________________

- Review this article on finding meaningful projects (www.aacn.org/docs/cemedia/C1563.pdf). This article is the first in a series of four articles about starting the quality improvement (QI) process. You may find the content informative.
- Discuss your thoughts with your DNP faculty.

REFERENCE AND RESOURCE

Stausmire, J., & Ulrich, C. (2015). Making it meaningful: Finding quality improvement projects worthy of your time, effort, and expertise. *Critical Care Nurse*, *35*(6), 57–62. doi: 10.4037/ccn2015232

Lesson 3.2

IDENTIFYING GLOBAL AND NATIONAL PROBLEMS

BACKGROUND

The first step of the DNP Project is to identify a problem of interest. Problems may have different contexts if they are examined at different levels. For example, the global priorities for vaccine-preventable diseases may be different from national priorities. What if vaccines were readily available in one country, but not in another? The problems and issues would be different.

Ultimately, the DNP Project is narrowed to a single focus. The goal here is not to solve the problems of the world. The point is to learn about the potential for global and national priorities to connect or inform your work. Examining global and national health agendas will give you a broad place to start, especially if you have no idea what you want to do your project on. Global issues filter to national issues, which trickle down to state and local issues.

LEARNING OBJECTIVES

- Identify several global and national health priorities.
- List three priorities of interest to you.

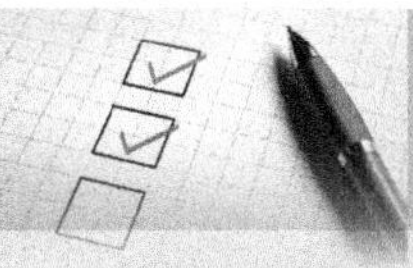

Activities

The World Health Organization (WHO) is a leader of global health. Visit the WHO website (www.who.int). Review the topics and explore those of interest to you. To look at a more focused list, examine the *Health-related Millennium Development Goals and Targets.* Take notes as you go. Remember, don't try to overanalyze. Go to what draws you in.

Topic:	**Notes:**
Topic:	**Notes:**
Topic:	**Notes:**

Topic:	Notes:
Topic:	Notes:

Highlight and list your three favorite global health topics.

1. ______________________________
2. ______________________________
3. ______________________________

Visit the Healthy People website (www.healthypeople.gov).

Review the Healthy People 2020 topics and the proposed Health People 2030 topics. Explore those of interest to you. Take notes as you go. Remember, don't try to overanalyze. Go to what draws you in.

Topic:	Notes:
Topic:	Notes:
Topic:	Notes:
Topic:	Notes:
Topic:	Notes:

NEXT STEPS

Highlight and list your favorite three national health topics.

1. ______________________________

2. ______________________________

3. ______________________________

We return to these lists at the end of the chapter. Remember that the global and national health agendas help to articulate needs. Healthcare organizations often set their goals to be in alignment with these. These sites are not comprehensive but are great places to start. To further explore global and national health priorities, see the suggested websites in the References and Resources section. You can adjust your list as needed.

REFERENCES AND RESOURCES

Centers for Disease Control and Prevention. (2019). Population health. Retrieved from https://www.cdc.gov/nccd php/dph/index.html

Centers for Medicare & Medicaid Services. (2019). Outcome measures. Retrieved from https://www.cms.gov/Medicare/Quality-Initiatives-Patient-Assessment-Instruments/HospitalQualityInits/OutcomeMeasures.html

World Health Organization. (2019a). Health-related millennium development goals and targets. Retrieved from https://www.who.int/gho/mdg/goals_targets/en

World Health Organization. (2019b). Topics. Retrieved from https://www.who.int

U.S. Department of Health and Human Services. (2019). Healthy people. Retrieved from https://www.healthypeople.gov

RELATED TEXTBOOK

Rosa, W. (2017). *A new era of global health.* New York, NY: Springer Publishing Company.

Lesson 3.3

IDENTIFYING STATE AND LOCAL PROBLEMS

BACKGROUND

This chapter is about brainstorming. We are gathering information to help solidify the idea for your DNP Project. The information being gathered is essentially a list of problems, conditions, and experiences that peak your interest. Later, we will make sense of the information.

In this lesson, we look around at our regional, state, and local environments. What are the pressing health problems? For example, I live in Kentucky. Tobacco abuse and misuse is a major health problem. The problem of tobacco abuse could result in a number of health-related problems such as asthma, chronic obstructive pulmonary disease (COPD), or a health risk factor. Are the local problems cultural? What populations live in your area? Is there a lack of resources? Are there problems with access to care? You are more likely to be aware of issues at this level, but we will still utilize online resources to explore further.

LEARNING OBJECTIVES

- Determine health priorities by visiting websites and writing down what you know.
- List the top three health problems of interest to you.

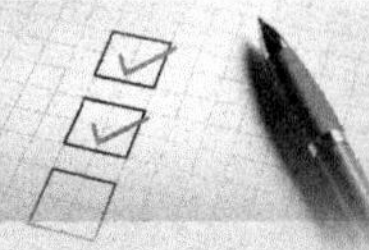

Activities

Start this session by visiting the Centers for Disease Control and Prevention (CDC) website (www.cdc.gov.). In the search bar, select your state and explore the information presented. Also visit your official state agency for health's website. Make a list of health problems of interest to you and take notes as you go. Remember, don't analyze the list yet. Just write down what piques your interest.

State: ____________________

Topic:	Notes:
Topic:	**Notes:**
Topic:	**Notes:**
Topic:	**Notes:**
Topic:	**Notes:**
Topic:	**Notes:**

Highlight and list three keywords from what you have written about a health-related problem.

1. ______________________________
2. ______________________________
3. ______________________________

Most likely you are already aware of local health problems. However, make sure that you fully explore the available information. First, see whether you can identify local agencies involved in healthcare. Make a list of the agencies and then, if they have websites, look at the sites. If you can visit the agencies in person, that may also be a great way to network and learn more about local health problems. Second, think about health in your communities—your schools, your place of worship, and your local government. Remember that healthcare does not always occur in a healthcare facility. Finally, talk to people: network. You may discover perspectives that you have not considered.

Local Agency Name: **Health Problems/Priorities:**	**Notes:**
Local Agency Name: **Health Problems/Priorities:**	**Notes:**
Local Agency Name: **Health Problems/Priorities:**	**Notes:**
Local Agency Name: **Health Problems/Priorities:**	**Notes:**
Local Agency Name: **Health Problems/Priorities:**	**Notes:**

NEXT STEPS

Circle the three agencies most of interest to you. Make a list of three local health problems of interest to you. At the end of this chapter, we return to this list. If you feel overwhelmed at this point, remember that we will analyze our work later. The goal at this time is to gather information. Analysis of information is discussed later. At the end of this chapter, we return to this list. If you feel overwhelmed at this point, remember that we will analyze our work later. The goal at this time is to gather information. Analysis of information is discussed later.

1. ______________________________

2. ______________________________

3. ______________________________

RELATED TEXTBOOK

Ervin, N. E., & Kulbok, P. (2018). *Advanced public and community health nursing*. New York, NY: Springer Publishing Company.

Lesson 3.4

PROBLEMS WITH THE HEALTHCARE SYSTEM, INFORMATION, AND TECHNOLOGY

BACKGROUND

When problems in healthcare arise, they are often a result of a faulty system (Institute of Medicine [IOM], 1999). To practice at the highest level, DNP graduates are skilled in identifying problems, making changes, and evaluating the impact of the change. Often, there are problems in the healthcare system that need to be changed. Changes might occur on different system levels.

Information and technology have a close relationship with health systems. Let's first consider information. As information is generated, it can be used to evaluate and improve practice. Information about patients must be communicated and passed from one healthcare team member to another. Patients must be able to access and interpret their health information. Next, consider the impact of technology. Ideally, technology should be a means to improve system issues like scheduling, communication, or access to information. Is that always the case? No, because technology is rarely perfect. It can improve some system issues and cause others.

In this exercise, you can take a few different approaches:

- Examine the system where you are currently employed.
- Examine the system of a place you have worked in the past.
- Examine the system where you hope to be employed in the future.
- Examine a system like your community: a school, place of worship, or club.
- Examine the system as if you were a patient with a given condition.
- Other: ______________________________

You can repeat this exercise in the future if needed. Highlight the option you select so that you can discuss it later with faculty.

LEARNING OBJECTIVES

- Identify the system you are going to examine in this exercise.
- Organize problems and challenges as either macro- or micro-system related.
- State the potential for impact by information.
- State the potential for impact by technology.

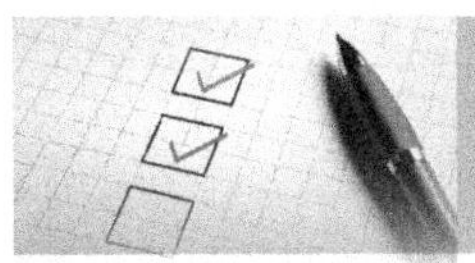

Activities

Systems thinking provides a good framework to begin problem identification (Figure 3.1). Write down potential problems for each level.

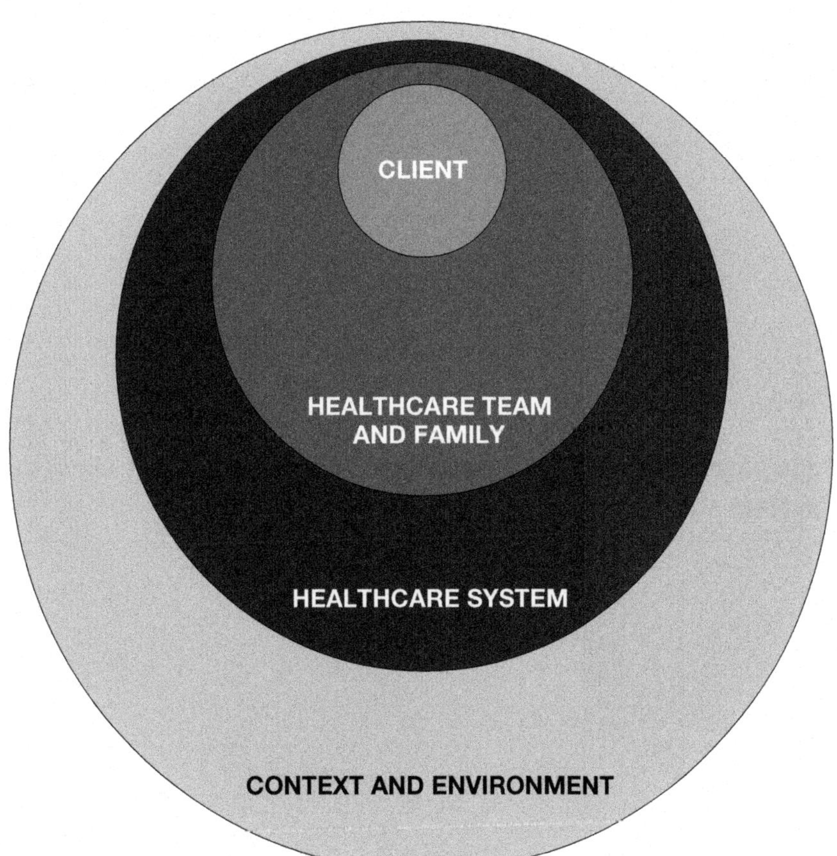

Figure 3.1 The levels of systems thinking.

Patient Level

Problem of Interest: ______________________________

Care-Team Level

Problem of Interest: ______________________________

Organizational Level

Problem of Interest: ______________________________

Environmental Level

Problem of Interest: ______________________________

Consider the potential impact of information. Write a statement about the impact of information on the system problems.

____

Consider the potential impact of technology. Write a statement about the impact of technology on the system problems.

____

Review your work on this activity to date. Highlight and list three key problems. List them here:

1. ______________________________

2. ______________________________

3. ______________________________

If you are following the workbook lessons in order, we are starting to gather several problems. You may or may not notice overlap. Remember, do not try to analyze anything yet. We are working toward a summary and synthesis. For now, continue to gather ideas and deepen your understanding of various problems. In a later chapter, we talk more about organizational assessment and workflow analysis. You are doing great! Keep going. Work hard.

NEXT STEPS

- Talk to your DNP faculty.
- Continue to be alert for opportunities to improve systems and technology use.

REFERENCES AND RESOURCES

Bisht, C., Mehrotra, D., & Kalra, P. (2019). To calculate the usability of healthcare mobile applications using cognitive walkthrough. Retrieved from https://link.springer.com/chapter/10.1007/978-981-13-1642-5_24

Institute of Medicine. (1999). *To err is human*. Washington, DC: National Academies Press.

Sheehan, B., & Bakken, S. (n.d.). Approaches to workflow analysis in healthcare settings. Retrieved from https://www.ncbi.nlm.nih.gov/pmc/articles/PMC3799136/pdf/amia_2012_ni_371.pdf

Stalter, A. M., Phillips, J. M., Ruggiero, J. S., Scardaville, D. L., Merriam, D., Dolansky, M. A., … Winegardner, S. (2017). A concept analysis of systems thinking. *Nursing Forum*, *52*(4), 323–330. doi: 10.1111/nuf.12196

The Office of the National Coordinator for Health Information Technology. (2019). Topics. Retrieved from https://www.healthit.gov/topics

RELATED TEXTBOOK

McBride, S., & Tietze, M. (2018). *Nursing informatics for the advanced practice nurse: Patient safety, quality, outcomes, and interprofessionalism* (2nd ed.). New York, NY: Springer Publishing Company.

Chapter 9: Workflow Redesign

Lesson 3.5

COGNITIVE WALKTHROUGH

BACKGROUND

Cognitive walkthrough is a technique used to evaluate process and determine ease of usability. It helps to identify problems. DNP students may or may not have access to the site where their DNP Projects will take place in the beginning of the planning process. If you do have access, you may find it more helpful to do a live, literal walkthrough of the workspace in this exercise. If you do not have access, just use experience, imagination, and critical thinking skills to do a "cognitive" walkthrough.

LEARNING OBJECTIVES

- Document potential problems in the context of your setting.

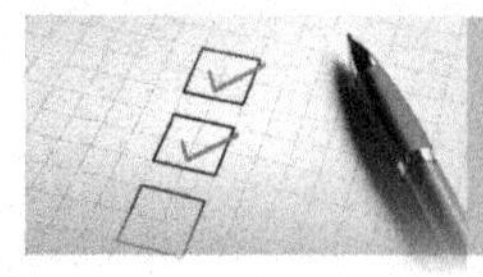

Activities

In this lesson, you will be guided through a series of prompts. As you complete the lesson, your goal is to focus on the perspective of the patient.

Describe the patient.

- Do they have a certain condition?
- Does the patient have any impairment?
- What does this patient need to improve his or her health?

Imagine that the patient has entered the health system.

- In what context: Community, outpatient, or inpatient?
- How does the patient find access?
- What is it like when the patient arrives?

Walk through the environment and the interactions the patient will have with staff.

- Have you identified any problems?

Now imagine the patient's care is in transition.

- In what context: Community, outpatient, or inpatient?
- What types of communications need to take place?
- Does the patient have the resources they need
- Have you identified any problems?

SUMMARY

In later chapters, we talk more about formal organizational assessment and process mapping. The point here is to critically think about what problems a patient might encounter. It is an informal strategy to get you thinking about potential problems. You will organize your chapter findings in the next activity.

Lesson 3.6

NETWORKING TO IDENTIFY AND DISCUSS PROBLEMS

BACKGROUND

Networking with others adds perspective. Just because you identify that something is a problem, it does not mean that others perceive it in the same way. Networking also creates connections that may lead to collaboration in the future. In this lesson, it may be helpful for you to utilize some of the tips we suggested in the beginning of the workbook. As you network, be sure to leave your business card with people. Organize information from the discussions by taking notes that include the time and date. Later, you may want to incorporate the discussion in your DNP Project proposal. The conversation can be recorded as a "personal communication."

Whom should I network with? To begin, we recommend starting with your faculty. Review the faculty profiles at your school. If possible, schedule a meeting with faculty who have expertise in your area of interest. Then, you may consider networking with a stakeholder in one or two of the organizations/systems you identified. Who are the leaders there whom you will need to know to make change?

We also recommend networking with others in your current or future nursing role. If you are a nurse executive, talk to other nurse executives. If you are a BSN–DNP student transitioning to a role as a pediatric nurse practitioner, talk to other pediatric nurse practitioners. Professional organizations often have outlets for connecting to online discussion forums. You can also join the Doctor of Nursing Practice Organization for free (www.doctorsofnursingpractice.org). This organization is the only national organization for DNP-prepared nurses, but it is not specific to nursing role.

LEARNING OBJECTIVES

- Engage in networking.
- Discuss problems of interest to colleagues, stakeholders, and others.

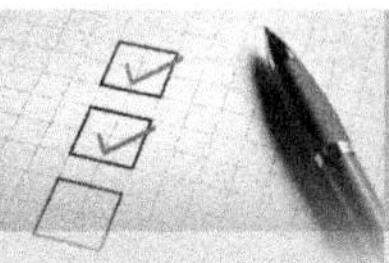

Activities

Use this outline to begin your networking journey. For the purposes of finding the problem you want to work on for your project, we recommend that you network with at least three people. Review the suggested questions which are all open ended to begin conversation. As you interact, you can ask more pointed questions. Remember to get contact information so that you can reach out again in the future. Be on time, gracious, and thank people for their input.

Start: I am a DNP student at ______________________. I am interested in ______________________.

- What have you observed related to ____?
- How does the system, information, technology, or policy impact ____?
- What has been done so far to address ____?
- Are there any discussions on improving ____?
- What are some problems you experienced ____?
- How are problems analyzed ____?

Networking Activity 1

Name:
Organization:

Notes:

Networking Activity 2

Name:
Organization:

Notes:

Networking Activity 3

Name:
Organization:

Notes:

Expert Commentary: Jill Cornelison, DNP, RN

As a faculty advisor for DNP students, I am astutely aware that identification of a clinical problem for a potential DNP Project is not a simple task for the student. Often, students choose a problem they feel passionate about or have become aware of through reading the healthcare literature. Conversely, I encounter students who have already decided what they want to implement for their project or what practice change they want to make without knowing whether a problem actually exists. Difficulties also arise when the clinical problem that the student has chosen does not align with an agency's needs and objectives or the clinical problem does not evolve into the implementation of a scholarly project.

Identifying a clinical problem requires early discussion and analysis of a potential agency's needs. The student should have conversations with leaders within the agency before making a final decision on a clinical problem for the DNP Project. In other words, the need to network. The effort spent on the front end to identify a viable, appropriate, and feasible clinical problem affords the student more opportunity to develop a scholarly DNP Project that impacts healthcare outcomes. Networking is purposeful. It is actively seeking and engaging others who may have common concerns, interests, and goals. You need to get out and put yourself out there. Take advantage of every opportunity to network.

NEXT STEPS

- Network to align your goals with the needs of the organization/agency.
- Determine the timelines for your project and the agency's need.

RELATED TEXTBOOK

Marshall, E. S., & Broome, M. E. (2016). *Transformational leadership in nursing*. New York, NY: Springer Publishing Company.

Chapter 5: Collaborative Leadership Contexts: Networks, Communication, Decision-Making, and Motivation

NOTES

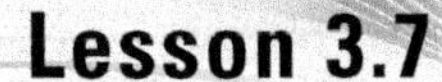

Lesson 3.7

ORGANIZING YOUR FINDINGS

BACKGROUND

As discussed earlier, brainstorming is a process of generating ideas without judgment. Problems are the foundation of DNP Projects. You have been completing a series of exercises to identify problems. Now we begin the process of organizing the information. After it is consolidated, we will begin critiquing the information and move toward selecting the problem for your DNP Project.

LEARNING OBJECTIVES

- List the top findings from each activity in its designated location.
- Analyze the information and select your two favorite problems.

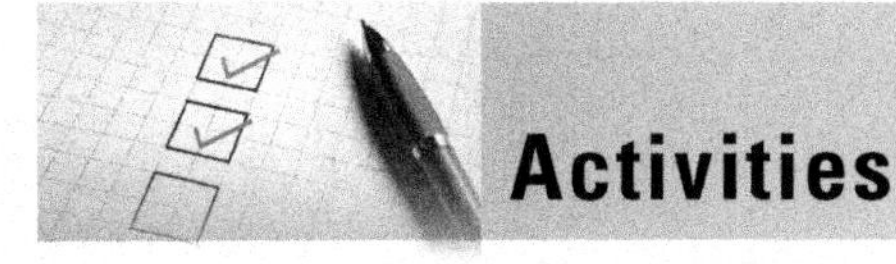

Activities

Reflection

Write a short summary of your new perspective of health-related problems after completing the previous activities.

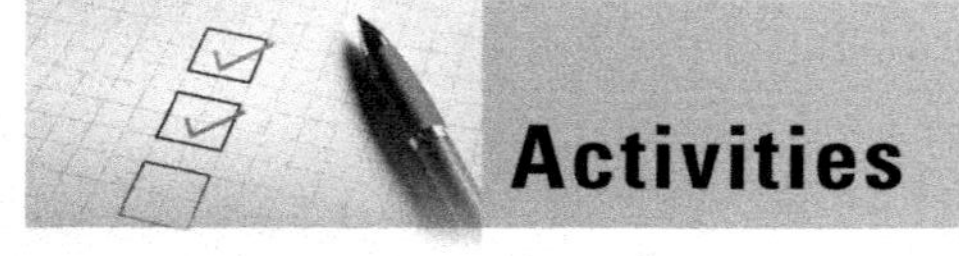

Activities

Transfer your lists from previous activities completed in this chapter to their designated locations here. Then, take some time to reflect on the content. After careful reflection, highlight the top two problems of interest to you and write them down.

ORGANIZING YOUR FINDINGS:

Problems I have Identified

Transfer your lists from each lesson to this page.

Initial Ideas:

Initial Thoughts, Subjects, and Experiences

1.

2.

3.

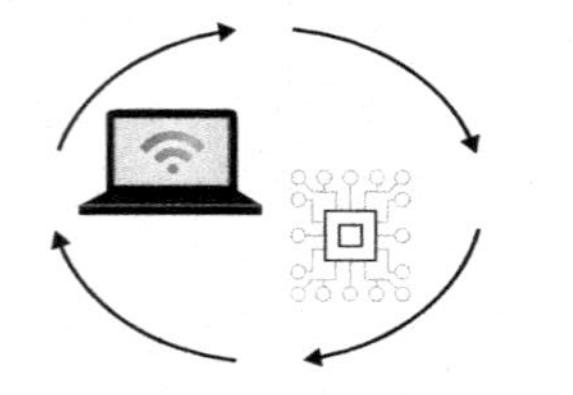

Problems With Systems, Information, and Technology:

1.

2.

3.

Global Problems:

1.

2.

3.

National Problems:

1.

2.

3.

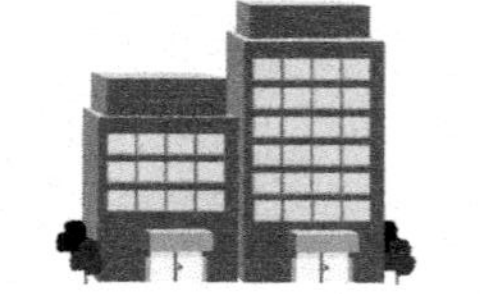

State and Local Problems:

1.

2.

3.

After Networking, These Problems Were Identified:

1.

2.

3.

Selection

1. Highlight similar problems in the same color.
2. Highlight your *favorite* problem.
3. Circle your top two choices and list them here.

Selected Problem A: ______________________

Selected Problem B: ______________________

Are you pleased with these topics?

Notes:

Write your selected problems here.

Problem A:

Problem B:

NEXT STEPS

- Discuss your top two ideas with your faculty.

Lesson 3.8

SELECTING THE PROBLEM AND DRAFTING THE PROBLEM STATEMENT

BACKGROUND

After completing the brainstorming process, you have identified two potential problems for your DNP Project. You must discuss them with your faculty or DNP Project chair. Complete the prompts that follow. Attempt a draft of your DNP Project problem statement.

LEARNING OBJECTIVES

- Discuss with your faculty the potential problems you have identified.
- Finalize your choice for the problem of interest in your DNP Project.
- Draft a problem statement.

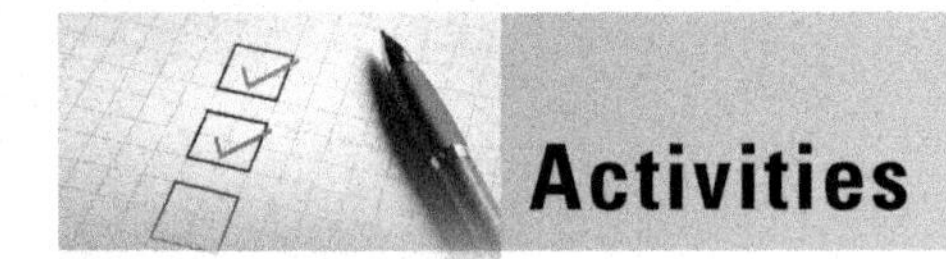

Activities

In this activity you will do a side-by-side comparison of the two problems you identified in the previous lesson. After listing each problem, complete the prompts to share with your DNP Faculty. This may also provide perspective if you are "torn" between two project ideas.

Problem A:	**Problem B:**
______________________	______________________
I selected this problem because:	I selected this problem because:
______________________	______________________
______________________	______________________
______________________	______________________
______________________	______________________
______________________	______________________
I know it's a problem because:	I know it's a problem because:
______________________	______________________
______________________	______________________
______________________	______________________
______________________	______________________
______________________	______________________

Tips From Faculty Experts

Finding the Middle Ground for the Student and Clinical Agency

Sharon Lock, PhD, APRN, FNAP, FAANP

Many students enter a DNP program without an idea about what they want to do their project on. They know they have to do a project but haven't put much thought into it. During initial discussions, I try to find out, in general, what topics students are interested in. If a clinical agency has a need for a quality-improvement (QI) study that a student could be a part of, that could be a win–win for both the agency and the student. However, the time frames of the clinical agency and the student may not coincide.

Typically, the time frame for DNP Projects is over a period of years, whereas a clinical agency will want a QI project to be completed in a much shorter time frame.

Often, the student's original idea is broad, and they need help narrowing down the project. I ask students to think about part of the problem that could be managed in a better way. Once the student has narrowed down the topic, I advise the student to go to the literature to see what has been published on the topic. Sometimes, the student finds a study or project that is very similar to what they were interested in doing and gets discouraged. When that happens, we brainstorm about ways to replicate or improve the project. How can it be translated into the context of the clinical agency the student is working at? The key is to find the middle ground—the project that a student can complete for an agency over a period of time that is reasonable for both.

Collaborate With an Open Mind

Maureen Anderson, DNP, APN, CRNA

Identifying a project topic takes an open mind and multiple levels of collaboration. A single idea has the ability to grow into a topic that can have a substantial impact on professional practice. As students start to navigate the DNP process and develop ideas, it is crucial to have conversations with experts in the area of interest. It is through these early conversations that a project truly evolves and takes on a life of its own. These conversations should begin with fellow classmates who share the same novice vantage point and then continue with expert faculty who can focus, validate, and vet an idea. Pairing a novice DNP student with an expert faculty member and clinician lends itself to fresh innovative ideas due to the difference in perspectives and level of experience.

As the project idea is being established and vetted, the conversations can and should continue with stakeholders at a local, state, and even national level. Examples include local private practice groups or state and national professional associations. Making these connections early in the process can set the stage for a DNP Project and create additional opportunities for reporting and dissemination. A project's success can be directly related to the level of collaboration, networking, and a student's open mind.

Problem Before Innovation

Patricia Hindin, PhD, CNM, RYT 200

The initial critical misstep that students often make is that after identifying a topic, they begin formulating their innovation. The proposed change is usually a teaching project with a pre- and posttest questionnaire. So I inquire. What do you really know about the most current literature? And why do you think that people have to be educated about it? What is the problem at your clinical site? You need to analyze the topic and focus the issue and find out what has been done in the literature to address the problem. How successful has the site been with the problem? Why? Why not? Your role as a DNP is to take evidence from the literature and translate that to your specific problem situation.

WARNING AND CRITICAL POINT: Before you begin the selection process, you must have a conversation with your faculty. We recommend against moving forward with the workbook unless you have assurance from your faculty that the problem is viable. Remind the faculty that our goal is to find problems. We have not performed official workflow analysis or explored the potential solutions yet. Bring your work from this chapter with you. Talk about the pros and cons of each problem and utilize this worksheet to help you.

PROBLEM A:	PROBLEM B:

PROS	CONS	PROS	CONS

After discussions with faculty and weighing pros and cons, my final selected problem for my DNP Project is:

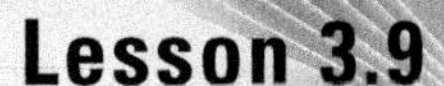

Lesson 3.9

WRITING A PROBLEM STATEMENT

BACKGROUND

The problem statement addresses the practice problem and provides continued direction throughout the duration of the project. It answers the questions of who, what, where, when, why, and how. A problem statement specific to a DNP Project offers the reader an understanding of the issues surrounding the practice problem and the reason the project was selected.

A properly constructed problem statement has four components: lead-in, declaration or presentation of originality, explanation, and indication of the central focus (Hernon & Schwartz, 2007). The lead-in will help to set the stage. The declaration or presentation of originality will substantiate the need for inquiry and document the gap in practice. The explanation will highlight the value and/or benefits of the intervention, and the indication of the central focus states what the project will accomplish.

LEARNING OBJECTIVES

- Draft a problem statement for the DNP Project.

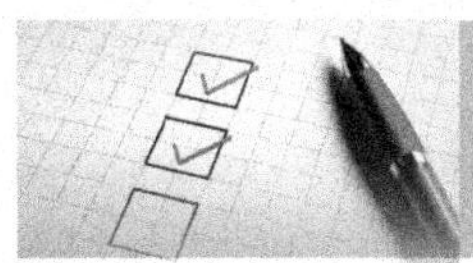

Activities

An exemplar problem statement is provided. After reading it, follow the prompts that break it down and use it to write your own problem statement.

What is the problem or gap in practice that you are planning to address?

1. Start with your lead-in (this will answer a reader's "why should I care" question):

Exemplar: Caregivers often experience negative psychological, behavioral, and physiological effects on their daily lives and health.

2. Next is your declaration or presentation of originality (this will answer a reader's "so what" question):

Exemplar: Many studies have documented the value of conducting interventions to decrease stress for those at risk for developing chronic stress due to being a caregiver. These studies have documented decreased stress outcome scores and increased self-rated health for this population. A needs assessment conducted within a parish setting has documented the need to implement these evidence-based interventions to reduce stress outcomes scores and to increase self-rated health in this population.

3. Next comes your explanation (this will answer a reader's "what will we gain from this" question):

Exemplar: Participation in this stress-reduction program will decrease stress outcome scores and the number of lost workdays and increase self-rated health in African American women experiencing caregiver stress.

4. End with the indication of the central focus (this will answer a reader's "how so" question):

Exemplar: The project implements and evaluates a care delivery model of stress reduction integrating the nurse in the parish setting to assist in achieving positive clinical and cost outcomes related to caregiver stress.

NEXT STEPS

- Take time to reflect on your problem statement.
- Revise the statement as necessary and with the input of your DNP team.
- Remember that this is only a first draft. You will continue to revise the problem statement as you go further in the process.

REFERENCES AND RESOURCES

Hernon, P., & Schwartz, C. (2007). What is a problem statement? *Library & Information Science Research*, *29*(3), 307–309. Retrieved from http://www.lis-editors.org/bm~doc/editorial-problem-statement.pdf

RELATED TEXTBOOK

Bonnel, W., & Smith, K. (2018). *Proposal writing for clinical nursing and DNP Projects.* New York, NY: Springer Publishing Company.

Chapter 3: Writing a Good Problem Statement and Putting the Problem in Context

CHAPTER SUMMARY

The focus of this chapter is to identify problems that could potentially translate into the topic of your DNP Project. Problems are broad. Identifying the problem gives you a starting point from which to further develop your project. It is to be hoped that the experience of working on a DNP Project related to this topic will advance your knowledge and skills toward your long-term goals. Solidifying the problem statement adds clarity to your DNP Project.

Reflections

What are two things that you have learned in this chapter?

1.

2.

If you were able to choose a problem for your project, what is your final selection? Why is working on this problem important to you?

____

____

____

If you were not able to select a problem to pursue, we recommend the following actions:

- Can you identify a reason why you are struggling?
- Consult with your faculty.
- Review the lessons and repeat activities as necessary.
- Examine the suggested list of problems in the Appendix.

You should have a problem identified before moving on to Chapter 4, Developing the DNP Project Background and Context. Realize that if the problem changes, you may need to repeat these lessons. Additional copies of the forms are located in the online resources of this textbook. If this is the case, do not be discouraged. This is a real-world project subjected to real-world circumstances. The only thing that you can count on is that things change and evolve. Continue to work the process.

NOTES

4

Developing the DNP Project Background and Context

Molly J. Bradshaw, Tracy R. Vitale, and Karen Gilbert

Lessons

OBJECTIVES

After selecting a problem to address for the DNP Project, a problem statement is written and finalized. The next step is to fully describe the background and context of the problem. What is the problem? Who is affected by it? Why is it a problem? In this chapter, students are guided through lessons to gather information about the problem in its local context. After a thorough investigation, students explore potential solutions to address the problem. By the end of this chapter, you will be able to:

- Refine the problem statement and describe what is currently known.
- Present the key points of policy, standards, and guidelines related to the problem.
- Examine the problem in its local context.
- List potential solutions to the problem.
- Organize findings in preparation for proposal writing.

INTRODUCTION

The DNP Project is centered on a problem. The problem of interest is both the starting point and the focal point. Starting today, if someone asks you this question, "What is your DNP Project about?" your reply should be, "The problem I am focused on is ________________." In this chapter, our goal is to gather information to ensure that you fully understand this problem in its local context. We will help you organize this information so that you are prepared to begin writing the first draft of your project proposal. Our goals for this chapter are to determine:

- What is the problem?
- Who is affected by the problem?
- Why it is a problem?

What questions do you have about your problem of interest? For some DNP students, the problem may be a topic with which you have a strong working knowledge and experience. Maybe there is more to learn. A spirit of inquiry will sharpen and broaden your perspective. There may be factors you have overlooked or were not aware of that influence the problem. For other DNP students, the problem may be new. For example, if you are a BSN–DNP student and your faculty is suggesting a problem to you for investigation, you may be starting with a more novice perspective. In either case, we are here to help you discover information and organize the findings to deepen your understanding.

The DNP graduate should be an expert in her or his project subject matter. At the doctoral level, this is very important. Remember that the American Association of Colleges of Nursing (AACN, 2015) suggests that this is a foundation of future scholarship. Is addressing this problem something that could advance your career, role, or future endeavors? Does addressing the problem add value to the community, organization, or healthcare system? Most importantly, will addressing this problem improve health outcomes for patients, families, and populations?

The lessons and activities in this chapter are the next logical steps of the DNP Project process.

- You are prepared for success.
- You are positioned for leadership.
- You have identified your problem of interest.
- You are moving toward comprehensive investigation of the problem in this chapter.

At the end of the chapter, we guide you toward resources to help you with the writing process. We recommend that you complete all of the lessons in this chapter *before* you begin formal writing. Think of this chapter as presenting an opportunity to gather all of the information you possibly can about this problem. You will then synthesize the information to help you assemble a DNP Project proposal. Let's begin.

REFERENCE

American Association of Colleges of Nursing. (2015). *The doctor of nursing practice: Current issues and clarifying recommendations.* Retrieved from https://www.aacnnursing.org/Portals/42/News/White-Papers/DNP-Implementation-TF-Report-8-15.pdf

Lesson 4.1

REVISING THE PROBLEM STATEMENT

BACKGROUND

The DNP Project begins by identifying a problem(s) that directly or indirectly impacts the health of patients (American Association of Colleges of Nursing, 2015). Patients generally belong to a larger group or population. To bring the DNP Project into focus, it is necessary to clearly define the problem and population of interest. You will have an opportunity to finalize the problem statement at the end of this chapter.

For our purposes, we use the following definitions:

- Problem of interest: The primary issue, focal point, and subject considered in the DNP Project.
- Population of interest: The patient and larger group that is impacted by the problem.

The problem statement is the one- to two-sentence key phrase that concisely describes what your project is based on. The problem statement must be clearly written. Review the lesson on the elements of a problem statement described in the introduction to this chapter.

LEARNING OBJECTIVES

- Further define the problem of interest.
- Identify the population(s) impacted by the problem.

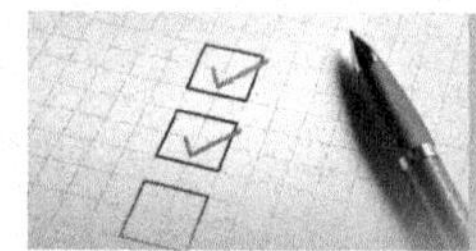

Activities

Complete the following questions and statements. Be concise. Write one to two sentences for each item.

What is the problem you have identified?
How do you know it's a problem?

What population(s) is affected by the problem? Make a list.
How do you know the population is impacted?

Where (context) does the problem occur?
Where is the affected population(s) located?

Why is the problem important?

Besides yourself, who else thinks it's important?

Off the top of your head, what do you think could be done about this problem?

Other notes:

Reflect on the content.

Problem of Interest

- Is there an official definition of your problem? Write it here and note the source.
- If the problem is a diagnosis/condition, answer the following and note the source:
  - How is the condition screened?
  - How is the condition diagnosed?
  - How is the condition treated?
    - Pharmacological treatments:
    - Nonpharmacological treatments:

Population of Interest

You will learn in your program that certain populations are vulnerable. Therefore, when doing projects or completing research (PhD), examination by an institutional review board (IRBs) is needed to protect these groups from harm. Some examples include pregnant women, children, prisoners, or the elderly. At some point, you will most likely get formal training offered through the Collaborative Institutional Training Initiative (CITI) Program. Check with your school and faculty regarding use of vulnerable populations and training requirements. We are making you aware of this for purposes of planning. It does not mean that you should necessarily avoid these groups. Rather, it means that you should plan appropriately and under the advisement of your faculty.

Here are some additional questions you will need to answer:

- Population descriptors: Age, gender, diagnosis, comorbid conditions, other?
- Where can you get access to this population (organization, community setting, other)?
  - Location 1:
  - Location 2:
  - Location 3:

SUMMARY

The goal of this lesson is to articulate the problem and examine the population it impacts. As you develop the project, you may or may not directly involve your population of interest. This will become clearer as you develop the methods of the project.

Example: Population of Interest—Patients aged 65 years and older with chronic obstructive pulmonary disease (COPD)

Direct Impact: "My project goal is to promote self-management of COPD."

Indirect Impact: "My project will ensure providers are increasing vaccination rates for COPD patients."

Now rewrite the problem statement for your project. Ensure you have the following four elements: Lead-in, declaration, explanation, and indication of central focus. Next steps:

- Discuss your school training requirements for dealing with vulnerable populations, ethics, and so on.
- Define your problem in a key phrase. Describe your population in one to two words.

REFERENCES AND RESOURCES

American Association of Colleges of Nursing. (2015). *The doctor of nursing practice: Current issues and clarifying recommendations.* Retrieved from https://www.aacnnursing.org/Portals/42/News/White-Papers/DNP-Implementation-TF-Report-8-15.pdf

CITI Program. (n.d.). Research ethics and compliance training. Retrieved from https://about.citiprogram.org/en/homepage/

RELATED TEXTBOOKS

Christenbery, T. (Ed.). (2018). *Evidence-based practice in nursing.* New York, NY: Springer Publishing Company.

Chapter 10: Identifying Significant Evidence-Based Practice Problems Within Complex Health Environments

Chapter 20: Evidence-Based Practice: Empowering Nurses

Hickey, J. V., & Brosnan, C. A. (Eds.). (2017). *Evaluation of health care quality for DNPs* (2nd ed.). New York, NY: Springer Publishing Company.

Chapter 12: Evaluating Populations and Population Health

Lesson 4.2

INITIAL INQUIRY AND INITIAL SEARCH

BACKGROUND

Nurses prepared with the DNP degree are committed to the use of evidence to guide and change when necessary (Christenbery, 2018). When problems are identified, change begins by asking questions. What is the problem? What impacts or influences the problem? The spirit of inquiry drives exploration of data, relationships, phenomena, and practice to better understand the problem's context.

In this lesson, we guide you through the initial inquiries that are necessary for the background of the project. You will need to complete some initial literature searches. The goal at this time is to gather information about the problem. We ask you to track your searches and keep a working reference list.

As the project develops, you will have additional questions that need clarification. What is the best method for __________? What strategies promote adoption of a clinical guideline? To answer these pointed, focused questions, a formal review of the literature, an integrative review, or a systematic review is completed. We discuss the differences in a later lesson. Ultimately, the DNP Project is guided by question(s) you ask (Christenbery, 2018) and the evidence you translate and implement to solve your problem of interest (Holly, 2019).

It is critical to mention the importance of working with librarians. Librarians are trained specifically to help identify and retrieve information. They know the nuances of keywords, Boolean phrasing, and databases. We *highly* recommend that you reach out to your university library and seek assistance *early*. Librarians are invaluable colleagues.

LEARNING OBJECTIVES

- Complete initial searches related to the problem.
- Compile a working reference list with a minimum of 10 references.

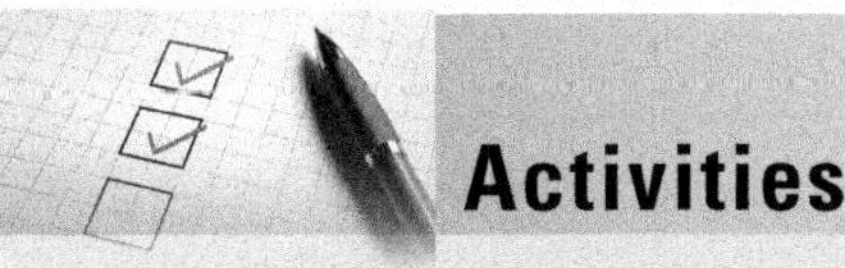

Activities

(Editable versions of these activities may be accessed in a supplemental forms document available at springerpub.com/dpw. This supplement is also available at connect.springerpub.com/content/book/978-0-8261-7433-8.)

Ground Zero. Ask yourself whether you are informed on your topic. In other words, do you routinely read and consume information on this topic? To become an expert, you need to begin by improving your general knowledge. Make a plan:

1. I will read two to three articles daily starting on: ______________________ (date)

2. I will explore podcasts on this topic starting on: ______________________ (date)

3. I will consume information daily on this topic starting on: ______________________ (date)

Search the literature on your own using the Internet. Gather as much information related to your problem as possible. Use this table to help you organize your findings.

Source Citation:	Notes:
1	
2	
3	
4	
5	
6	
7	
8	
9	
10	

Write a short summary of what you have discovered about your problem. Why is it a problem?

Now let's focus on your database searches. Develop a series of keywords based on your problem and population.

SUMMARIZE YOUR PROBLEM IN ONE SENTENCE	SELECT THREE KEYWORDS RELEVANT TO THE PROBLEM
	1. ______________________ 2. ______________________ 3. ______________________

My population of interest is: ____

Boolean logic is a symbolic method of combining keywords to focus searches (Digital Literacy, 2010; Kate the Librarian, 2011). Here, we focus on the use of "OR." When you type the keywords in a search box with OR (in all caps) between the key terms, the database will produce results with _(Key Term)_ OR _(Key Term)_ (Figure 4.1). The OR operator can be effective when there are terms that are synonymous (or nearly synonymous) to your keywords, saving a second search. For example, kidney disease OR renal disease. The next approach is to use AND (in all caps) between key terms. This will cause the database to combine results that contain both key terms (Figure 4.2).

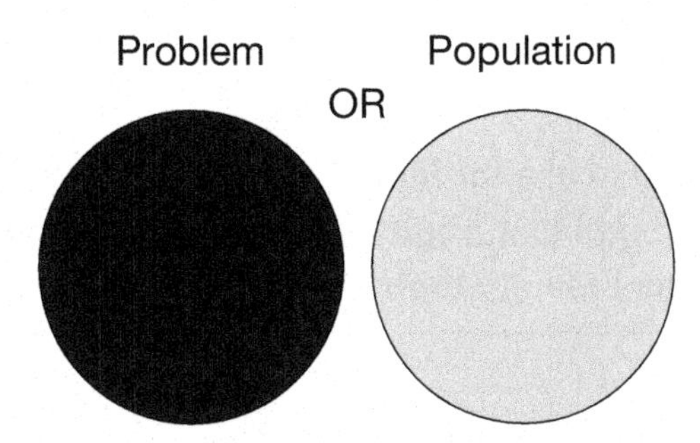

Figure 4.1 Booleanlogic: The use of "OR."

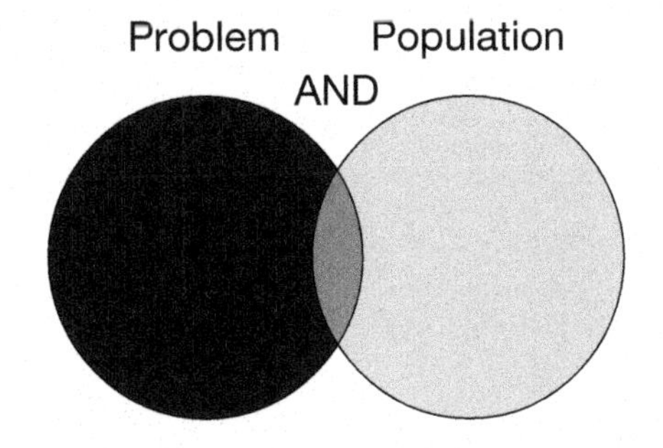

Figure 4.2 Booleanlogic: The use of "AND."

Attempt this search in three to four databases. Document the number of results you get with each search. Review the titles and begin to review information you feel is relevant. Are you finding different information compared to your first searches?

DATABASE	SEARCH COMBINATION	# OF RESULTS	# OF ITEMS REVIEWED
For example, CINAHL	COPD OR elderly/ COPD AND elderly	110	27
		658	256

CINAHL, Cumulative Index to Nursing and Allied Health Literature; COPD, chronic obstructive pulmonary disease.

Suggested Databases:

- CINAHL
- PubMed
- PsycINFO
- Google Scholar
- Other:

Another great strategy to use for initial searches is to review the reference lists of completed DNP Projects or articles that align with your problem/population. Find two DNP Projects related to your topic and review their reference lists.

Project #1: Title ____

Key References:

Project #2: Title ____

Key References:

Additional Suggestions

Is there a key journal that deals with your problem? Search this journal.

Is there an author who writes frequently about your problem? Search the author's work.

SUMMARY

The initial inquiry and searches are meant to improve your knowledge and discover basic information about your problem. A tip for students: As a faculty member, I personally want to see the reference list, formatted using the seventh edition of the American Psychological Association (2020) style manual, that a student has complied for an initial search. I generally recommend that it contain 10 references minimum, often more. Students will often say, "I have reviewed the literature and ..." I stop them immediately. I want to see the reference list. *Exactly*, what have you found so far? It helps me guide students in a more precise way. Next steps:

- Work toward goals set to routinely consume information about your problem.
- Keep a record of your searches and findings to present to faculty.

REFERENCES AND RESOURCES

American Psychological Association. (2020). *Publication manual of the American Psychological Association* (7th ed.). Washington, DC: Author.

Christenbery, T. (Ed.). (2018). *Evidence-based practice in nursing*. New York, NY: Springer Publishing Company.

Digital Literacy. [Screen name]. (2010, May 14). Boolean logic [Video file]. Retrieved from https://youtu.be/YlghuxGjHok

Holly, C. (2019). *Practice-based scholarly inquiry and the DNP capstone*. New York, NY: Springer Publishing Company.

Kate the Librarian [Screen name]. (2011, July 11). Boolean searching basics [Video file]. Retrieved from https://youtu.be/jMV7X3W_beg&feature=youtu.be

Sliante Department of Health. (2013). How to conduct a literature search. Retrieved from https://health.gov.ie/wp-content/uploads/2015/01/conducting_a_literature_search_2013.pdf

RELATED TEXTBOOKS

Christenbery, T. (Ed.). (2018). *Evidence-based practice in nursing*. New York, NY: Springer Publishing Company.

Chapter 5: Using Nursing Phenomena to Explore Evidence

Chapter 6: Evidence-Based Practice: Success of Practice Change Depends on the Question

Holly, C. (2019). *Practice-based scholarly inquiry and the DNP capstone*. New York, NY: Springer Publishing Company.

Chapter 2: Practice-Based Scholarly Inquiry

Lesson 4.3

FINDING EVIDENCE AND DATA TO DOCUMENT THE PROBLEM

BACKGROUND

To solve a problem, you need proof that the problem exists. You need evidence and data to document the problem and plan for intervention and evaluation. This exercise helps you begin to gather evidence and data. Hickey and Brosnan (2017) outline common sources of evidence used by DNPs:

- Print and electronic resources (including databases).
- Guidelines and protocols
- Standards for practice
- Observations
- Interviews
- Surveys
- Comparisons
- Personal experiences
- Reflections

You will need to discuss this lesson with your faculty. Determine the policies at your school on interviews, focus groups, needs assessments, and surveys *prior* to conducting them. Ensure that you are compliant with the institutional review board (IRB).

Having data about a problem is compelling. Our world is exploding with data. Electronic health records, personal health records, mobile technology, wearable devices, and public health data are just a few of the data sources that might provide context to your problem. Explore the potential data sources for your problem of interest.

LEARNING OBJECTIVES

- Gather evidence and data to inform the problem of interest.

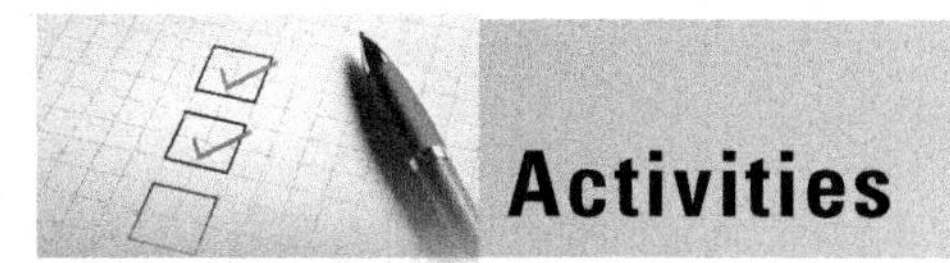

Activities

In this lesson, we are building on the information you found in Lesson 4.2. Some information may be redundant, but that may indicate its importance. We try to use multiple lenses in approaching these activities. Using this table, gather data, information, and evidence related to your problem of interest. Document the source and key points from each. Remember to bookmark them for later reference in writing the DNP Project proposal. Setting this up electronically may be most helpful.

TYPE OF EVIDENCE	SOURCE	KEY POINTS
Print/electronic		
Guidelines/protocols		
Standards of practice		
Observations		
Interviews		
Surveys		

Data

As you partner with an organization to plan for your DNP Project, ask about what data and information the organization has collected to document a problem. The agency may be willing to partner with you to collect information. Ask about its systems for collecting information on process improvement and quality. This will be important later as you plan for your intervention and evaluation of process/outcomes. Identify potential data sources and explore them.

NEXT STEPS

- Continue to explore and collect evidence and data to document your problem.
- Ensure that you explore public databases.

REFERENCES AND RESOURCES

Community Action Toolbox. (n.d.). Collecting information about a problem. Retrieved from https://ctb.ku.edu/en/table-of-contents/assessment/assessing-community-needs-and-resources/collect-information/main

Hickey, J. V., & Brosnan, C. A. (Eds.). (2017). *Evaluation of health care quality for DNPs* (2nd ed.). New York, NY: Springer Publishing Company.

RELATED TEXTBOOKS

Hickey, J. V., & Brosnan, C. A. (Eds.). (2017). *Evaluation of health care quality for DNPs* (2nd ed.). New York, NY: Springer Publishing Company.

Chapter 2: The Nature of Evidence as a Basis for Evaluation

Chapter 10: Evaluation of Patient Care Based on Standards, Guidelines, and Protocol

Chapter 11: Healthcare Teams

McBride, S., & Tietze, M. (2019). *Nursing informatics for the advanced practice nurse.* New York, NY: Springer Publishing Company.

Chapter 10: Evaluation Methods for Electronic Health Records

Chapter 11: Electronic Health Records and Health Information Exchanges Providing Value and Results for Patients, Providers, and Healthcare Systems

Chapter 13: Public Health Data to Support Healthy Communities in Health Assessment Planning

Chapter 18: Data Management and Data Analytics: The Foundations for Improvement

Chapter 27: Big Data and Advanced Analytics

Lesson 4.4

STRATEGIC AGENDAS RELATED TO THE PROBLEM

BACKGROUND

A strategic agenda is a set of goals or principles that guide the activity of an organization. For example, Healthy People is a strategic agenda that drives healthcare in the United States. An organization might have goals that help it achieve its mission statement. A healthcare team might develop a strategic plan for a patient, family, or population. In this lesson, you investigate strategic agendas that are related to your problem of interest.

LEARNING OBJECTIVES

- Locate related strategic agendas.
- Explain how they relate to your problem of interest.

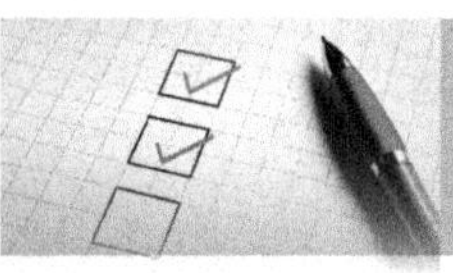

Activities

Recall our discussion of the Institute of Medicine (IOM) reports *To Err Is Human* (1999), *Crossing the Quality Chasm* (2001), *The Future of Nursing* (2011), and Healthy People. From the perspective of your problem and population of interest, write down the relationships.

STRATEGIC AGENDA:	RELATIONSHIP TO YOUR PROBLEM/POPULATION OF INTEREST
Future of Nursing Report	
Healthy People	
Other IOM report:	
Other:	

At the organizational level, are there strategic agendas that relate to your problem? If so, describe.

From the perspective of the healthcare team, are there strategic agendas for patients or populations that are related to your problem? If so, describe.

NEXT STEPS

- Be alert to strategic agendas at all levels that are related to your problem/populations of interest.
- Continue to build on your findings.

REFERENCES AND RESOURCES

Institute of Medicine. (1999). *To err is human: Building a safer healthcare system*. Washington, DC: National Academies Press.
Institute of Medicine. (2001). *Crossing the quality chasm*. Washington, DC: National Academies Press.
Institute of Medicine. (2011). *The future of nursing: Leading change, advancing health*. Washington, DC: National Academies Press.

RELATED TEXTBOOK

Hickey, J. V., & Brosnan, C. A. (Eds.). (2017). *Evaluation of health care quality for DNPs* (2nd ed.). New York, NY: Springer Publishing Company.
Chapter 3: Conceptual Models for Evaluation in Advanced Nursing Practice

Lesson 4.5

CLINICAL GUIDELINES RELATED TO THE PROBLEM

BACKGROUND

The DNP degree is practice focused (American Association of Colleges of Nursing [AACN], 2015). Variation in clinical practice creates potential for risk and ultimate harm to the patient. To streamline practice, utilize evidence, and promote patient safety, use of clinical practice guidelines (CPGs) makes logical sense (Christenbery, 2018). If the CPG is well developed, it can be used as a cornerstone, guide, and benchmark for the DNP Project.

CPGs are usually developed by an organization to streamline practice and reduce potential harm (Institute of Medicine [IOM], 2011). To best utilize them in a DNP Project, it will be necessary to identify a guideline, understand its context, and formally appraise the content. The IOM (2011) published a document to assist health professionals in determining the quality of guidelines called *Clinical Practice Guidelines We Can Trust*. We use those standards to frame the work of this activity. Nurses may also be in contact with variations of CPGs—protocols, clinical pathways, and care plans—in their work settings. In the book by Christenbery, Table 9.3, Clinical Practice Guideline Terms, outlines and clarifies the differences among guidelines.

LEARNING OBJECTIVES

- Identify a CPG related to your problem of interest.
- Appraise the guideline using the IOM standards.

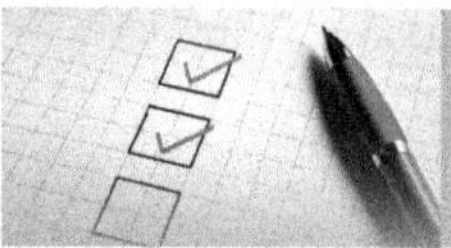

Activities

Use this worksheet to appraise the guideline you have identified. For more details on each standard, refer to the IOM document (http://data.care-statement.org/wp-content/uploads/2016/12/IOMGuidelines-2013-1.pdf).

Problem: ______________________________

Official Title of Selected Guideline: ______________________________

Developer/Source: ______________________________

IOM STANDARD	IS THE STANDARD MET?
Established Transparency: Is the process used to develop the guideline identified?	Yes/No Notes:
Conflict of Interest: Are the relationships (personal/financial, etc.) of the guideline developers fully disclosed?	Yes/No Notes:
Group Composition: Do the credentials of the guideline developers represent a diverse group of expertise?	Yes/No Notes:
Systematic Review: Is there a process for methodical review of evidence identified?	Yes/No Notes:
Rating of Recommendations: Is there a system for rating the recommendations and is it described?	Yes/No Notes:
Articulation of Recommendations: Are the recommendations clear?	Yes/No Notes:
External Review: Is the process for external review sound?	Yes/No Notes:
Updating: Is the guideline reviewed and updated?	Yes/No Notes:

IOM, Institute of Medicine.

In your own words, describe how this guideline is related to:

Population of interest:

Problem of interest:

Describe three specific recommendations in the guideline that are related to your problem:

1. ______________________________

2. ______________________________

3. ______________________________

Do you think this guideline is being following in clinical practice?

List the potential barriers and facilitators of guideline use:

BARRIERS	FACILITATORS

SUMMARY

The purpose of a CPG is to reduce variation in practice. However, guidelines do not replace the importance of critical thinking and individualization of patient care (Christenbery, 2018). When you have identified an agency/organization to partner with for your project, further explore the protocols and clinical guidelines used in the institution to consider how they impact your project. Next steps:

- Explore the partnering organization's use of guidelines, protocols, and pathways.
- If there is more than one guideline relevant to the same problem, use the AGREE II Instrument to compare them (www.agreetrust.org/agree-ii/).

REFERENCES AND RESOURCES

American Association of Colleges of Nursing. (2015). *The doctor of nursing practice: Current issues and clarifying recommendations.* Retrieved from https://www.aacnnursing.org/Portals/42/News/White-Papers/DNP-Implementation-TF-Report-8-15.pdf

Appraisal of Guidelines for Research & Evaluation II. (2017). AGREE II instrument. Retrieved from https://www.agreetrust.org/wp-content/uploads/2017/12/AGREE-II-Users-Manual-and-23-item-Instrument-2009-Update-2017.pdf

Christenbery, T. (Ed.). (2018). *Evidence-based practice in nursing.* New York, NY: Springer Publishing Company.

Institute of Medicine. (2011). *Clinical practice guidelines we can trust.* Washington, DC: National Academies Press. Retrieved from http://data.care-statement.org/wp-content/uploads/2016/12/IOMGuidelines-2013-1.pdf

RELATED TEXTBOOK

Christenbery, T. (Ed.). (2018). *Evidence-based practice in nursing.* New York, NY: Springer Publishing Company.

Chapter 9: Clinical Practice Guidelines

Lesson 4.6

POLICIES RELATED TO THE PROBLEM

BACKGROUND

Now that you have identified a problem, it is important to consider how health policy fits into the picture. It is also important to remember that most of what we do and how we practice is guided, in some way, by health policy. This may include local, state, or national policies, but clearly there is an impetus behind why we do what we do that is grounded in health policy. This means that it is important that nurses, especially doctorally prepared nurses, are not merely reacting to the health policy, but rather play an active role in developing and evaluating health policy.

> *"Nurses must see policy as something they can shape rather than something that happens to them."*
> ~Institute of Medicine (IOM, 2011), *The Future of Nursing: Leading Change, Advancing Health*

The American Association of Colleges of Nursing's (2006) Essential V outlines how the DNP graduate can influence healthcare policy through advocacy in healthcare. Consider the reach of health policy and its influences on health disparities, ethics, access to and quality of care, and equity and social justice. Being aware and taking an active role in advocating for health policy issues is part of being a responsible nurse leader and is necessary as part of our professional practice. Remember, these policies are guiding the way we practice; therefore, we should not only be aware, but we should have a voice and seat at the table. The IOM (2011) also reminds us that DNP graduates can frame healthcare financing, practice regulation, access, safety, quality, and efficacy of care through their ability to design, influence, and implement healthcare policies.

Never underestimate your ability to influence health policy on any level. Your DNP education has provided you with the skills to be leaders and advocates who can not only advance your own practice but also protect your patients.

LEARNING OBJECTIVES

- Learners will be able to analyze their own contribution to health policy.
- Learners will be able to identify existing health policy pertaining to their problem of interest.

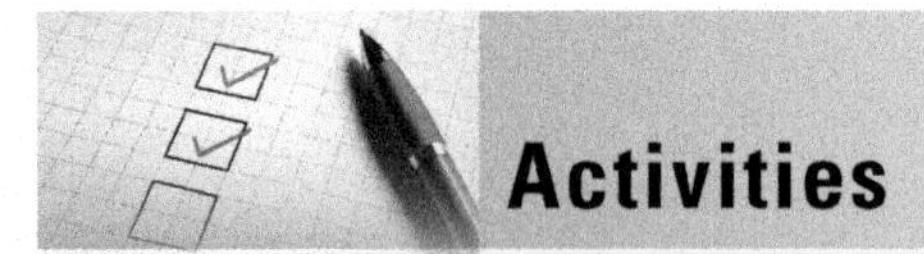

Activities

Understanding Your Contribution to Health Policy

As a novice DNP nurse, you are able to review the literature and research supporting certain health policies. As a result, you are able to develop a new and unique awareness of issues of which you may have previously been unaware. This eye-opening exposure is the first step in recognizing your potential to influence policy. As you become more knowledgeable about the health policy process, you can increase your involvement in issues important to you and be a contributor to health policy.

ORGANIZATION	ISSUES/EFFORTS	RESULT
Example: Student representative on university's School of Nursing curriculum committee (*local influencer*)	• Need for reevaluation due to student evaluations/updated DNP requirements/variations across programs • Have an active voice in providing student perspectives on course sequencing, concurrent courses, facilitators/challenges, and course deliverables	• Awareness of process and influencers on curriculum development within the school • Input on institutional policy for curriculum plans of study
Local organizational influencer		
State organizational influencer		
National organizational influencer		

Consider your problem of interest. Is there any existing health policy associated with this problem? Consider larger pieces of work that can also impact the problem of interest, including IOM reports, Centers for Medicare & Medicaid Services guidelines/requirements, Joint Commission Standards, and so on. Complete the following table. Be concise. Write one to two sentences for each item.

Problem of Interest:

Organizational policy	
State policy	
National policy	

SUMMARY

The goal of this lesson is to allow you to consider how you can influence health policy. This lesson also allows you to focus on how your problem of interest is influenced by health policy at various levels. Reflect with your faculty or DNP chair on what you have identified about how your project is influencing or being influenced by health policy.

REFERENCES AND RESOURCES

American Association of Colleges of Nursing. (2006). The essentials of doctoral education for advanced nursing practice. Retrieved from https://www.aacnnursing.org/Portals/42/Publications/DNPEssentials.pdf

Institute of Medicine. (2001). *Crossing the quality chasm: A new health system for the 21st century*. Washington, DC: National Academies Press.

Institute of Medicine. (2011). *The future of nursing: Leading change, advancing health.* Washington, DC: National Academies Press.

RELATED TEXTBOOKS

Hickey, J. V., & Brosnan, C. A. (Eds.). (2017). *Evaluation of healthcare quality for the DNP* (2nd ed.). New York, NY: Springer Publishing Company.

Chapter 13: Translating Outcomes From Evaluation to Health Policy

Zalon, M., & Patton, R. (2018). *Nurses making policy* (2nd ed.). New York, NY: Springer Publishing Company.

Unit II: Analyzing Policy

Chapter 4: Identifying a Problem and Analyzing a Policy Issue

Chapter 5: Harnessing Evidence in the Policy Process

Lesson 4.7

USING THE QUADRUPLE AIM TO EXAMINE THE PROBLEM

BACKGROUND

The Institute for Healthcare Improvement (IHI) advocates for the Triple Aim. The Triple Aim describes a goal. It states that healthcare should work toward (a) improving the patient experience, (b) improving the health of populations, and (c) reducing the cost of healthcare (IHI, 2019). Recently, a fourth goal has been added (IHI, 2017). It asserts that to care for patients, we, the healthcare team, must also care for ourselves (Bodenheimer & Sinsky, 2014). Thus, the Triple Aim is now being referred to as the *Quadruple Aim* (Figure 4.3). In this lesson, we use this IHI model to examine the relationship of these goals to your problem of interest.

LEARNING OBJECTIVES

- List factors that impact the problem of interest.
- Explore the relationships between the problem of interest and the Quadruple Aim.

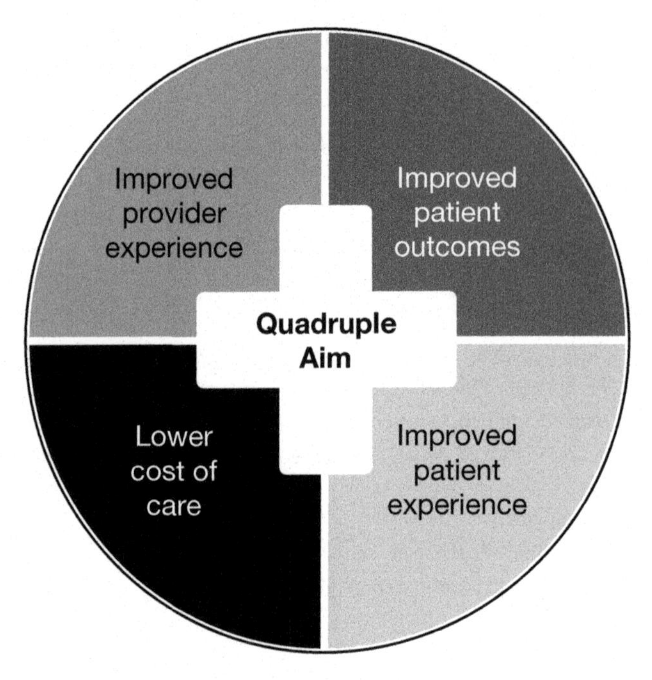

Figure 4.3 The Quadruple Aim.

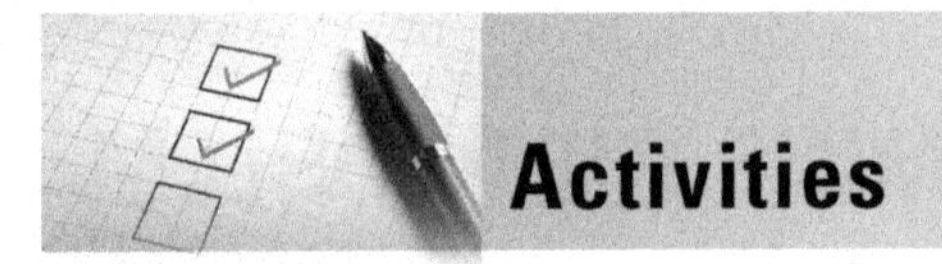

Activities

Under each column, list key points, information, and facts related to the problem of interest.

COST	POPULATION HEALTH	PATIENT EXPERIENCE	PROVIDER EXPERIENCE
What are the issues related to cost for both the system and the patients?	What are the issues that impact the collective health of the population?	What are the issues related to patient satisfaction? What are the issues related to quality of care and safety of the patients?	What are the issues that impact the healthcare providers and healthcare team?

In reflecting of this information, how does it collectively relate to your problem of interest?

___

___

___

What are the key takeaway points?

Takeaway 1:

___

___

Takeaway 2:

___

___

NEXT STEPS

- Talk to your DNP faculty about your findings.
- Continue to talk to colleagues and organizational stakeholders.

REFERENCES AND RESOURCES

Bodenheimer, T., & Sinsky, C. (2014). From triple to quadruple aim: Care of the patient requires care of the provider. *The Annals of Family Medicine, 12*(6), 573–576.

Institute for Healthcare Improvement- IHI [Screen name]. (2017, November 28). IHI's position on the Quadruple Aim [Video file]. Retrieved from https://youtu.be.d1uX0WFcAY

Institute for Healthcare Improvement. (2019). The IHI Triple Aim. Retrieved from https://www.marquette.edu/center-for-teaching-and-learning/interprofessional-education.php

RELATED TEXTBOOK

Hickey, J. V., & Brosnan, C A. (2017). *Evaluation of health care quality for DNPs* (2nd ed.). New York, NY: Springer Publishing Company.

Chapter 5: Economic Evaluation

Chapter 6: Evaluation of Organizations

Chapter 7: Evaluation of Healthcare Information Systems and Patient Care

Chapter 11: Healthcare Teams

Lesson 4.8

IMPACT OF THE PROBLEM ON PATIENTS, FAMILIES, AND COMMUNITIES: SOCIAL DETERMINANTS OF HEALTH

BACKGROUND

At the heart of nursing is a desire to serve our patients, their families, and communities. The problems they experience provide a starting point to initiate change. Our goal in this exercise is to fully explore the impact of a problem on these entities through the lens of social determinants of health (Healthy People, n.d.-c).

To start, consider talking to people. Talk to your patients about how their health problems affect them. Remember, you are trying to understand, not to collect official project data. What challenges do they have navigating the health system? How does their family cope? In the literature, you may identify qualitative research studies that will help you. Qualitative research helps to describe the lived experiences of patients and families. For example, what is it like to experience fatigue with multiple sclerosis? Try to better understand your problem of interest from a patient's perspective. Then, try to relate to their family.

To better assess community, Healthy People (n.d.-a, n.d.-b) offers a framework called "MAP-IT" (mobilize, assess, plan, implement, track). We use their suggested activities under "assess" to ensure that you are fully examining the impact of your problem of interest on the community. The tools will also help you set priorities.

LEARNING OBJECTIVES

- Outline the impact of the problem on patients.
- Trace the impact of the problem on the patient's family.
- Report the impact of the problem on the larger community.

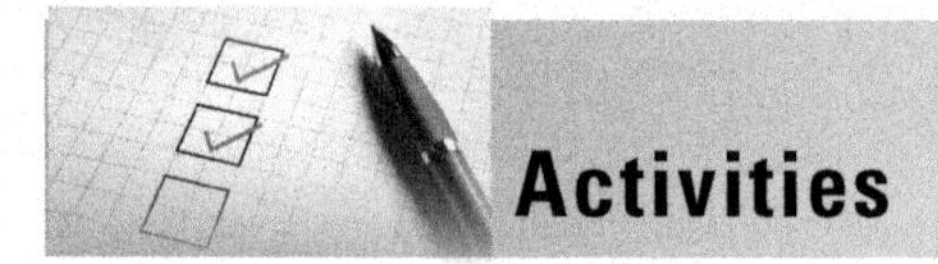

Activities

Impact on Patients

Use qualitative literature or personal communications to answer the following questions:

- How does the problem impact your activities of daily living?
- How does the problem impact your coping ability?
- How does the problem impact your finances?
- How does the problem impact your spirituality?
- How does the problem impact your relationships with others?
- What is the most difficult thing about your condition/problem/diagnosis?
- Is there anything about the situation that could be improved?

Impact on Families

Use qualitative literature or personal communications to answer the following questions.

- How does the problem impact your relationship with your family member?
- What challenges do you personally have with the situation?
- Is there anything about the situation that could be improved?

Impact on Community

Consider the impact of the problem on the community to answer these questions.

- Who is affected and how?
- What resources do we have in the community?
- What resources do we need in the community?

To pull these concepts together, consider the Healthy People 2020 social determinants of health (Healthy People, n.d.-c). How do the five social determinants of health mentioned in Healthy People impact your problem?

---

1. Economic stability:

   ____

   ____

2. Education:

   ____

   ____

3. Social and community context:

   ____

   ____

4. Health and healthcare:

   ____

   ____

5. Neighborhood and built environment:

____

____

Explore additional resources on community assessment for more detailed analysis.

NEXT STEPS

- Explore additional resources on community assessment for more detailed analysis.
- Summarize and organize your findings for later use.

REFERENCES AND RESOURCES

CDC, CHANGE Tool. (n.d.). Building a foundation of knowledge to prioritize community needs: An action guide. Retrieved from https://www.cdc.gov/nccdphp/dch/programs/healthycommunitiesprogram/tools/change/pdf/changeactionguide.pdf

Community Tool Box. (n.d.). Chapter 3: Assessing community needs and resources. Retrieved from https://ctb.ku.edu/en/table-of-contents/assessment/assessing-community-needs-and-resources

Healthy People. (n.d.-a). MAP-IT Framework: ASSESS. Retrieved from https://www.healthypeople.gov/2020/tools-and-resources/program-planning/Assess

Healthy People. (n.d.-b). Program Planning: MAP IT Framework. Retrieved from https://www.healthypeople.gov/2020/tools-and-resources/Program-Planning

Healthy People. (n.d.-c). Social determinants of health. Retrieved from https://www.healthypeople.gov/2020/topics-objectives/topic/social-determinants-of-health

RELATED TEXTBOOK

Hickey, J. V., & Brosnan, C. A. (2017). *Evaluation of health care quality for DNPs* (2nd ed.). New York, NY: Springer Publishing Company.

Chapter 8: Program Evaluation

Chapter 12: Evaluation of Populations and Population Health

Lesson 4.9

IMPACT OF THE PROBLEM ON ORGANIZATIONS

BACKGROUND

Although you have been focusing on understanding the problem and its impact on others, it is just as important to be aware of how the problem impacts the organization and how to properly assess an organization in order to facilitate improvements. Keep in mind that if the problem is not a priority for the organization, you will likely face many roadblocks in your ability to successfully implement your project.

Understanding the organization and the impact of the problem on it is necessary in order to obtain buy-in from the organization and recognition of the importance of the problem. The first step is to properly assess the organization and analyze workflow. This includes systematically reviewing key indicators, requiring all parts of the organization to work together, and recognizing the need for resources and support (Hickey & Brosnan, 2017). This requires you to think not only internally about the unit in which you plan to conduct your project but also about the larger organization. Our goal in this exercise is to look at the impact of the problem through the lens of a nurse leader.

First, understand the organization. Recognize that, depending on your role within the organization, there is more going on than you may realize. What do you know about the organization? What type of organization is it? How does it generate revenue? What is the reach of the organization? For example, what is the size and location of the organization and how does that impact the type and scope of services it provides? A small, community-based hospital that offers routine obstetrical services and low-risk deliveries may rely on referral services for high-risk obstetrical care rather than treat in-house. As a result, a project focusing on the preeclamptic patient may not be feasible at this organization.

You will also want to understand the leadership structure and mission/vision/values of the organization. Having an understanding of the decision-makers and the fundamental beliefs driving the organization is also important as they guide how decisions are made and where to focus efforts. If an organization's mission is to serve the underprivileged, certainly a project that looks to address this would at least pique its interest. Who are the players who make decisions? Certainly the C-suite, but who else? Specific to your project, you will want to know who oversees projects/research. Including them is pertinent and necessary. Knowing what initiatives are on their radar will also help identify whether your problem is equally as important to them.

Once you have completed an organizational assessment, you will conduct a workflow analysis, which will ensure that the outcomes you were hoping for actually occur. Depending on the nature of your project, this may include productivity or efficiency in the process, customer/patient satisfaction, compliance, and even employee engagement. It's important to recognize that workflow analysis is the review of how the work *actually* gets done, not the protocols/methods in place that guide how it *should* be done.

According to the Agency for Healthcare Research and Quality (AHRQ, 2015), redesigning workflows has two goals: (a) improving performance and (b) increasing efficiency. After you outline actual practice, you can then work with other stakeholders in redesigning the workflow to incorporate the desired improvements/processes and then test these changes.

LEARNING OBJECTIVES

- Identify key components of the organizational structure and basic factors influencing decision-making efforts.
- Utilize workflow analysis to identify opportunities for improvement in care delivery processes.

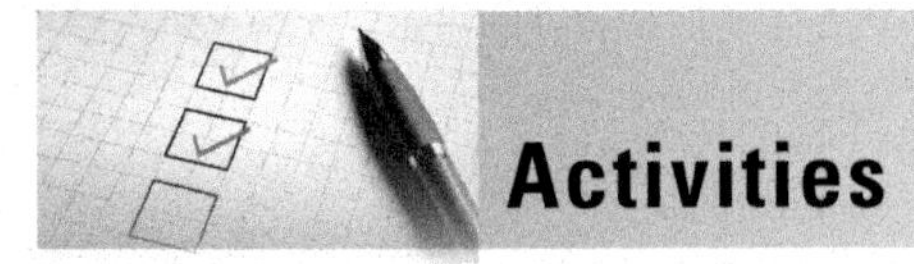

Activities

Conduct an organizational assessment of the intended project site. Use these prompts based on the content outlined by Hickey and Brosnan (2017), Table 6.1, Key Components of Organization and System Evaluation.

The Basics of the Organization

ORGANIZATIONAL COMPONENT	NOTES
History and overview	
Type of organization	
Funding/revenue sources	
Governance	
Mission, vision, and values	
Strategy and goals	
Size and scope of services	
Culture	
Organizational structure	
Authority and decision-making	
Reputation	
Outcomes, quality, and patient satisfaction	
Role of nursing	

Does the organization agree that your problem of interest is a priority?

____

____

____

What is the gap in this organization? Why is this problem occurring? What does the organization want to improve?

Within organizations, there are complex processes. Workflow analysis is a broad process and might include looking at the flow of a patient who is transitioning, the process of prescribing and filling a medication, or the flow of information between healthcare team members. List three workflows or processes related to your problem or population of interest.

1.

2.

3.

Now, select the process that is most likely to have the biggest impact on your problem or population. Review the IHI content on improving workflow and removing waste, available at www.ihi.org/resources/Pages/Changes/ImproveWorkFlowandRemoveWaste.aspx. Then, read through the content on workflow redesign from the HealthIT.gov website (www.healthit.gov/faq/what-workflow-redesign-why-it-important).

On a separate sheet of paper, complete a workflow analysis of the identified problem using one of the suggested tools:

- Root-cause analysis
    - https://videos.asq.org/asking-why-with-root-cause-and-5-whys
    - https://asq.org/quality-resources/root-cause-analysis
- AHRQ (2015)
    - https://pcmh.ahrq.gov/sites/default/files/attachments/pcpf-module-10-workflow-mapping.pdf
- Other:

NEXT STEPS

- Discuss your findings with stakeholders and your faculty.
- Take note of opportunities for improvement that you identify.

REFERENCES AND RESOURCES

Agency for Healthcare Research and Quality. (2015). Primary care practice facilitation curriculum. Module 10: Mapping and redesigning workflow. Retrieved from https://pcmh.ahrq.gov/sites/default/files/attachments/pcpf-module-10-workflow-mapping.pdf

Hickey, J. V., & Brosnan, C. A. (Eds.). (2017). *Evaluation of health care quality for DNPs* (2nd ed.). New York: Springer Publishing Company.

RELATED TEXTBOOK

Hickey, J. V., & Brosnan, C. A. (Eds.). (2017). *Evaluation of health care quality for DNPs* (2nd ed.). New York, NY: Springer Publishing Company.

Chapter 6: Evaluation of Organizations and Systems

Chapter 7: Evaluation of Health Care Information Systems and Patient Care Technology

Chapter 8: Program Evaluation

Chapter 9: Quality Improvement

Lesson 4.10

CATALOGING OUTCOMES, POTENTIAL SOLUTIONS, AND VALUE OF THE DNP PROJECT

BACKGROUND

You have been working hard gathering information to better understand and describe your problem of interest. Based on all of this new knowledge, what do you think needs to change? What could be done to improve health outcomes for the patients and population you serve? Could you make a list of what others have tried to do to improve these health outcomes? What would work best in your situation? How can you add value to the organization? This is our next task: to list information and ideas.

LEARNING OBJECTIVES

- Catalog outcomes.
- List potential solutions.
- Consider the value added by the DNP Project.

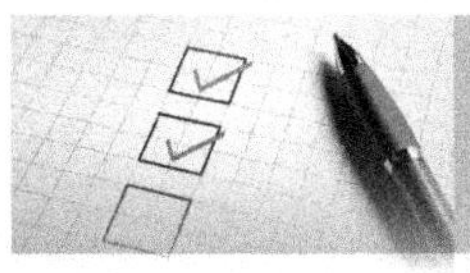

Activities

Based on your problem, catalog the outcomes that would improve the health of your patients/population. Then, explore the solutions others have tried to achieve that outcome. Think of outcomes in terms of clinical outcomes, safety and quality, leadership, and policy.

The problem of interest for my project is: ______________________________

____

The population of interest for my project is: ______________________________

To improve the health of my population, I would like to see these outcomes:

Outcome #1: ______________________________

Potential ways this outcome could be achieved:

1.

2.

Outcome #2: ______________________________

Potential ways this outcome could be achieved:

1.

2.

Outcome #3: ______________________________

Potential ways this outcome could be achieved:

1.

2.

Interventions and solutions to improve health outcomes should be evidence based. White, Dudley-Brown, and Terhaar (2020) discuss the top methods for evidence translation. Review the information in this table and highlight the three methods that could work best in the context of your DNP Project.

Academic detailing	Audit and feedback	Bundles	Decision support	Order sets
Practice guidelines	Process redesign	Protocols	Quality improvement	Scorecards and dashboards
Teaming	Technology-based solutions	Tool kits (practice resources)	Other:	Other:

According to the Institute of Medicine (IOM), education alone as an intervention will change practice only 4% of the time (IOM, 2011). Therefore, we recommend that you think beyond just "educating" on a topic. How can you help people apply, utilize, or engage with the information?

A DNP Project must be valued by an organization, population, or entity. Review the 30 Elements of Value shown in Figure 4.4. According to the author, the more the elements of value are added, the better the product or services. (Read more at: https://hbr.org/2016/09/the-elements-of-value.)

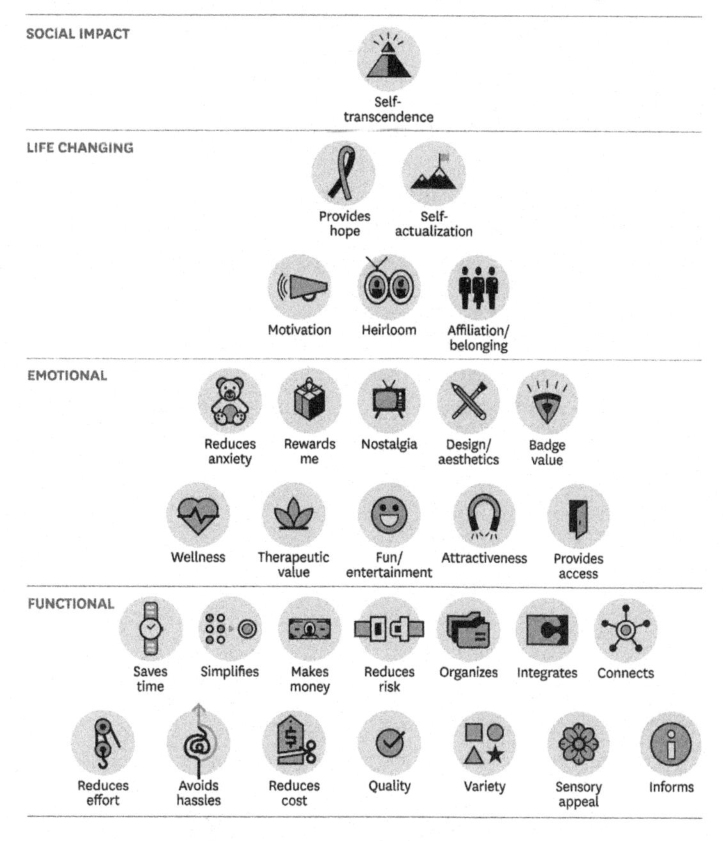

Figure 4.4 The elements of value pyramid.
Source: Almquist, E., Senior, J., & Bloch, N. (2016). The elements of value. *Harvard Business Review, 94*(9), 47–53.

List five elements from Figure 4.4 that your DNP Project could add:

1.

2.

3.

4.

5.

NEXT STEPS

- Review this information with your faculty.
- Determine your most viable project options.
- Find literature documenting interventions others have done to achieve the outcomes you want to achieve.

REFERENCES AND RESOURCES

Almquist, E., Senior, J., & Bloch, N. (2016). The elements of value. *Harvard Business Review, 94*(9), 47–53.
Institute of Medicine. (2011). *Clinical practice guidelines we can trust.* Washington, DC: National Academies Press.
White, K. M., Dudley-Brown, S., & Terhaar, M. F. (Eds.). (2020). *Translation of evidence into nursing and healthcare* (3rd ed.). New York, NY: Springer Publishing Company.

RELATED TEXTBOOK

White, K. M., Dudley-Brown, S., & Terhaar, M. F. (Eds.). (2020). *Translation of evidence into nursing and healthcare* (3rd ed.) New York, NY: Springer Publishing Company.
Chapter 4: Translation of Evidence to Improve Clinical Outcomes
Chapter 5: Translation of Evidence for Improving Safety and Quality
Chapter 6: Translation of Evidence for Leadership
Chapter 7: Translation of Evidence for Health Policy
Chapter 8: Methods for Translation

Lesson 4.11

PUTTING IT ALL TOGETHER—THE DNP PROJECT OUTLINE: DRAFT #1

BACKGROUND

The DNP Project starts with a problem. As the student, you are the leader of the DNP team. In order to implement an intervention(s) that will change practice, you need to offer a proposal describing how you plan to accomplish that goal. What is the problem? Who is affected by the problem? Why is it a problem?

Bonnel and Smith (2018) describe the process of writing a good clinical problem statement. They offer strategies on how to put the clinical problem in context. We help you organize your information from this chapter to make an outline, which will be the first draft of your DNP problem statement and background.

LEARNING OBJECTIVES

- Prepare a draft of the DNP problem statement.
- Outline the elements of the background for the DNP Project proposal.

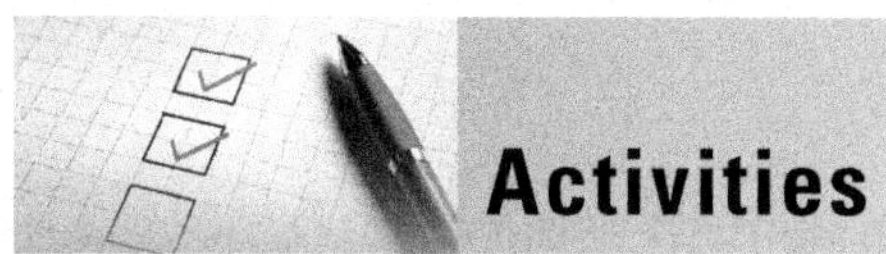

Activities

Reflect on the information that you have gathered about your problem of interest. Begin to narrow and funnel the information to focus the problem.

Problem of interest: ____

Population it impacts: ____

I know it is a problem because: (List your top three key points from your gathering of information.)

1.

2.

3.

Why is it important to address this problem?

Now, put this information into a sentence format. Example:

______ (condition/disease) _______ is a significant health problem for _______ (population of interest) _______. ______ (key point #1) _____, _____ (key point #2)______, and _____ (key point #3) _____ are all factors that contribute to the problem. As a result, these patients experience negative health outcomes, such as ______ (outcome #1) ______ and ______ (outcome #2) ______.

Example:

"COPD is a significant health problem for Kentucky residents. Tobacco abuse, medication noncompliance, and poor self-management of the disease are all factors that contribute to the problem. As a result, these patients experience negative health outcomes such as hospitalization and decreased quality of life."

Write a draft of your final problem statement:

- ☐ Did you state the problem? (What is the problem?)
- ☐ Did you identify the population of interest? (Who is affected?)
- ☐ Did you include key points that contribute to the problem? (Why is it a problem?)
- ☐ Did you identify the outcomes that need improvement?

Outline the first draft of your DNP Project proposal in context using the information you have collected. Refer to your school's requirements and discuss with your faculty before you begin. Modify as required.

DNP Project Outline: Draft #1

Title page

Abstract (always written last, hold a spot but skip this for now)

Introduction

Background

- Problem of interest
- Population of interest
- Relevant definition(s)
- Results of initial inquiries and searches: Demographics, incidence, prevalence
- Strategic agendas related to the problem
- Policies related to the problem
- Clinical guidelines related to the problem
- Quadruple aim
- Impact on patients, families, and community: social determinant of health
- Impact on healthcare systems and organizations
- Desired outcomes and potential solutions
- Value added by the DNP Project

Remember to consult with your faculty and review the DNP Project proposal guidelines for your school. Students often ask, "How long should a DNP Project proposal be?" This cannot be consistently quantified. We would *roughly* suggest one to two paragraphs for each component in the preceding list depending on the situation. Additional content may be needed. Seek help early in the writing process. Get someone to proofread what you write. Remember that many people will read this document, so you have to explain things, provide definitions, and make the sections flow logically.

NEXT STEPS

- Present your problem statement and outline to your faculty.
- Discuss and finalize the project goals and desired outcomes.

REFERENCE AND RESOURCE

Bonnel, W., & Smith, K. (2018). *Proposal writing for clinical nursing and DNP Projects.* New York, NY: Springer Publishing Company.

RELATED TEXTBOOK

Bonnel, W., & Smith, K. (2018). *Proposal writing for clinical nursing and DNP Projects.* New York, NY: Springer Publishing Company.
Chapter 1: Introduction: Why a Scholarly Proposal for the Clinical Project Proposal?
Chapter 2: Using the Writing Plan as a Developmental Tool for the Advanced Clinical Project
Chapter 3: Writing a Good Clinical Problem Statement and Placing the Clinical Problem in Context

CHAPTER SUMMARY

The purpose of this chapter was to fully investigate your problem of interest:

- What is the problem?
- Who is affected by the problem?
- Why is it a problem?

Briefly you began to explore:

- Where is this problem occurring (context)?
- What needs to be improved?
- How could it be improved?

You have gathered information, prepared a problem statement, outlined content for the background of the proposal, and considered your desired outcomes for the project. The next step depends on the layout of your DNP curriculum. The order of Chapter 5, Skills for Formal Review of Literature and Evidence Appraisal and Chapter 6, Framing the DNP Project—Taking Aim and Being SMART could be interchanged. After consultation with your faculty, your next goal will be to:

- Complete a formal review of literature on a focused question (Chapter 5).
- Frame the project using defined aims and objectives (Chapter 6).
  OR
- Frame the project using defined aims and objectives (Chapter 6).
- Complete a formal review of literature on a focused question (Chapter 5).

Reflections

What are two things you have learned in this chapter?

1.

2.

What questions or concerns do you still have at this point? How will you reconcile them?

1.

2.

Be open-minded. DNP Projects evolve. The project may take shape in a way that you did not originally consider. These are real-world projects with real-world problems. Stay the course and communicate with your faculty. Don't spend too much time in your own mind. Involve your DNP team. Seek information beyond this workbook using the suggested resources and reading the suggested Springer Publishing Company texts.

Continue to work hard!

NOTES

5

Skills for Formal Review of Literature and Evidence Appraisal

Molly J. Bradshaw, Tracy R. Vitale, Margaret Dreker,
Irina Benenson, and Marilyn Oermann

Lessons

OBJECTIVES

Formal review and appraisal of literature is a skill. It is different from gathering information for the project background. For our purposes, formal review of literature describes the process where by a specific question is formulated, a methodical literature search is completed, and findings are documented, appraised, and communicated. Recommendations are made for constructing an evidence table and writing a synthesis of the literature. By the end of this chapter, you will be able to:

- Develop an answerable question using PICOT (patient/problem, intervention, comparison, outcome, time) format.
- Complete a literature review and document your search.
- Explore options for evidence appraisal.
- Construct an evidence table.
- Write a synthesis of findings from your review of the literature.

INTRODUCTION

At this point, you have identified a problem and population of interest. You have written a problem statement. Write that statement on a piece of paper and tape it up on the wall. Keep it in front of you to keep your work focused. You should have a solid understanding of the background and context of the problem. Now it is time to ask a more focused question(s).

Reviewing and appraising evidence is a skill. In the process of gathering information for your background understanding, you certainly looked at literature and evidence. However, it is unlikely that you used a formal process. You were gathering information to better understand a situation. With that knowledge in hand, what else do you need to know? Do you need to know more about a certain outcome? Do you need to know more about the evidence-based solutions to improve that outcome? Do you need to know more about instruments to measure the outcome? Take some time to think very carefully about this. Talk to your faculty.

In this chapter, we are going to hone a spirit of inquiry (Melnyk, Fineout-Overholt, Stillwell, & Williamson, 2019). Then, we will guide you through the skills of scholarly inquiry. For purposes of this workbook, we use the phrase "formal review of literature" to describe a pointed strategy for developing a question, searching the literature, appraising the literature, and making sense of the findings. It's not just looking around. We present a lesson on the different types of literature reviews and their working definitions. The point to appreciate is that we are talking about more in-depth searching and analysis of literature than discussed before. Your school may have requirements regarding the type of literature review required for the DNP program.

Depending on the structure of your program, you may benefit from reversing the order of this chapter and Chapter 6, Framing the DNP Project—Taking Aim and Being SMART. This is the point at which you develop the specific aims and objectives of the project. You will write a purpose statement. The reason we offer skills on review of literature first is because we feel that you will need to use them prior to developing aims and objectives. Discuss the approach with your faculty to ensure alignment with the process for DNP Projects at your school. Again, this is a skill to learn. A review of literature is simply a methodical approach to identification, appraisal, and synthesis of evidence to answer a specific question. This chapter introduces these skills at a fundamental level to get you started.

Keep in mind that this chapter offers a basic overview. We cannot emphasize enough the importance of developing relationships with librarians and other colleagues with this skill set. Additional training beyond coursework is often required, especially for completion of systematic reviews using Cochrane or Joanna Briggs Institute methodologies (Cochrane Training, n.d.; Joanna Briggs Institute, n.d.). It is very appropriate for DNPs to develop these skills, according to the DNP Essentials (American Association of Colleges of Nursing [AACN], 2015).

It is important to mention that your DNP Project will not end with integrative or systematic review. The DNP Project also needs an implementation component. You must take action. You must make a practice change. You must do something with the information from the review. The heart of DNP scholarship is translation and utilization of evidence into practice.

There will be one overarching question that drives your project and inquiry process. Get familiar with the skills required to develop a question, search and appraise the literature, then synthesize your findings. Then work with your faculty to determine their best fit to your project. If your school offers an option for systematic review as a DNP Project type, you will still need to plan for implementation, evaluation, and sustainability to meet AACN recommendations. Let's begin.

REFERENCES AND RESOURCES

American Association of Colleges of Nursing. (2015). *The doctor of nursing practice: Current issues and clarifying recommendations* [White paper]. Retrieved from https://www.aacnnursing.org/Portals/42/News/White-Papers/DNP-Implementation-TF-Report-8-15.pdf

Cochrane Training. (n.d.). Retrieved from https://training.cochrane.org

Joanna Briggs Institute. (n.d.). Education and learning. Retrieved from http://joannabriggs.org/education

Melnyk, B. M., Fineout-Overholt, E., Stillwell, S. B., & Williamson, K. M. (2019). Evidence based practice. A step by step guide. Igniting a spirit of inquiry. Retrieved from http://forces4quality.org/af4q/download-document/3517/Resource-Evidence_Based_Practice__Step_by_Step__Igniting_a.28.pdf

RELATED TEXTBOOK

Holly, C., Salmond, S., & Saimbert, M. (Eds.). (2017). *Comprehensive systematic review for advanced practice nursing* (2nd ed.). New York, NY: Springer Publishing Company.

MY GOALS FOR SKILLS FOR FORMAL REVIEW OF LITERATURE AND EVIDENCE APPRAISAL ARE TO:

Lesson 5.1

TYPES OF EVIDENCE AND LITERATURE REVIEWS

BACKGROUND

Fundamentally, evidence is information that is found to be credible based on standards of science. Evidence is generated from a scientific study designed to answer a question or describe a phenomenon of interest. The study is appraised to determine its quality. A nurse must then decide whether that information should be used in the practice setting. The goal is to integrate the best evidence into practice (Christenbery, 2018).

LEARNING OBJECTIVES

- Understand primary versus secondary literature.
- Distinguish between quantitative and qualitative.
- Examine the evidence pyramid.
- Articulate the differences in types of literature reviews.

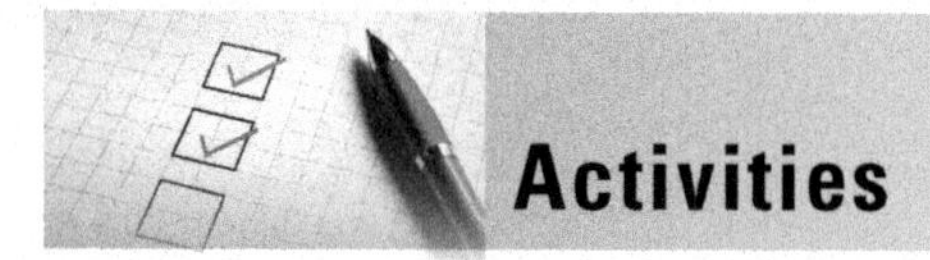

Activities

There are different types of literature. Review the following basic terms.

- Primary literature: This refers to an original experiment or first-hand account describing a phenomenon; sometimes called a "primary study."
- Secondary literature: This is a summary or synthesis of primary literature; for example, meta-analysis or meta-synthesis.
- Tertiary literature: This is a summary of primary and secondary literature; for example, a textbook.
- Filtered literature: This refers to literature that is reviewed and pooled to explore common outcomes in similar circumstances (Holly, Salmond, & Saimbert, 2017).

Literature is also broken down by the type of research study that took place: a quantitative study, a qualitative study, or a mixed-method study. "Mixed method" simply means there was both a quantitative and qualitative component to the research. To distinguish between quantitative and qualitative research, review the following table.

QUANTITATIVE RESEARCH (EXPERIMENTAL)	QUALITATIVE RESEARCH (OBSERVATIONAL)
Purpose: Describe, explain, predict, and determine probability of cause–effect relationships Research designs: Descriptive, correlational, quasi-experimental, experimental	Purpose: Describe, explore, discover, and seek understanding of phenomena Research designs: Ethnography, phenomenology, grounded theory, case study, narrative inquiry, historical review
Research setting: Controlled to the highest degree possible	Research setting: As natural as possible, observations made in natural environment
Measurements: Produce numbers—precise, based on valid, reliable instruments	Measurements: Produce words—narrative, words, images, artifacts

Source: Data from Christenbery, T. (2018). *Evidence-based practice in nursing.* New York, NY: Springer Publishing Company.

Evidence is often visually organized into a "evidence pyramid" (Figure 5.1). The information that is higher on the pyramid is often more compelling. Observational (qualitative) studies form the pyramid's foundation, followed by experiential (quantitative) studies. At the top, there is filtered or synthesized information. It makes sense that when you critically appraise multiple pieces of evidence, the final recommendation is based on multiple studies, not just one piece of primary research.

REFLECTION

- Can you find where background information and expert opinion fall on the pyramid? Think of these as the information you gathered for the project background. Now, you must ask a more specific question and try to find the best evidence to answer that question.
- The question you ask will often determine the type of evidence you find. Based on your question, do you anticipate finding more observational (qualitative) studies or experimental (quantitative) studies?

A literature review involves the process of collecting pieces of evidence to answer a specific question. Consider the basic differences between review types in the table following Figure 5.1.

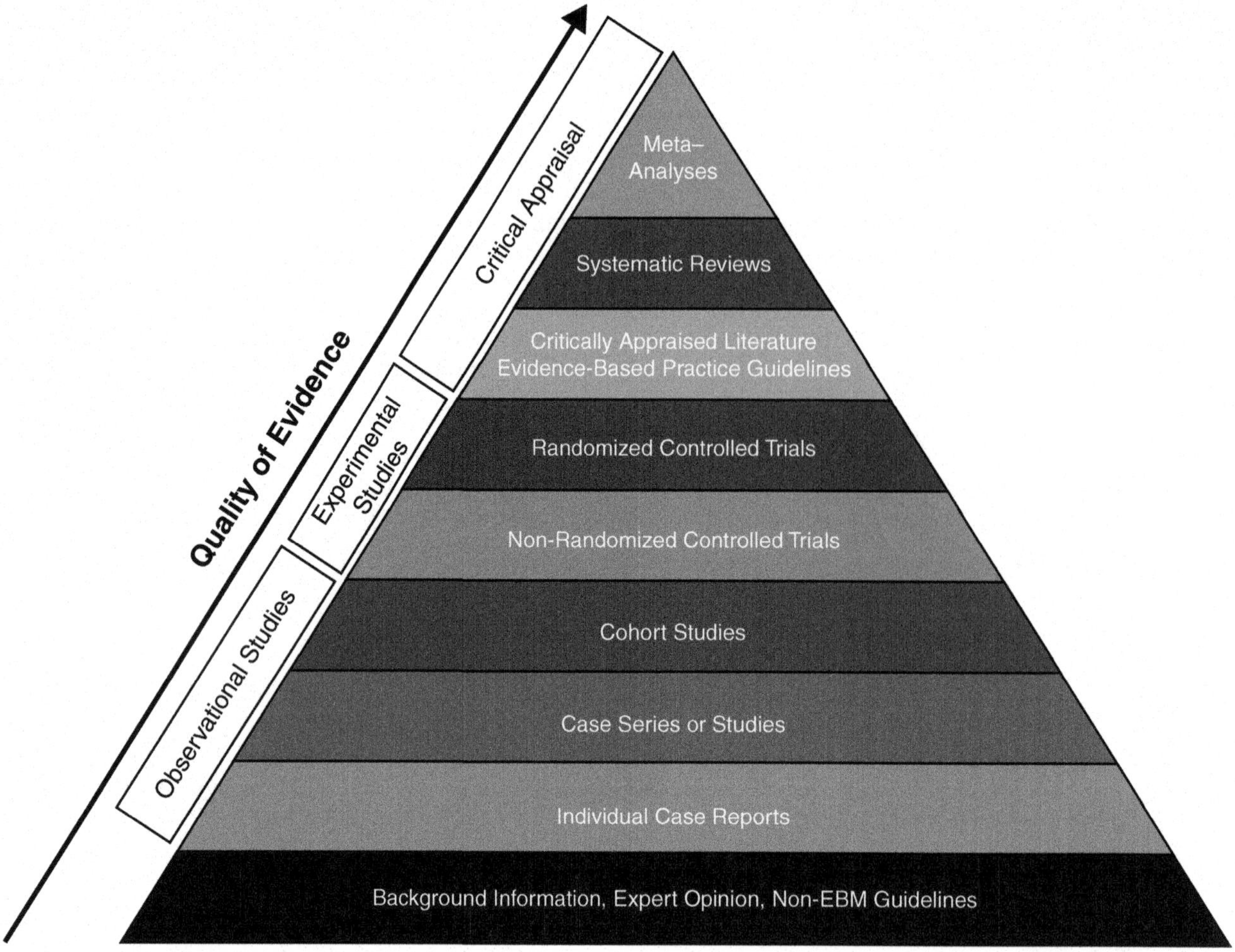

Figure 5.1 The Evidence Pyramid.

EBM, evidence-based medicine.

Source: Central Michigan University. (n.d.). Evidence-based medicine: Resources by levels of evidence. Retrieved from https://libguides.cmich.edu/cmed/ebm/pyramid

	FORMAL LITERATURE REVIEW	INTEGRATIVE REVIEW	SYSTEMATIC REVIEW
Focus	**Broad**	**Defined**	**Precise**
Search strategy	Based on keywords; may search 2–3 databases and limit to past 5 years	Based on keywords and MeSH terms; searches for pivotal papers (research or theory) in 2–6 databases or search engines	Exhaustive, including hand searches and searches for unpublished (grey) literature; uses explicit strategy

(*continued*)

	FORMAL LITERATURE REVIEW	INTEGRATIVE REVIEW	SYSTEMATIC REVIEW
Focus	**Broad**	**Defined**	**Precise**
Appraisal	Rapid appraisal if any; performed to establish support for the question Recommendations by: Melnyk & Fineout-Overholt Johns Hopkins	May be rigorous; generally done by one reviewer: Recommendations by: Whittemore & Knalf (2005)	Rigorous; completed by two independent reviewers; uses valid and reliable tools for appraisal based on the design of the study. Recommendations by: Cochrane Joanna Briggs Institute
Outcome	Support; not generally considered a good source for clinical decision-making	Offers a recommendation; selected literature should be analyzed, not just summarized—articles and groups of articles compared, themes identified, gaps noted, and so on	Suggests a best practice; the purpose of a systematic review is to reach some conclusion regarding the topic: e.g., the selection of high-quality studies to be used in a meta-analysis, the gaps in current research, or the best clinical evidence for determining evidence-based practice
DNP Project considerations	Answers a question, supports some component of the project, and is more focused than the project background	Answers a question, makes project-related recommendations, and should be rigorous	Answers a question, precisely articulates the best practice, and is rigorous

MeSH, Medical Subject Headings.

Source: Adapted from Holly, C. (2014). *Scholarly inquiry and the DNP capstone.* New York, NY: Springer Publishing Company.

Expert Commentary: Marilyn Oermann, PhD, RN, ANEF, FAAN

There are many different types of reviews of research and literature that you can do. Three common types are systematic, integrative, and literature reviews. Use of these terms varies, but all reviews answer questions or describe what is known (and gaps) about a topic. The goal of a systematic review is to answer a specific clinical or research question by carefully searching for and selecting studies based on predetermined criteria and critically appraising them. Systematic reviews use an explicit and reproducible methodology for searching relevant bibliographic databases, such as MEDLINE and Cumulative Index to Nursing and Allied Health Literature (CINAHL); including selected studies in the review; evaluating the quality of individual studies; and synthesizing the findings. With some systematic reviews, the researchers also do a meta-analysis, which uses statistical techniques to integrate the results.

Integrative reviews are broad reviews that include both research and theoretical literature. Because of the various types of studies in these reviews, they provide a more comprehensive summary of a topic than a systematic review, which is focused on answering a specific question. An integrative review includes various types of literature, making it difficult to critically appraise studies as done in a systematic review. A literature review searches for current information on a topic to reveal what is known and gaps in our understanding.

NEXT STEPS

- Think about the question you need to answer.
- Consider what type of evidence would be needed to support the question/intervention/outcome.
- Discuss with your faculty the best approach to your review of literature.
- If integrative review is selected, pull and read the article by Whittemore and Knalf (2005).

REFERENCES AND RESOURCES

Central Michigan University. (n.d.). Evidence-based medicine: Resources by levels of evidence. Retrieved from https://libguides.cmich.edu/cmed/ebm/pyramid

Christenbery, T. (Ed.). (2018). *Evidence-based practice in nursing*. New York, NY: Springer Publishing Company.

Cochrane Review. (n.d.). Training and events. Retrieved from https://us.cochrane.org/training-and-events

Holly, C. (2014). *Scholarly inquiry and the DNP capstone*. New York, NY: Springer Publishing Company.

Holly, C., Salmond, S., & Saimbert, M. (Eds.). (2017). *Comprehensive systematic review for advanced practice nursing* (2nd ed.). New York, NY: Springer Publishing Company.

Hopia, H., Latvala, E., & Liimatainen, L. (2016). Reviewing the methodology of an integrative review. *Scandinavian Journal of Caring Sciences, 30*, 662–669. doi: 10.1111/scs.12327

Joanna Briggs Institute. (n.d.). Education. Retrieved from http://joannabriggs.org/education

Johns Hopkins. (n.d.). Center for evidence-based practice. Retrieved from https://www.hopkinsmedicine.org/evidence-based-practice/ebp_education.html

Melnyk, B. M., & Gallager-Ford, L. (n.d.). Fuld Institute for Evidence-Based Practice. Retrieved from https://fuld.nursing.osu.edu/

Toronto, C., Quinn, B., & Remington, R. (2017). Characteristics of reviews. Published in nursing literature. *Advances in Nursing Science, 41*(1), 30–40. doi: 10.1097/ANS.0000000000000180

Whittemore, R. & Knalf, K. (2005). The integrative review: Updated methodology. *Journal of Advanced Practice Nursing, 52*, 546–553. doi: 10.1111/j.1365-2648.2005.03621.x

RELATED TEXTBOOKS

Christenbery, T. (Ed.). (2018). *Evidence-based practice in nursing*. New York, NY: Springer Publishing Company.
- Chapter 3: Integrating Best Evidence Into Practice
- Chapter 8: How to Read and Assess for Quality of Research

Holly, C. (2019). *Practice-based scholarly inquiry and the DNP Project*. New York, NY: Springer Publishing Company.

Holly, C., Salmond, S., & Saimbert, M. (Eds.). (2017). *Comprehensive systematic review for advanced practice nursing* (2nd ed.). New York, NY: Springer Publishing Company.

Oermann, M., & Hays, J. C. (2019). *Writing for publication* (4th ed.). New York, NY: Springer Publishing Company.
- Chapter 6: Review and Evidence-Based Practice Articles

Lesson 5.2

FORMALIZING A QUESTION USING PICOT

BACKGROUND

What information do you need for your DNP Project? With your background information complete, now we can formulate a question that needs to be answered. The question must be designed in a way that makes it easy to search for relevant literature. It must be a question that can be answered.

LEARNING OBJECTIVES

- Use PICO to develop a question.
- Organize the components of the question into categories.
- Develop a list of synonyms for use in the search.

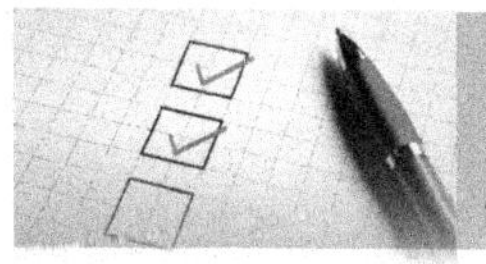

Activities

Recall your problem, population of interest, potential intervention, and desired outcomes for your DNP Project. Formulate a draft of the question.

P: Population of Interest + Problem = ______________________________

I: Potential Intervention = ______________________________

C: Comparison = ______________________________

O: Outcome(s) = ______________________________

PATIENT	INTERVENTION	COMPARISON	OUTCOME
What are the patient's most important characteristics? • Primary problem • Disease state • Coexisting condition **Describe your patient specifically:** • Sex • Age • Ethnicity • Socioeconomic factors	**What do you want to do for the patient?** • Order a test • Prescribe a drug • Order a procedure • Other considerations: • Main intervention • Prognostic factors • Exposures	**What is the alternate intervention, if any?** • A different drug • No medication • A placebo • A different test • A different procedure	**What are you hoping to achieve, measure, or change for the patient?** • Alleviate symptoms • Improve test results • Reduce adverse events • Improve function Could also seek a *not desired* result.
ALWAYS include this piece in your search.	**ALMOST ALWAYS** include this piece in your search.	It is **LESS COMMON** to include this piece in a search.	**SOMETIMES** include this piece in your search.

To start, keep this simple. For the comparison, just say "usual care" or "current practice." If you are making a change in practice, the comparison is the current way things are being done. As you become more adept, you can add in comparisons.

Your question may have more than one outcome. In such a circumstance, you still develop the question the same way, just list all the outcomes.

Depending on the nature of your project, it may be important to avoid biasing your question by including what you *want* to happen. Keep in mind we are not testing hypotheses. Example: Instead of stating, "Among nurses caring for patients with perinatal loss (P), *does* a simulation learning experience (I), compared to usual training (C), *improve* confidence levels in caregiving," you could ask, "Among nurses caring for patients with perinatal loss (P), *how does* a simulation learning experience (I), compared to usual training (C), *impact* confidence levels in caregiving."

When you see "PICOT," the letter *T* stands for "time." What period of time is involved? We recommend adding this later. Focus now on the skill of formulating a PICO question.

Example: "Among patients with COPD (P), what is the impact of a COPD action plan (I), compared to usual care (C), on hospital readmission (O)?"

P (Patient/population)	Patients with COPD
I (Intervention/indicator)	COPD action plan
C (Comparison/control)	Usual care or standard of care (what is currently happening)
O (Outcome)	Hospital readmission

Draft your PICO question:

Now, identify the keywords of each component and write them in each box. Then, try to think of different ways that word might appear in the literature. Make a list.

	KEYWORDS	SYNONYMS
P		
I		
C		
O		

Search databases are complex. We remind you to seek help from your librarian to achieve the best results and utilize the appropriate Medical Subject Headings (MeSH).

Ensure that your question is a good question. Be prepared to answer these "FINER" questions (Christenbery, 2018; Holly, 2019):

F: Is the question feasible?

I: Is the question interesting?

N: Is the question novel?

E: Is the question ethical?

R: Is the question relevant?

NEXT STEPS

- Consult with your faculty.
- Consult with the librarian to prepare for database searching.

REFERENCES AND RESOURCES

Christenbery, T. (Ed.). (2018). *Evidence-based practice in nursing.* New York, NY: Springer Publishing Company.
Holly, C. (2019). *Practice-based scholarly inquiry and the DNP Project* (2nd ed.). New York, NY: Springer Publishing Company.
Asking the clinical question. Retrieved from https://youtu.be/PJhnN7sjPBg
Introduction to EBP. Retrieved from https://youtu.be/GZWkh-gpC8U

RELATED TEXTBOOKS

Christenbery, T. (Ed.). (2018). *Evidence-based practice in nursing.* New York, NY: Springer Publishing Company.

Chapter 6: EBP: Success of Practice Change Depends on the Question

Holly, C. (2019). *Practice-based scholarly inquiry and the DNP Project* (2nd ed.). New York, NY: Springer Publishing Company.

Chapter 2: Practice-Based Scholarly Inquiry

Lesson 5.3

DATABASE SELECTIONS

BACKGROUND

After formulating your question using the PICO format, continue to keep track of synonyms for each component of your question. The elements of the PICO question are the key terms that are entered into the databases to help retrieve your literature. A database is simply a large electronic collection of information organized and cataloged for efficiency in searching. You must make a decision about which databases you will look in and determine which ones are the most likely to house the information you seek.

Depending on the type of review you are doing, you will need to explore multiple databases. The question and purpose of the review drive the type of review: (a) review of literature, (b) integrative review, or (c) systematic review (see table in Lesson 5.1).

LEARNING OBJECTIVES

- Review your question, purpose of review, key terms, and potential synonyms.
- Read the descriptions of commonly used databases.
- Select databases most likely to yield information of interest.

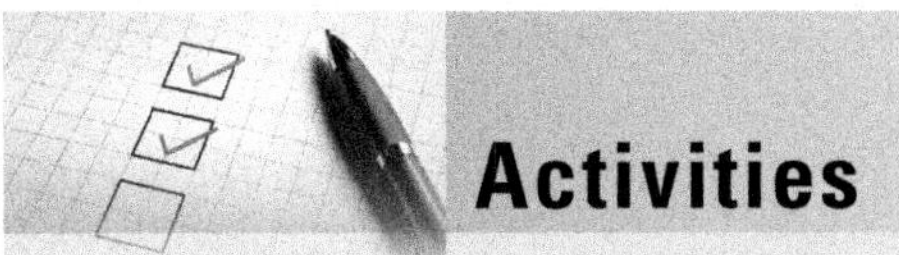

Activities

Complete the following prompts.

Your Problem Statement

____

____

____

Your PICO Question

P
I
C
O

What types of reviews will you complete? Circle your answer.

- Formal review of literature
- Integrative review
- Systematic review

Commonly Used Databases

Review the descriptions and highlight databases you will utilize.

DATABASE	DESCRIPTION
Cumulative Index to Nursing and Allied Health Literature (CINAHL)	The world's most comprehensive nursing and allied health research database. It provides indexing of the top nursing and allied health literature available, including nursing journals and publications from the *National League for Nursing* and the *American Nurses Association*. It also includes references and abstracts on nursing, biomedical, allied health, and consumer health literature; healthcare books; nursing dissertations; selected conference proceedings; standards of practice; educational software; audiovisuals; and evidence-based care sheets. Full text is provided for hundreds of journals, plus legal cases, clinical innovations, critical paths, drug records, research instruments, and clinical trials. **User tools:** Journal alerts, search-history alerts, saved search with personalized account, and compatible with most reference management software.
Cochrane Library	A collection of six databases that contain different types of high-quality, independent evidence to inform healthcare decision-making, and a seventh database that provides information about Cochrane groups. All include full-text Cochrane systematic reviews. **User tools:** Journal alerts, search history alerts, saved search with personalized account, and compatible with most reference management software.
Joanna Briggs Institute	Database of systematic reviews that complement those found in the Cochrane Library. Includes a comprehensive range of resources, including >3,000 records across seven publication types, including literature reviews, recommended practices and procedures, information guideline sheets, comprehensive systematic reviews and protocols, consumer information sheets, and technical reports. **User tools:** Tools to create manuals, consumer information pamphlets, and to adapt existing guidelines for local use. Tools to help users appraise individual papers using a checklist, conduct clinical audits, and develop systematic reviews of multiple papers.
MEDLINE	Widely recognized as the premier source for bibliographic and abstract coverage of biomedical literature. Provides information from the fields of medicine, nursing, dentistry, as well as coverage in the areas of allied health, biological and physical sciences, humanities, and information science as they relate to medicine and healthcare, communication disorders, population biology, and reproductive biology. Contains >25 million citations from 5,200 biomedical journals published in the United States and other countries. Utilizes MeSH indexing with tree, tree hierarchy, subheadings, and explosion capabilities to search citations. **User tools:** Journal alerts, search-history alerts, saved search with personalized account, and compatible with most reference management software.

(*continued*)

DATABASE	DESCRIPTION
PsycINFO	Provides abstracts and citations from the scholarly literature in the behavioral sciences and mental health. Includes articles in psychology, medicine, psychiatry, education, social work, criminology, social science, business, and organizational behavior. This American Psychological Association database includes material of relevance to psychologists and professionals in related fields, such as psychiatry, management, business, education, social science, neuroscience, law, medicine, and social work. Includes citations and summaries of peer-reviewed journal articles, book chapters, books, dissertations, and technical reports. Indexes >2,000 journals, 98% of which are peer reviewed. **User tools:** Journal alerts, search-history alerts, saved search with personalized account, and compatible with most reference management software.
PubMed	Free search engine primarily accessing the MEDLINE database of references and abstracts on life sciences and biomedical topics. Comprises more than 29 million citations for biomedical literature from MEDLINE, life science journals, and online books. Citations may include links to full-text content from PubMed Central and publisher websites. The U.S. National Library of Medicine at the National Institutes of Health maintains the database. Most universities allow full-text holdings to be linked to citations. Indexed using MeSH. **User tools:** Journal alerts, search-history alerts, saved search with personalized My NCBI account, and compatible with most reference management software.
ScienceDirect (Elsevier)	Subscription-based access to a large database of scientific and medical research. Hosts >12 million pieces of content from 3,500 academic journals and 34,000 e-books. Journals are grouped into four main sections: physical sciences and engineering, life sciences, health sciences, and social sciences and humanities. **User tools:** Journal alerts, search-history alerts, saved search with personalized account, and compatible with most reference management software.
Scopus (Elsevier)	Citation and abstract database of peer-reviewed literature that can be used by researchers to determine the impact of specific authors, articles/documents, and journals. Contains >70 million records in the areas of science, technology, medicine, social sciences, arts, and humanities, with coverage strongest in the physical sciences (7,200+ titles) and health sciences (6,800+ titles), followed by the life sciences (4,300+ titles), and finally the social sciences and humanities (5,300+ titles). Titles are selected based on journal policies, content, journal standing, regularity of publication, and online availability. More than 25,000 titles (including open-access journals) from around the world are included. **User tools:** Journal alerts, search-history alerts, saved search with personalized account, and compatible with most reference management software, integrated with ORCID.

(*continued*)

DATABASE	DESCRIPTION
Web of Science (Clarivate Analytics)	Core Collection includes nine indexes containing information gathered from >20,000 scholarly journals, books, book series, reports, conferences, and more. The "cited reference" search is a main feature of Web of Science search capabilities. Provides complete bibliographic data, searchable author abstracts, and cited references. Coverage is strongest in the sciences, followed by social sciences, and arts and humanities. **User tools:** Journal alerts, search-history alerts, saved search with personalized account, and compatible with most reference management software.
UpToDate	A point-of-care clinical evidence-based medicine database, providing coverage of >10,000 topics in 25 medical specialties. Integrates drug information (Lexi-Comp) and clinical images (Visual Dx). In addition to searching the entire resource or viewing topics by specialty, there are options to view the newest updates (What's New), practice-changing updates, drug information, and patient education information. **User tools:** Bookmarks, history, most viewed. Other features include standard medical calculators, and a drug interactions analysis tool. Registered users can earn CME/CE/CPD credit.

CE, continuing education; CME, continuing medical education; CPD, continuing professional development; EBP, evidence-based practice; JBI, Joanna Briggs Institute; MeSH, Medical Subject Headings; NCBI, National Center for Biotechnology Information.

We recommend that you discuss your search strategy with a librarian. Understand that different databases use different terms and MeSH for different concepts. Databases may also use different symbols for their truncation techniques. Completing this prework will make your meeting with a librarian more productive. Many librarians will help you remotely if you can send them this information.

NEXT STEPS

- Arrange to consult the librarian, in person or remotely.
- Prepare to keep track of your findings as you search.

REFERENCES AND RESOURCES

ISU Libraries [Screen name]. (2015, May 26). Evidence-based practice, Step 2 (part 1): searching [Video file]. Retrieved from https://www.youtube.com/watch?v=799zn5gv_GM&feature=youtu.be

ISU Libraries [Screen name]. (2015, May 26). Evidence-based practice, Step 2 (part 1): searching [Video file]. Retrieved from https://www.youtube.com/watch?v=tqQ94s-3dCc&feature=youtu.be

RELATED TEXTBOOKS

Christenbery, T. (Ed.). (2018). *Evidence-based practice in nursing*. New York, NY: Springer Publishing Company.
Chapter 3: Integrating the Best Evidence into Practice

Holly, C. (2019). *Practice-based scholarly inquiry and the DNP Project* (2nd ed.). New York, NY: Springer Publishing Company.

Oermann, M., & Hays, J. C. (2019). *Writing for publication in nursing* (4th ed.). New York, NY: Springer Publishing Company.

Lesson 5.4

DOCUMENTING YOUR SEARCH, ANNOTATION, AND CITATION MANAGEMENT

BACKGROUND

According to the National Institutes of Health (NIH), it is important to document your search strategy when reviewing literature. The information should be detailed enough that the search could be recreated (NIH, 2018). This adds to the credibility and transparency of your project. The search strategy is fully described in the text of the document and often visually presented in a diagram.

Annotation is sometimes referred to as "close reading." It's the part where you highlight and make notes in the margins about what you are reading. Does this information answer your PICO (patient/population, intervention, comparison, outcome) question? To stay organized in a doctoral program, we are warning you now: You need to formulate a strategy for your approach to reading. You will read so much that, without annotation, you will not remember what you read. In my own experience, I read so much over such a long period that I forgot exactly where I read things and could not cite things properly. Be smarter than I was! We will review the pros and cons of manual annotation versus technology-based annotation.

The product of your literature search is evidence. Evidence is referred to with a citation. Most nursing programs use the style manual of the American Psychological Association (APA, 2020). The citation of the evidence should be cataloged. Technology is available to help you combine annotation and citation management. These software options are vital when working with large amounts of information. Check with your school to see whether these software items are offered as part of your technology package. Details of common software options are reviewed.

LEARNING OBJECTIVES

- Utilize Boolean logic to search.
- Document searches and results of each.
- Begin an organized process for annotation.
- Consider use of software to better organize annotation and citation management.

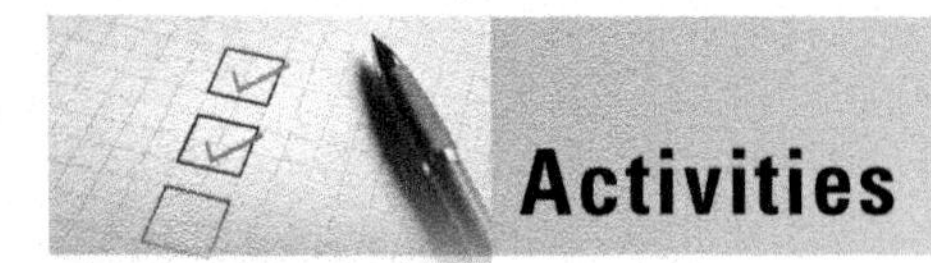

Activities

Add your PICO question to your problem statement and always keep these in front of you as you work. Begin to search in the databases you identified.

Keywords Versus Subject Terms (CINAHL Headings or MeSH)

- Keywords are a good way to start a search. Keyword searching is how you typically use search engines. Think of important words or phrases and type them in the search field to get results. Keyword searching may return many unrelated results.
- Generate keywords by describing important concepts in your own words. Make a list.
- Subject headings are assigned words or phrases used to label materials (similar to hashtags). Subject headings describe the content of each item in a database. Use these headings to find relevant items on the same topic. Searching by subject headings (a.k.a. descriptors) is the most precise way to search article databases. Searches run using subject heading usually return very relevant results.
- Whenever you find an article, look for the subject terms associated with it to use it in your subsequent searches.
- You can also search for subject terms within databases.

Connecting Your Terms

- Join similar concepts or alternate terms with "OR." Use **OR** to broaden your search by connecting two or more synonyms.
- Link different parts of your topic with "AND." Use **AND** to narrow your search: All of your search terms will present in the retrieved records.
- Exclude concepts with "NOT." Use **NOT** to exclude term(s) from your search results.

Use Limiters Within Databases

- Depending on what you are looking for you can use specific limiters to filter your results and make searches more precise.
- The most common limiter is whether the articles are from peer-reviewed journals, which limits your results to scholarly journals that count on experts in disciplines to review drafts of articles prior to publishing them.
- Limiters are specific to databases, and each one has numerous valuable limiters such as evidenced based, clinical queries, age groups, sex, and publication type, among others.

Narrow the Date Range

- When looking for current research or evidence-based practices, limit your date range to the past 3 to 5 years.

Personal Accounts

- Each database allows you to set up a personal account. With a personal account, you can save preferences, organize your research with folders, share your folders with others, view others' folders, save and retrieve your search history, create email alerts and/or RSS (rich site summary) feeds, and gain access to your saved research remotely.

Documentation

The NIH (2018) recommends documentating the following search information:

- Complete, reproducible strategies
- Databases searched with range of dates
- Dates the searches were run, including any updates
- Number of results from each search
- Number of duplicates removed
- Grey literature sources searched
- Other techniques:
  - Hand-searching
  - Bibliography/reference list review
  - Journal search
  - Author search

Keeping track of what progress you have made in your research is an important part of the research process. What databases have you tried? What search terms and limiters have you used? Did you discover new keywords that you would like to try in future searches? What search techniques have been successful and unsuccessful? Knowing the answers to questions such as these can help prevent you from conducting duplicate research or from overlooking valuable resources. This can be done by keeping a simple research log in a word-processing or spreadsheet program (Exhibit 5.1).

Exhibit 5.1 Sample Research Log

QUESTION	DATE	DATABASE NAME	SEARCH TERMS	SEARCH LIMITS	RESULTS
Does handwashing among healthcare workers reduce hospital-acquired infection?	April 12, 2019	MEDLINE (Ovid): 1946 to April 2, 2019	(handwashing OR hand hygiene OR hand disinfection) AND (cross-infection OR hospital-acquired infection)	English, Humans Last 10 years Adults Only randomized controlled trails or meta-analysis	76 results

Grey Literature

Literature that is "semipublished," is not published, and/or is not available through the usual bibliographic sources, such as databases or indexes, is known as "grey literature." It is often information that has been conveyed by another route such as an oral presentation or an internal report. *Grey literature* takes many different forms but is essentially documentation that has not been formally published and has commonly not been peer reviewed. Examples of grey literature include conference abstracts, presentations, and proceedings; regulatory data; unpublished trial data; government publications; reports (such as white papers, working papers, and internal documentation); dissertations/theses; patents; and policies and procedures. Sources can also be oral, in print form, and increasingly, electronic formats.

Searching the grey literature can be an overwhelming task. You should search those resources that make the most sense for your research question. At a minimum, consider searching abstracts and conferences. If your question involves drugs and interventions, check trial registries and pharma data. Also check out the papers and reports of relevant stakeholder organizations. Online repositories, dissertations, and thesis are also examples of where grey literature can be found. Sources for gray literature are consolidated in the table that follows.

GREY LITERATURE TYPES	GREY LITERATURE SOURCES
Abstracts and Conferences	• Conference Papers Index • Embase • F1000 Research Posters • NLM Gateway • Papers First • Scopus • Web of Science
Repositories or Reports	• Google Scholar • Grey Literature Report • The Joanna Briggs Institute • OAIster • Open DOAR • PROSPERO—International Register of prospective systematic reviews • Virginia Henderson Repository
International Grey Literature	• Centre for Reviews and Dissemination (United Kingdom) • International Network of Agencies for Health Technology Assessment (INAHTA) • Institute for Scientific and Technical Information (INstitut de l'Information Scientifique et Technique—INSIST) of the French National Center for Scientific Research (CNRS; Centre national de la recherche scientifique) • International Clinical Trials Registry Platform (ICTRP) • Lenus (The Irish Health Repository) • National Academic Research and Collaborations Information System (NARCIS; the Netherlands) • Open Grey • RIAN (Pathways to Irish Research) • UK Clinical Research Network Study Portfolio • Virtual Health Library • World Health Organization (WHO)

(continued)

GREY LITERATURE TYPES	GREY LITERATURE SOURCES
Clinical Trials	• ClinicalTrials.gov • WHO • International Clinical Trials Registry Platform (ICTRP) • International Standard Randmomised Controlled Trials Number (ISRCTN)
Regulatory Agencies	• Drugs@FDA • Devices@FDA • Health Canada Drug Product Database (DPD) • European Public Assessment Reports
Government	• NIH RePORTER (National Institutes of Health) • HSRProj (NLM; National Library of Medicine) • AHRQ (Grants On-Line Database) • Health Services and Sciences Research Resources (HSRR) • National Technology Information Service (NTIS)

Expert Commentary: Marilyn Oermann, PhD, RN, ANEF, FAAN

All searches need to be done using a carefully developed and documented process. The Preferred Reporting Items for Systematic Reviews and Meta-Analyses (PRISMA) reporting method was developed to guide a systematic review. Although not developed for other types of reviews, PRISMA can be used to conduct these reviews, document what was done, and report the review process and findings in a DNP Project and manuscript later.

Link: PRISMA Explanation and Elaboration. Retrieved from http://www.prisma-statement.org/documents/PRISMA%20EandE%202009.pdf

Link: PRISMA Checklist (PDF). Retrieved from http://prisma-statement.org/documents/PRISMA%202009%20checklist.pdf

Annotation: Review the abstracts first. If selected, print the article or source. Read the item and highlight key information. Then consider adoption of one or several of the suggested strategies.

Suggestion #1: On an index card, transcribe the key points and list the in-text APA citation you would use at the top. Staple to the article.

Suggestion #2: Open a document and list the selected citation. Then write a summary of key points under the citation. Keep a running list. This is sometimes called an "annotated bibliography."

Suggestion #3: Download citation management software (see the following list). Use the annotation feature to electronically highlight and annotate your selected citations.

Suggested citation management software:

- EndNote, Product Details. Retrieved from https://www.endnote.com/product-details
- Zotero, Meet Zotero. Retrieved from https://www.zotero.org
- RefWorks. Retrieved from https://proquest.libguides.com/refworks

Remember to ask whether this software is provided by your school. Video demonstrations of each are linked in the resource list. Explore additional options on your own.

NEXT STEPS

- Experiment and select your preferred annotation and citation management style.
- Complete your searches with assistance from faculty and librarians, if needed.

REFERENCES AND RESOURCES

Alberani, V., Pietrangeli, P. D. C., & Mazza, A. M. (1990). The use of grey literature in health sciences: A preliminary survey. *Bulletin of the Medical Library Association, 78*(4), 358.

American Psychological Association. (2020). *Publication manual of the American Psychological Association* (7th ed.). Washington, DC: Author.

EndNote Training [Screen name]. (2018, July 31). How to use EndNote in 6 minutes: Windows [Video file]. Retrieved from https://www.youtube.com/watch?v=7e6-6QkcYm0&feature=youtu.be

Kyle Denlinger [Screen name]. (2012, November 12). Ready, set, Zotero! [Video file]. Retrieved from https://www.youtube.com/watch?v=7FOu94Ah85Y&feature=youtu.be

National Institutes of Health. (2018). Documenting your work. Retrieved from https://www.nihlibrary.nih.gov/services/systematic-reviews/documenting-your-work

RELATED TEXTBOOK

Oermann, M., & Hays, J. C. (2019). *Writing for publication in nursing* (4th ed.). New York, NY: Springer Publishing Company.

Chapter 4: Reviewing the Literature

Lesson 5.5

OPTIONS FOR EVIDENCE APPRAISAL

BACKGROUND

After completing your literature search, reading and selecting the items to be included, it is time to critically appraise your findings. How do you know that this is "good" research? Was it well conducted? Does it help answer your original question? Our goal is to integrate the best evidence into practice (Christenbery, 2018).

The approach to evidence appraisal is determined by the purpose of the review and the type of evidence you are examining. For example, if your question warranted quantitative studies, it will be appraised in a different way than those needing qualitative studies. There is also a difference in appraisal of evidence that has been synthesized already (i.e., systematic review, clinical guideline) versus primary studies (i.e., randomized controlled trial [RCT], cohort study). In this lesson, we focus on appraisal of primary studies. There will be a later lesson on appraisal and reconciliation of clinical guidelines. To fully embrace the approach to systematic review, training beyond this workbook is warranted.

Discuss your options with your faculty. Keep in mind that sometimes schools adopt a particular method of evidence appraisal that you will be required to use for your DNP Project. In coursework, you may learn about different methods. But be clear about your schools' preferences for the approach used in the DNP Project.

In this lesson, a broad overview of two commonly used approaches is presented. Review the content, explore online, and then talk to your faculty. Methods are not mixed. You will need to select one strategy for the DNP Project and clearly articulate which strategy was used.

LEARNING OBJECTIVES

- Explore two commonly used approaches to rapid appraisal of primary studies.
- Select the strategy to be used in the DNP Project.

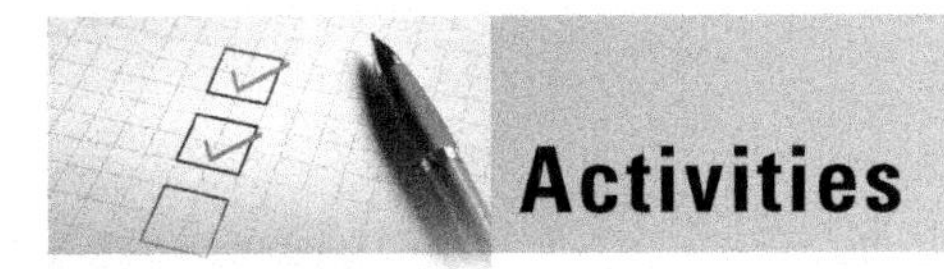

Activities

We have discussed three basic types of literature reviews: systematic, integrative, and formal. The approach to literature appraisal largely depends on the type of review you are conducting. Completing a systematic review requires additional training. Systematic review can be a component of the DNP Project, but there must be an implementation component (AACN, 2015).

- Cochrane Review. (n.d.). Training information. Retrieved from https://us.cochrane.org/training-and-events
- Joanna Briggs Institute. (n.d.). Training information. Retrieved from http://joannabriggs.org/education

The majority of DNP Projects will include an integrative review or formal review of literature as a component of the evidence-based practice process. Review the following evidence-based practice models, which offer approaches for rapid appraisal of evidence. Compare and contrast each approach; discuss with faculty.

- Evidence-Based Practice Process (Melnyk, Fineout-Overholt, Stillwell, & Williamson, 2010a, 2020b, 2010c):

  Critical Appraisal of the Evidence: Parts 1–3

- The Johns Hopkins Evidence-Based Practice Model:

  Appendix D: Evidence Level and Guide

  Appendix E: Research Evidence Appraisal Tool

  Appendix F: Non-research Evidence Appraisal Tool

SIMILARITIES	DIFFERENCES

NEXT STEPS

- Select the approach you will use for evidence appraisal.
- Begin the appraisal of your selected literature.

REFERENCES AND RESOURCES

American Association of Colleges of Nursing. (2015). *The doctor of nursing practice: Current issues and clarifying recommendations* [White paper]. Retrieved from https://www.aacnnursing.org/Portals/42/News/White-Papers/DNP-Implementation-TF-Report-8-15.pdf

Christenbery, T. (Ed.). (2018). *Evidence-based practice in nursing.* New York, NY: Springer Publishing Company.

Dang, D., & Dearholt, S. (2017). *Johns Hopkins nursing evidence-based practice: Model and guidelines* (3rd ed.). Indianapolis, IN: Sigma Theta Tau International.

Johns Hopkins Evidence-Based Practice Model. (2017). Sample of tools. Retrieved from https://www.hopkinsmedicine.org/evidence-based-practice/ijhn_2017_ebp.html

Melnyk, B. M., Fineout-Overholt, E., Stillwell, S. B., & Williamson, K. M. (2009). Igniting a spirit of inquiry: An essential foundation for EBP. *American Journal of Nursing, 109*(11), 49–52. Retrieved from http://forces4quality.org/af4q/download-document/3517/Resource-Evidence_Based_Practice__Step_by_Step__Igniting_a.28.pdf

Melnyk, B. M., Fineout-Overholt, E., Stillwell, S. B., & Williamson, K. M. (2010a). Critical appraisal of the evidence: Part 1. *American Journal of Nursing, 110*(7), 47–52. Retrieved from http://download.lww.com/wolterskluwer_vitalstream_com/PermaLink/NCNJ/A/NCNJ_541_516_2011_01_13_DFGD_5161_SDC516.pdf

Melnyk, B. M., Fineout-Overholt, E., Stillwell, S. B., & Williamson, K. M. (2010b). Critical appraisal of the evidence: Part 2. *American Journal of Nursing, 110*(9), 41–48. doi: 10.1097/01.NAJ.0000388264.49427.f9

Melnyk, B. M., Fineout-Overholt, E., Stillwell, S. B., & Williamson, K. M. (2010c). Critical appraisal of the evidence: Part 3. *American Journal of Nursing, 110*(11), 43–51. doi: 10.1097/01.NAJ.0000390523.99066.b5

RELATED TEXTBOOKS

Christenbery, T. (Ed.). (2018). *Evidence-based practice in nursing.* New York, NY: Springer Publishing Company.

Chapter 3: Integrating Best Evidence Into Practice

Chapter 6: EBP: Success of Practice Change Depends on the Question

Chapter 8: How to Read and Assess for Quality of Research

Holly, C., Salmond, S., & Saimbert, M. (Eds.). (2017). *Comprehensive systematic review for advanced practice nursing* (2nd ed.). New York, NY: Springer Publishing Company.

Lesson 5.6

APPRAISAL, COMPARISON, AND RECONCILIATION OF CLINICAL GUIDELINES

BACKGROUND

Clinical guidelines are synthesized pieces of evidence. But are they the best evidence? In a study of 4,000 clinical guidelines, only 14% were based on randomized controlled trials and 55% on expert opinion (White, Dudley-Brown, & Terhaar, 2020). Have the guidelines been updated to reflect the most recent evidence? As discussed in a previous chapter, the International Organization for Migration (IOM, 2011) sets standards for guideline development. Assuming the guideline is well developed, it could be considered good evidence for translation to practice.

Nurses will often find that there is more than one clinical guideline on a given topic. Remember that the AGREE II tool can help you compare and contrast the differences between two guidelines. But what if there are more than two guidelines to consider. For example, on the topic of obesity, there are more than six well-known clinical guidelines. What strategies can you use to reconcile the content of the guideline? How can the information be translated to your practice situation?

LEARNING OBJECTIVES

- Build on the clinical guideline previously selected for the background.
- Appraise the individual guideline(s) based on the IOM standards.
- Compare two guidelines using the AGREE II tool.
- Reconcile guidelines for translation to your DNP Project.

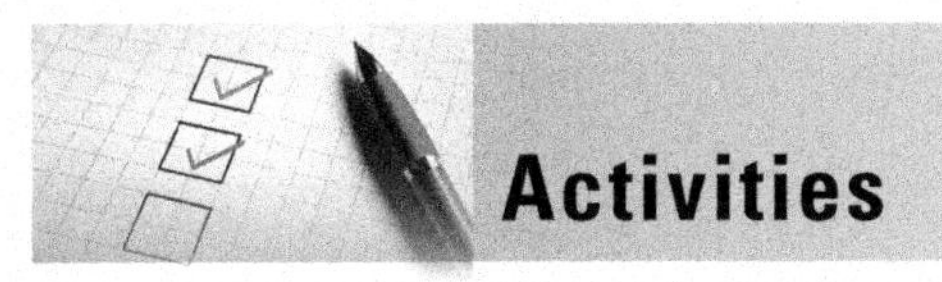

Activities

1. Name the clinical guideline you previously selected as part of your DNP Project background.

____

2. Name at least one additional guideline on the same topic.

____

3. Are there any other guidelines available on the same topic? List them here.

____

____

____

Evaluate each guideline. Do they meet these IOM standards?

- Transparency
- Conflict of interest
- Diverse group composition
- Systematic review of literature
- Foundations for rating strength of recommendations
- Articulation of recommendations
- External review
- Updating

Select two guidelines for comparison. Use the AGREE II tool to evaluate each guideline.

SIMILARITIES	DIFFERENCES

Use the AGREE II tool to evaluate additional guidelines if necessary.

Collectively, what are the recommendations made by all?

What are the key differences in the recommendations?

Why do you think these discrepancies exist?

What are the key recommendations, regardless of guideline, that should be applied or translated to your practice situation?

Expert Commentary: Guideline Reconciliation in Hypertension: Irina Benenson, DNP, FNP-C, CEN

Appreciation for evidence-based clinical guidelines has grown during the past two decades. However, many guidelines provide conflicting recommendations on the same clinical issue, such as "hypertension" or "high blood pressure." It becomes challenging to adopt contradicting guidelines to the clinical practice or scholarly work. Inconsistent guidance commonly occurs when data are inconclusive and sparse and when guideline developers differ in their approach to evidence interpretation and synthesis.

For example, two sets of guidelines published in 2017 are aimed to address management of hypertension in older individuals (Qaseem et al., 2017; Whelton et al., 2017). Recommendations from the American College of Cardiology and American Heart Association (ACC/AHA) and the American College of Physicians and American Academy of Family Physicians (ACP/AAFP) guidelines have many similarities. However, there is a substantial variation in guidance on blood pressure treatment goals (Benenson, Waldron, & Bradshaw, 2019). The ACC/AHA authors support systolic blood pressure targets of less than 130 mmHg for older adults. On the other hand, the ACP/AAFP developers endorse a more conservative goal, below 150 mmHg, that is grounded in the total amount of evidence. What is the best guideline for your project, patient, or population?

This example illustrates how differences in the approach to data synthesis may impact treatment recommendations. No system is currently in place for reconciling differences. The solution here is for the DNP student, with faculty and preceptors, to carefully examine evidence, choosing recommendations that are applicable to the focus population, and allowing options for decisions when the evidence is mixed or insufficient. That is, if the practice differences are unlikely to harm the quality of care. It is important to remember that decision-making regarding the care of the individual patient should always incorporate patients' personal preferences and perspectives.

When developing the DNP Project, the goal is to apply the best evidence that is aligned to the population of interest and desired outcomes.

NEXT STEPS

- Continue to discuss the development of your review of literature with faculty.
- Engage the assistance of the librarian, if necessary.
- Stay organized as you review content using annotation and citation management.

REFERENCES AND RESOURCES

Benenson, I., Waldoron, F., & Bradshaw, M. (2019). Treating hypertension in older adults: Beyond the guidelines. *Journal of the American Association of Nurse Practitioners.* doi: 10.1097/JXX.0000000000000220

Institute of Medicine. (2011). Clinical guidelines we can trust. Retrieved from https://www.nap.edu/read/13058/chapter/1

Qaseem, A., Wilt, T. J., Rich, R., Humphrey, L. L., Frost, J., & Forciea, M. A. (2017). Pharmacologic treatment of hypertension in adults aged 60 years or older to higher versus lower blood pressure targets: A clinical practice guideline from the American College of Physicians and the American Academy of Family Physicians. *Annals of Internal Medicine, 166*(6), 430–437. doi: 10.7326/M16-1785

Whelton, P. K., Carey, R. M., Aronow, W. S., Casey, D. E., Jr., Collins, K. J., Dennison Himmelfarb, C., ... Williamson, J. D. (2017). 2017 ACC/AHA/AAPA/ABC/ACPM/AGS/APhA/ASH/ASPC/NMA/PCNA guideline for the prevention, detection, evaluation, and management of high blood pressure in adults: A report of the American College of Cardiology/American Heart Association Task Force on Clinical Practice Guidelines. *Journal of the American College of Cardiology (JACC), 70*(19). doi: 10.1016/j.jacc.2017.11.006

White, K. M., Dudley-Brown, S., & Terhaar, M. F. (Eds.). (2020). *Translation of evidence into nursing and healthcare* (3rd ed.). New York, NY: Springer Publishing Company.

RELATED TEXTBOOK

Christenbery, T. (Ed.). (2018). *Evidence-based practice in nursing.* New York, NY: Springer Publishing Company.

Chapter 9: Clinical Practice Guidelines

Lesson 5.7

CONSTRUCTING AN EVIDENCE TABLE

BACKGROUND

The purpose of an evidence table is to organize, outline, and present the findings of appraised literature in a succinct way. Consult with your faculty to determine whether they have preferences for content to be included. Faculty may also set criteria for the number of studies to be included, again depending on the question and purpose of the review.

In our experience, we find that students tend to be too wordy when constructing the table. Keep wording concise. The table should present key, abbreviated information. (Melnyk, Fineout-Overholt, Stillwell, and Williamson, 2010, offer a solid example of a completed evidence table.) We recommend that your evidence table be included as part of the DNP Project proposal and final academic paper. It catalogs and demonstrates your work.

LEARNING OBJECTIVES

- Review Melnyk et al.'s (2010) example.
- Organize your findings into a table based on the suggestions of your faculty and school requirements for the DNP Project.

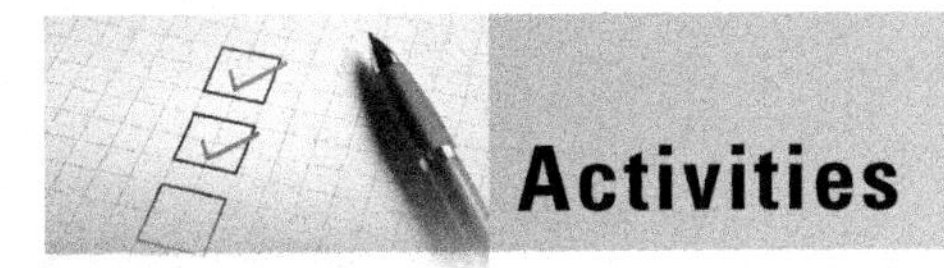

Activities

1. Review the article by Melnyk et al. (2010). Retrieved from https://www.nursingcenter.com/nursingcenter_redesign/media/EBP/AJNseries/Critical3.pdf
2. Create the outline for your table using their suggested headings:
   - First author, year
   - Conceptual framework
   - Design/method
   - Sample/setting
   - Major variables studied (and their definitions)
   - Measurement
   - Data analysis
   - Findings
   - Level of evidence
3. Insert your information, in a concise way, into the designated columns.

NEXT STEPS

- Review your work with your faculty and make revisions as needed.
- Prepare to write a synthesis of your findings in paragraph format.

REFERENCES AND RESOURCES

Melnyk, B. M., Fineout-Overholt, E., Stillwell, S. B., & Williamson, K. M. (2010). Critical appraisal of evidence: Part III. *American Journal of Nursing, 110*(11), 43–51. doi: 10.1097/01.NAJ.0000390523.99066.b5

National Institute for Clinical Excellence. (2014). Examples of evidence tables. Retrieved from https://www.nice.org.uk/process/pmg15/chapter/appendix-c-examples-of-evidence-tables

RELATED TEXTBOOK

Christenbery, T. (Ed.). (2018). *Evidence-based practice in nursing*. New York, NY: Springer Publishing Company.

Lesson 5.8

WRITING A SYNTHESIS OF FINDINGS

BACKGROUND

As a DNP student, you have to make sense of the body of literature you have collected and appraised. You need to identify relationships, understand what is known, and describe any identified gaps (Oermann & Hayes, 2019). Altogether, what does it mean? How does it relate to your problem and population of interest? How will it guide your project?

The evidence table first will help you get organized as you begin to write up the synthesis of the findings. Generally, you start the literature review section by stating the question you are trying to answer, followed by your search strategy. The strategy should be described in such a way that it could be reproduced. It should include databases, key terms used, inclusion/exclusion criteria, and the number of results. If the results are further narrowed, describe how you approached that process.

Next, present the findings. There are several ways to approach this. Some authors take a chronological approach, discussing findings on a continuum. Others organize the studies into groups, perhaps each group addressing each outcome mentioned in the PICO (patient/population, intervention, comparison, outcome) question. Determine your approach before you write. Also, remember that you are not simply regurgitating the content of the studies. You are synthesizing, making connections, and showing the relationships to your problem/population of interest. Make that very clear to your reader.

LEARNING OBJECTIVES

- Construct a paragraph describing your search strategy and findings.
- Outline an approach to a synthesis of findings.

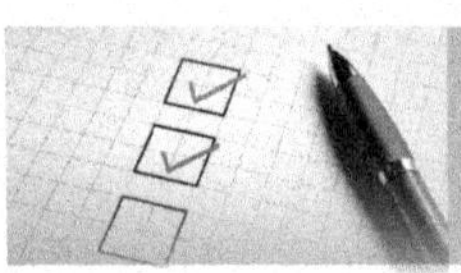

Activities

Use these prompts as an example of how to write an introductory paragraph for a review of literature.

The purpose of this ______________________________ (type of review) is to answer the question (PICOT), "______________________________?" Selected databases for this review included (list databases) ______ ______________________________. Using the key terms (list key terms), ______________________________ ____________________ a combination was entered _______ and tracked resulting in a total of (#) __________ results. The results were further narrowed by (inclusion/exclusion criteria) ______________________________ _________. After applying those limitations, a total of (#) _______ articles were selected for review and the synthesis of findings is presented here.

Additional descriptors are required if you did hand-searching as well. Inserting a diagram illustrating the search strategy and results is also a good idea.

Determine your approach to your synthesis of the findings. Write an outline here.

As you write any component of the DNP Project Proposal, we strongly recommend that you use antiplagiarism software to ensure that you are compliant.

NEXT STEPS

- Enlist a classmate or support person to read your paper.
- Ensure that someone else can follow your process and understand your findings.

REFERENCE AND RESOURCE

Oermann, M., & Hays, J. (2019). *Writing for publication in nursing* (4th ed.). New York, NY: Springer Publishing Company.

RELATED TEXTBOOK

Oermann, M., & Hays, J. (2019). *Writing for publication in nursing* (4th ed.). New York, NY: Springer Publishing Company.

Chapter 4: Reviewing the Literature

Exhibit 4.7: Analyzing Nursing Literature

Exhibit 4.12: Preventing Plagiarism

CHAPTER SUMMARY

Your DNP Project is under development. A full description of the problem of interest is contained in the background and context section of your DNP Project proposal. Again, depending on your school requirements, the order of this chapter and Chapter 6, Framing the DNP Project—Taking Aim and Being SMART, may be interchangeable. Regardless, at some point, you will deploy your skills and complete some type of review of literature for the project— a formal review of literature, integrative review, or systematic review. The DNP Project should utilize the recommendations of your findings in practice. Reflect on your work at this point:

What challenges are you experiencing?

____

____

____

____

What are two actions that you can take to resolve your challenges and move forward?

1.

2.

Remember to keep in regular communication with your faculty as this work is introductory and intended to give you a jump start. At the doctoral level, deeper engagement into evidence and literature is expected and required. Work hard.

NOTES

____

____

____

____

____

____

6

Framing the DNP Project: Taking Aim and Being SMART

Molly J. Bradshaw and Mercedes Echevarria

Lessons

OBJECTIVES

The aim(s) and objectives of the DNP Project set the tone for project methodology. In this chapter, students build upon their problem statement. They add a purpose statement, aim(s), and objectives for the project. The chapter concludes with a brief introduction to change theory and ends with a worksheet to prepare for the project methodology. By the end of this chapter, you will be able to:

- Build on the problem statement.
- Write a clear project purpose statement.
- Articulate the main project aim(s).
- Draft specific, measurable, achievable, realistic, and time-bound (SMART) objectives.

INTRODUCTION

This chapter is pivotal. In previous chapters, you wrote a problem statement (Lesson 3.8 of Chapter 3, Identifying Problems and Project Topics) and revised it (Lesson 4.1 of Chapter 4, Developing the DNP Project Background and Context). In this chapter, you will be writing the purpose statement, aim, and objectives that will help drive your project methodology. Depending on the design of your DNP program, you may find the order of Chapter 5, Skills for Formal Review of Literature and Evidence Appraisal and this chapter interchangeable. In some programs, the purpose statement, aim(s), and objectives are written before the formal review of literature. In others, review of literature is done first. You can decide with your faculty the best approach to use.

To review, a DNP Project starts with a problem that impacts patients or populations, either directly or directly. What is the problem? What is the gap in practice? For this chapter, we will the terms "problem" and "practice gap" interchangeably. We ask you to identify what the standard of care, or current best practice is to address the problem or close this practice gap. This becomes the basis of your intervention. Being able to clearly articulate this information will make you an effective champion of the practice change that is necessary.

First, we guide you through some exercises to help make sure you have thought carefully about the potential intervention(s) and project feasibility. These points must be clarified before you write a purpose statement. The purpose statement builds on your problem statement. When you talk to others about the project, these statements will help you articulate with precision.

- "I have identified ______________________________ problem that affects ____________________ population. The purpose of my project will be to ______________________________."
- "I have identified a problem with ______________________________ (gap in practice that isn't fitting best practices). The standard of care is ____________________."
- "The purpose of my project will be to ______________________________ ______________________________."

The aim of the project is meant to reflect the project vision. In what direction do you want your project to go? The objectives are specific, measurable ways in which you will demonstrate that you met the aim. It is helpful to think of a bow-and-arrow analogy. The aim is the direction that you are aiming the arrow. The objective is the target. With its numbers and concentric circles, it lets you know precisely how close you get to the bull's-eye. Aim first, then hit your objective. We will help you with the structure and writing of these components to make sure that you are on target.

The chapter concludes with a brief discussion of common change theories. Students will need to think about how theory may help with identification of project barriers and assist with facilitation of certain project components. We will revisit your DNP Project outline and prepare a worksheet that will kick off the organization of the methodology. Let's begin.

You will need to arrange for a meeting and discussion with your project faculty when you have completed the work of this chapter. Do *not* move onto Chapter 7, Project Methodology: Develop, Implement, Evaluate, without faculty approval of your DNP Project purpose statement, aim(s), and objectives.

MY GOALS FOR FRAMING THE DNP PROJECT ARE TO:

Lesson 6.1

YOU ARE THE CHAMPION OF CHANGE

BACKGROUND

You have identified a problem. There is a practice gap. In other words, something should be happening (best practice); in short, it is not. During the background investigation and perhaps the formal review of literature, you should have explored what the standard of care is (current best practice). Based on what is in the literature and what is going on in the context of the organization/agency, do you see the implementation of this best practice as a fit for the organization to address the problem (practice gap)?

You need to make an argument for your intervention(s) of choice. What are you planning to do, and why would it work? What evidence exists to support your planned intervention? To lead this DNP Project, you must become the champion of change. The process starts by being able to clearly articulate your problem, the standards of care (best practices) related to that problem, and the reason that it is a fit for the organization or local context.

LEARNING OBJECTIVES

- List the possible interventions that may be used to address the identified problem/practice gap.
- Document the standard of care (current best practice) to address the problem/gap.

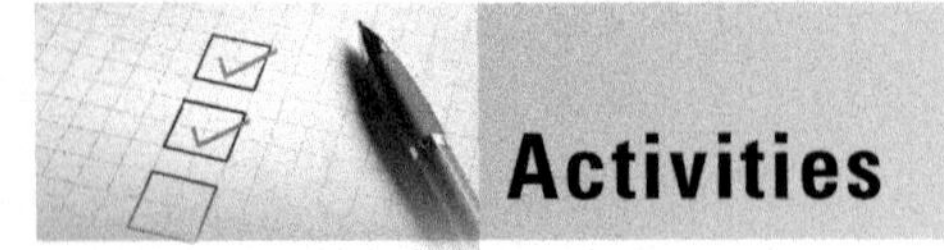

Activities

Record your project's problem statement:

____

____

Based on your background, review of literature, and/or other sources, list the potential standard of care (best practice) that you can implement to address the identified problem/practice gap. Cite the source.

STANDARD OF CARE (BEST PRACTICE)	FIT TO ORGANIZATION OR LOCAL CONTEXT
1.	
2.	
3.	
4.	

Notes:

NEXT STEPS

- Discuss your list with your faculty.
- Continue to reflect on use of this best practice in the project context.

RELATED TEXTBOOK

White, K. M., Dudley-Brown, S., & Terhaar, M. F. (Eds.). (2020). *Translation of evidence into nursing and healthcare* (3rd ed.). New York, NY: Springer Publishing Company.

Chapter 8: Methods for Translation

Lesson 6.2

CONSIDERATIONS FOR PROJECT FEASIBILITY

BACKGROUND

DNP students often have big dreams and big ideas. *This is wonderful*! However, we need a reality check. First, you have to graduate. Your project is meant to be a foundation of future scholarship (American Association of Colleges of Nursing [AACN], 2015). It must be designed in a way that it can be completed in a reasonable amount of time. Second, you will be working on a timeline in a real-world organization or situation. Your sense of urgency to get a project done for school may or may not align with the needs of the organization or context of the project. The project feasibility must be discussed before you finalize your purpose statement, aim(s), and objectives. You need to involve your faculty and project stakeholders in this conversation.

LEARNING OBJECTIVES

- Outline considerations for project feasibility.
- Discuss these considerations with faculty and stakeholders.

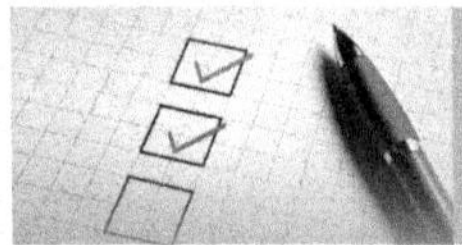

Activities

Reflect on the following:

1. What are your personal considerations for this project?
   - What do you hope to learn?
   - What do you want to change?
   - How does this build a platform for your future?
2. What are the DNP program considerations for this project?
   - Tentative graduation date:
   - Key school requirements:
3. What are the organizational/agency/context considerations for this project?
   - What is the tentative timeline for implementation of this project?
   - Are there any specific concerns?

Every project has challenges and potential barriers. You should complete an organizational, environmental, or community assessment to identify barriers and facilitators for successful implementation of your planned change. What barriers will you face? Ask yourself:

Q: Is the organization even ready for this change?

A: Consider using the Organizational Readiness to Change Assessment instrument (Helfrich, Li, Sharp, & Sales, 2009) to assess this.

Q: What are some of the reasons standards of care (best practice) are not currently being utilized?

A: Consider using the BARRIERS Scale (Williams, Brown, & Costello, 2015) to assess.

COMMONLY IDENTIFIED BARRIERS	COMMONLY IDENTIFIED FACILITATORS
Characteristics of intervention: • Cost • Time • Lack of precision • Not developed for users' need • Not designed to be self-sustaining Context of intervention: • Lack of organizational support • Competing demands • Lack of time/resources • Prevailing practice against the innovation Design of intervention: • Irrelevant to practice • Failure to evaluate cost, adoption, or sustainability • Low participation • Not aligned with organizational mission	* Facilitators largely depend on the organization. Research/evidence is more likely to be used in environments where: • Staff development is frequent • There is low emotional exhaustion • Positive leadership What facilitators in your project context will help you? List them here based on your organizational assessment:

* Not all inclusive.
Source: Adapted from White, K. M., Dudley-Brown, S., & Terhaar, M. F. (Eds.). (2020). *Translation of evidence into nursing and healthcare* (3rd ed., p. 306). New York, NY: Springer Publishing Company.

What are your top three concerns/challenges for project feasibility? What can be done in the planning phases to address these concerns?

Concern 1:

Plan for minimizing/addressing this concern:

Concern 2:

Plan for minimizing/addressing this concern:

Concern 3:

Plan for minimizing/addressing this concern:

NEXT STEPS

- Revisit this lesson if needed.
- Revise your plans for your project to ensure feasibility.
- Consult with your DNP Project chair and/or DNP team.

REFERENCES AND RESOURCES

American Association of Colleges of Nursing. (2015). *The doctor of nursing practice: Current issues and clarifying recommendations* [White paper]. Retrieved from https://www.aacnnursing.org/Portals/42/News/White-Papers/DNP-Implementation-TF-Report-8-15.pdf

Helfrich, C. D., Li, Y. F., Sharp, N. D., & Sales, A. E. (2009). Organizational readiness to change assessment (ORCA): Development of an instrument based on the Promoting Action on Research in Health Services (PARIHS) framework. *Implementation Science: IS, 4*, 38. doi:10.1186/1748-5908-4-38

White, K. M., Dudley-Brown, S., & Terhaar, M. F. (Eds.). (2020). *Translation of evidence into nursing and healthcare* (3rd ed.). New York, NY: Springer Publishing Company.

Williams, B., Brown, T., & Costello, S. (2015). A cross-cultural investigation into the dimensional structure and stability of the Barriers to Research and Utilization Scale (BARRIERS Scale). *BMC Research Notes, 8*, 601. doi:10.1186/s13104-015-1579-9

RELATED TEXTBOOKS

Christenbery, T. (Ed.). (2018). *Evidence-based practice in nursing.* New York, NY: Springer Publishing Company.

Chapter 15: EBP: A Culture of Organizational Empowerment

White, K. M., Dudley-Brown, S., & Terhaar, M. F. (Eds.). (2020). *Translation of evidence into nursing and healthcare* (3rd ed.). New York, NY: Springer Publishing Company.

Chapter 9: Project Planning and the Work of Translation

Chapter 13: Interprofessional Collaboration and Practice for Translation

Chapter 15: Best Practices in Translation: Challenges and Barriers in Translation

Chapter 16: Legal and Ethical Issues in Translation

Lesson 6.3

ARTICULATING DESIRED PROJECT OUTCOMES

BACKGROUND

All stakeholders in a DNP Project have goals—something they want to see happen as a result of the project. The goals vary depending on the perspective of the stakeholder. There is overlap and competing priorities. For example:

- Student goals: Graduation, leadership development, mastery of DNP Essentials
- Faculty goals: Meet curriculum requirements, prepare for new roles in nursing
- Organizational goals: Implement change to bridge a practice gap, improve safety/quality
- Patient goals: Improve health

The point here is for DNP students to appreciate that the DNP Project is not solely based on what you want as a student. A part of leadership development is learning to lead and execute projects in a way that satisfies the needs of multiple stakeholders.

Goals can be translated into outcomes. Outcomes must be measurable in order to assess the impact of the change that was implemented. When developing the DNP Project, the goals may be diverse. However, the DNP Project outcomes must be tied back, either directly or indirectly, to the patient (American Association of Colleges of Nursing, 2015). Again, the purpose is to improve health outcomes.

LEARNING OBJECTIVES

- List the project goals based on stakeholder perspective.
- Translate the goals to specific project outcomes.
- Provide rationales for direct or indirect impact on health outcomes.

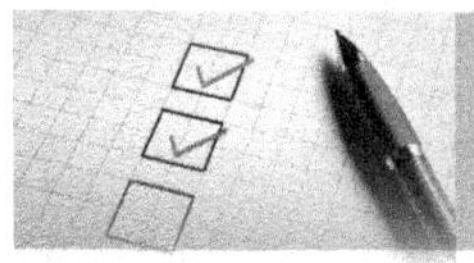

Activities

1. Reflect on your problem statement and your overall work up to this point. List the goals of this project for the identified stakeholders. Then translate those goals into specific outcomes for your project. State the relationship (direct or indirect) the goal has to patient outcomes. Determine whether this outcome is measurable.

Student goals:	Faculty goals:
Organizational goals:	Patient/population goals:

2. Target specific goals and translate them to potential project outcomes.

Outcome:	Rationale: (How does it relate to patient/population?)

Is this outcome measurable? Yes No Unsure

Outcome:	Rationale: (How does it relate to patient/population?)

Is this outcome measurable? Yes No Unsure

Outcome:	Rationale: (How does it relate to patient/population?)

Is this outcome measurable? Yes No Unsure

3. Complete this process until you have listed all the outcomes for your project. The number of outcomes for each project may vary. Confirm that all stakeholders are satisfied with this plan.

NEXT STEPS

- Discuss the project outcomes with your DNP team.
- Ensure that the organization/agency supports your project goals and outcomes.

REFERENCE AND RESOURCE

American Association of Colleges of Nursing. (2015). *The doctor of nursing practice: Current issues and clarifying recommendations* [White paper]. Retrieved from https://www.aacnnursing.org/Portals/42/News/White-Papers/DNP-Implementation-TF-Report-8-15.pdf

RELATED TEXTBOOKS

Hickey, J. V., & Brosnan, C. A. (Eds.). (2017). *Evaluation of health care quality for DNPs* (2nd ed.). New York, NY: Springer Publishing Company.

Chapter 4: Evaluation and Outcomes

White, K. M., Dudley-Brown, S., & Terhaar, M. F. (Eds.). (2020). *Translation of evidence into nursing and healthcare* (3rd ed.). New York, NY: Springer Publishing Company.

Chapter 4: Translation of Evidence for Improving Clinical Outcomes

Lesson 6.4

WRITING A PURPOSE STATEMENT

BACKGROUND

The DNP Project begins with a problem. You were instructed on how to develop a problem statement (Lesson 3.9 of Chapter 3, Identifying Problems and Project Topics) and refine that statement (Lesson 4.1 of Chapter 4, Developing the DNP Project Background and Context). We now build on that work by drafting a purpose statement.

The DNP Project moves in a linear direction to: (a) identify a problem/practice gap, (b) explore solutions based on evidence and best practice, (c) determine stakeholder goals and desired outcomes, and (d) state the purpose of the project. A purpose statement logically follows the problem statement. What does the DNP team want to accomplish? Think of it as your mission statement, the objective of the work. After completing this activity, we recommend that you keep your problem statement and purpose statement on an index card in front of you as you work. This helps keep you focused.

LEARNING OBJECTIVES

- Build on the problem statement.
- Add your purpose statement.

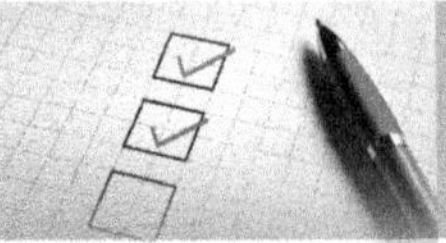

Activities

Complete these prompts to formulate the purpose statement.

1. Restate your problem statement:

____

____

____

2. List your project outcomes (as defined by the project question and the input of the DNP team in Lesson 6.3):

   1.

   2.

   3.

3. Ask yourself, "If I conduct this project, will the problem/practice gap be addressed or resolved?" The purpose statement will need to include the following elements:
   - The population who will be participating in the intervention
   - The proposed method or intervention
   - The setting the method will be implemented in
   - The outcomes to be measured
   - The time frame of the project

Example: Effective Purpose Statements

"The purpose of this DNP Project is to implement an evidence-based protocol within a community health clinic on the use of the teach-back method to newly diagnosed diabetics to optimize self-care management over a 3-month period."

"The purpose of this DNP Project is to implement the COPD Action Plan offered by the American Lung Association to all patients diagnosed with COPD on the unit prior to hospital discharge to improve medication compliance, self-management, and prevent readmission over a period of 30 days."

4. Draft your purpose statement:

___

___

___

The purpose statement will follow the problem statement. Although it would be nice for purpose statements to answer every who, what, when, where, and how question, it is not always feasible. Make sure that you have included the pivotal transition phrases like:

"The purpose of this DNP Project is to ..."
"The DNP team will ..."
"The goal of the DNP Project is to ..."

Write the problem statement followed by the final purpose statement here.

Problem statement:

____

____

____

Purpose statement:

____

____

____

NEXT STEPS

- Engage a classmate to review your work; revise as necessary.
- Discuss with your faculty, DNP chair, and DNP team.

REFERENCE AND RESOURCE

University of Arkansas. (n.d.). Creating a purpose statement. Retrieved from https://walton.uark.edu/business-communication-lab/Resources/downloads/Creating_a_Purpose_Statement.pdf

RELATED TEXTBOOK

Bonnel, W., & Smith, K. (2018). *Proposal writing for clinical nursing and DNP Projects.* New York, NY: Springer Publishing Company.

Chapter 9: Guiding the Advanced Clinical Project: The Purpose of a Purpose Statement

Lesson 6.5

DRAFTING THE AIMS AND OBJECTIVES

BACKGROUND

To review, the American Association of Colleges of Nursing (AACN, 2015) articulated several minimum expectations for DNP Projects:

- Focus on a change that impacts healthcare outcomes (directly or indirectly).
- Have a system or population focus.
- Demonstrate implementation in practice.
- Include an evaluation plan for process and outcomes.
- Include a plan for sustainability.
- Provide a foundation of future scholarship.

These standards can be used to guide the development of the aim(s) and objectives of the DNP Project. The purpose of the objectives is to precisely describe how the aim will be accomplished. In essence, the DNP Project will require development of an evidence-based intervention that is then implemented and evaluated. The project should be designed in a way that plans for sustainability, dissemination, and future scholarship of the students.

The aim of the DNP Project is to (project vision):

To achieve this aim, the DNP Project objectives are to:

- Develop ...
- Implement ...
- Evaluate ...
- With plans for:
    - Sustainability
    - Dissemination
    - Future scholarship

LEARNING OBJECTIVES

- Outline the DNP Project aim(s).
- Draft the DNP Project objectives.

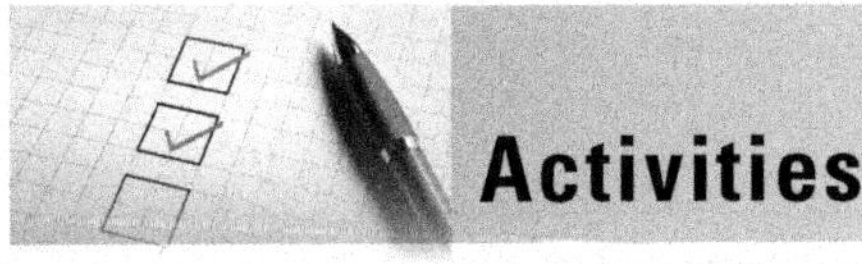

Activities

Apply the verbs *develop, implement,* and *evaluate* from the AACN (2015) criteria to the planning process for your DNP Project.

Project Aim:

We envision the aim of the project as one key sentence. It is meant to be visionary and all-encompassing. It could be considered a broader version of the purpose statement. Most likely, it will contain language about improving health outcomes for a population.

Write a Draft of the Project Aim:

For clarity and to streamline effort, we recommend using the verbs from the AACN (2015) recommendations to write the project objectives:

Objective—Develop: What intervention will you use?	List the steps necessary to accomplish this:
Objective—Implement: How will you implement the intervention?	List the steps necessary to accomplish this:
Objective—Evaluate: **a.** How will the outcomes be evaluated? **b.** How will the process be evaluated?	**a.** List the steps necessary to evaluate each outcome: **b.** List the steps necessary to evaluate the process:

Describe your thoughts on:

Sustainability:

Dissemination:

____

____

Future scholarship:

____

____

The statement of the aim(s) and objectives should be brief but focused. You should not go into explicit detail; that is reserved for the project methodology (Key Differences, n.d.). In the next lesson, we will streamline each objective to ensure that SMART (specific, measurable, achievable, relevant, time-bound) criteria are met. Depending on the requirements at your school, the focus and formatting of your DNP Project aim(s) and objectives might be slightly different. The goal here is to prepare a draft, which will help you develop your project methodology. The project methodology is a more detailed description of how you will execute the work of the project.

NEXT STEPS

- Review a draft with your DNP Project chair/team.
- Prepare to revise your objectives to ensure that SMART criteria are met (next lesson).

REFERENCES AND RESOURCES

American Association of Colleges of Nursing. (2015). *The doctor of nursing practice: Current issues and clarifying recommendations* [White paper]. Retrieved from https://www.aacnnursing.org/Portals/42/News/White-Papers/DNP-Implementation-TF-Report-8-15.pdf

Key Differences. (n.d.). Difference between aim(s) and objectives. Retrieved from https://keydifferences.com/difference-between-aim-and-objective.html

RELATED TEXTBOOK

White, K. M., Dudley-Brown, S., & Terhaar, M. F. (Eds.). (2020). *Translation of evidence into nursing and healthcare* (3rd ed.). New York, NY: Springer Publishing Company.

Chapter 9: Project Management for Translation

Lesson 6.6

SMART OBJECTIVES

BACKGROUND

Objectives speak to the action that must be taken to achieve the project aim. Verbs indicate action, and Bloom's taxonomy is a method of categorizing action verbs (Figure 6.1). Reflect on the verbs listed and gauge your project intervention. Your goal for the intervention is to *apply* evidence, *analyze* and *evaluate* outcomes, and *create* an improved healthcare outcome.

The SMART strategy for writing objectives is applied in multiple disciplines. The letters represent a required component of a good objective. Use the SMART strategy to ensure that your project objectives are well developed (Smart Sheet, n.d.). Define each term below, then use this checklist to ask yourself, "Are your objectives SMART?":

S: Specific

M: Measurable

A: Achievable

R: Realistic

T: Time-bound

LEARNING OBJECTIVES

- Review your DNP Project objectives.
- Ensure that each objective meets the SMART criteria.

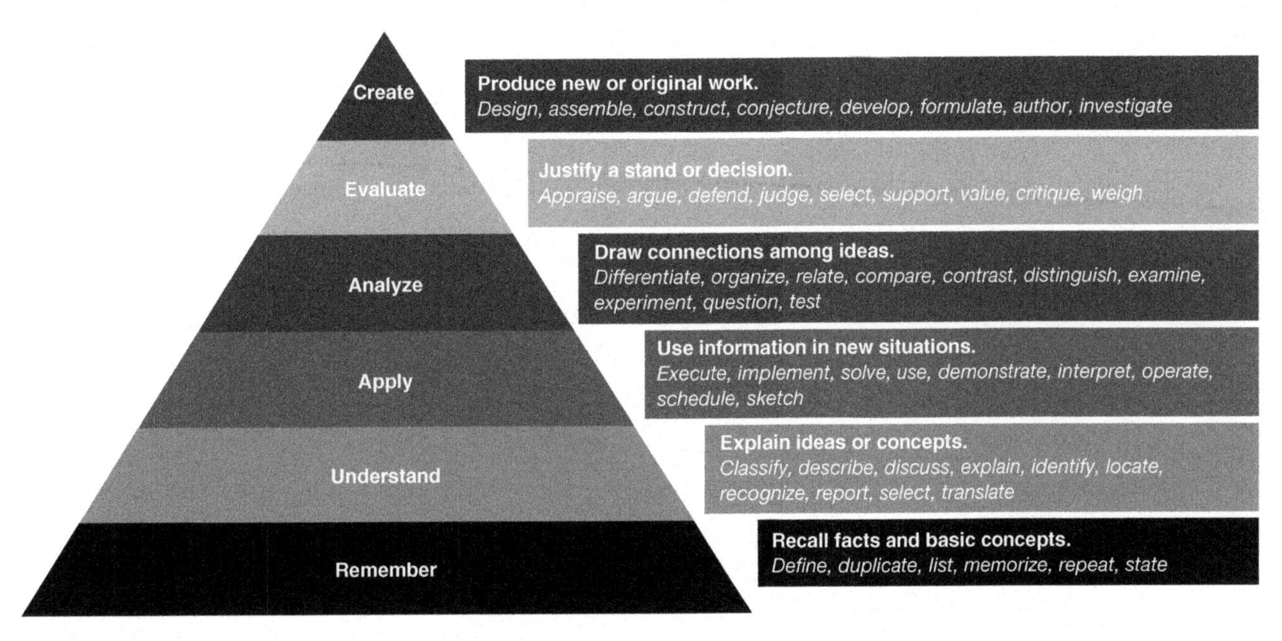

Figure 6.1 Bloom's taxonomy.
Source: From Vanderbilt University Center for Teaching (n.d.). Bloom's taxonomy. Retrieved from https://cft.vanderbilt.edu/guides-sub-pages/blooms-taxonomy

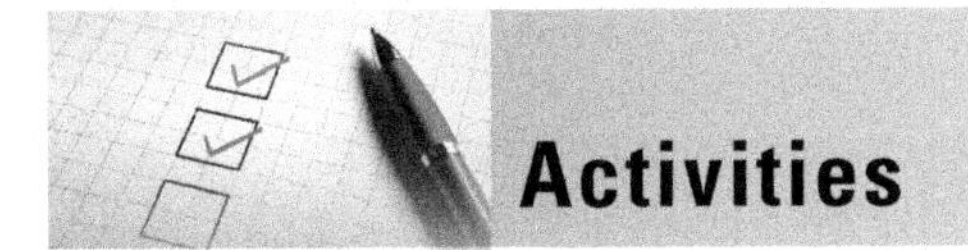

Activities

State your aim and objectives. Then review the objectives using the SMART checklist. Adapt the concept to meet your needs and school requirements.

Aim (Visionary statement of the project goal):

____

____

____

Objective 1: Develop (State the key components.)

____

____

Objective 2: Implement (State the key components.)

____

____

Objective 3: Evaluate (State the key components.)

____

____

NEXT STEPS

- Review your final versions with your faculty, DNP chair, or DNP team.
- Do *not* proceed onto project methodology without approval of this content.

REFERENCES AND RESOURCES

SmartSheet. (n.d.). How to write S.M.A.R.T. project objectives. Retrieved from https://www.smartsheet.com/how-write-smart-project-objective

Vanderbilt University Center for Teaching. (n.d.). Bloom's taxonomy. Retrieved from https://cft.vanderbilt.edu/guides-sub-pages/blooms-taxonomy/

RELATED TEXTBOOK

White, K. M., Dudley-Brown, S., & Terhaar, M. F. (Eds.). (2020). *Translation of evidence into nursing and healthcare* (3rd ed.). New York, NY: Springer Publishing Company.

Chapter 9: Project Management for Translation

Lesson 6.7

DNP PROJECT THEORY

BACKGROUND

Theories are often used to inform and guide project development. A single DNP Project may contain both a theory and an implementation framework. The purpose of the project theory is to explain, predict, or understand the problem, population of interest, or some element of the project. The theory helps the DNP student envision barriers and opportunities to facilitate obstacles. Then, the methodology of the project is designed based on an evidence-based practice implementation framework.

It is beyond the scope of this workbook to fully engage in discussing each and every possible theory. However, since the DNP Project is focused on change, we examine some change theories. This will be helpful in getting you started so that you can discuss it further with your DNP chair and DNP team.

LEARNING OBJECTIVES

- Determine the best options to guide your DNP Project.
- Sketch a conceptual framework for the project using the selected theory or framework.

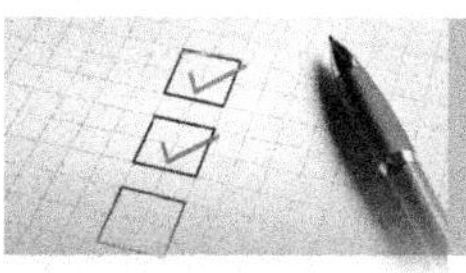

Activities

Research the following theories and consider how they apply to your DNP Project. Try to align the theory to your project context. Highlight your top two selections and discuss with faculty, the DNP chair, and DNP team.

- Lewin's Theory of Planned Change
- Roger's Diffusion of Innovations
- Lippitt's Phases of Change Theory
- Havelock's Stages of Planned Change
- Stages of Change Theory
- Social Cognitive Theory

Create a concept map that aligns the elements of the theory with your DNP Project.

NEXT STEPS

- Discuss your findings with your faculty, DNP chair, or DNP team.
- Revise your visual representation and use it to help you develop components of your project.

RELATED TEXTBOOKS

Christenbery, T. (Ed.). (2018). *Evidence-based practice in nursing*. New York, NY: Springer Publishing Company.

Chapter 7: Change Theories: The Key to Knowledge Translation

Utley, R., Henry, K., & Smith L. (2018). *Frameworks for advanced nursing practice and research*. New York, NY: Springer Publishing Company.

White, K. M., Dudley-Brown, S., & Terhaar, M. F. (Eds.). (2020). *Translation of evidence into nursing and healthcare* (3rd ed.). New York, NY: Springer Publishing Company.

Chapter 2: The Science of Translation and Major Frameworks

Chapter 3: Change Theories for Translation

Lesson 6.8

WORKSHEET: PREPARING FOR PROJECT METHODOLOGY

BACKGROUND

Before writing the DNP Project methodology, you need to prepare a document to kick off that process.

LEARNING OBJECTIVES

- Complete a worksheet to prepare for your project methodology.

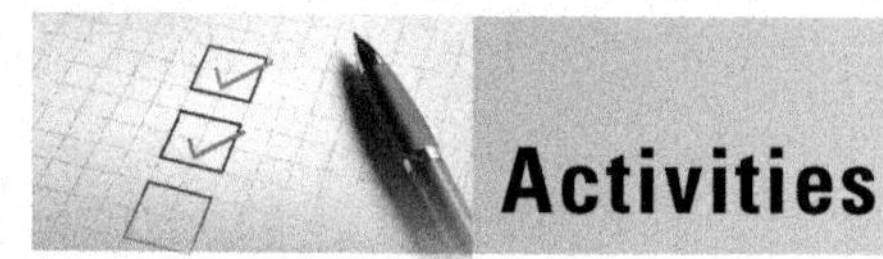

Activities

PREPARING FOR PROJECT METHODOLOGY

DNP Project Title: ______________________________
(fewer than 12 words)

DNP Team:

Student: ____________________

Chair: ____________________

Team Member(s):

List as appropriate to your school

- ______________________________
- ______________________________
- ______________________________

Problem Statement:

PURPOSE STATEMENT: ______________________________

____

____

Aims & Objectives:

(Remember: Develop, Implement, & Evaluate Using SMART Criteria)

Partnering Agency: Address: Phone: Email:	Contact at Agency: ○ Project support is verified in writing.
Plans for Sustainability, Dissemination, and Future Scholarship	Project Theory/Framework: Key Concepts. Attach the Conceptual Framework.

RELATED TEXTBOOK

White, K. M., Dudley-Brown, S., & Terhaar, M. F. (Eds.). (2020). *Translation of evidence into nursing and healthcare* (3rd ed.). New York, NY: Springer Publishing Company.

Chapter 9: Project Management for Translation

CHAPTER SUMMARY

This chapter builds on the problem statement. It guided you through the development of the purpose statement, aim(s), and SMART objectives. You have selected a project theory and/or framework. You have created a concept map based on the theory and/or framework. You are now ready to begin developing the Project methodology. Remember to communicate with your DNP chair and DNP team as you continue to work through this process. Reflect on your thoughts at this point:

List two "Aha" moments while developing your purpose statement, aim(s), and objectives:

1.

____

____

2.

What are your priorities as you move into the Project methodology? Make a list.

1.

2.

3.

4.

5.

Keep working hard!

NOTES

7

Project Methodology: Develop, Implement, and Evaluate

Molly J. Bradshaw, Tracy R. Vitale, Debra Bingham, Nancy Owens, and Gina Purdue

Lessons

OBJECTIVES

The DNP Project methodology is the road map of the project. It describes what will be done and how the outcomes and processes will be evaluated. In this chapter, you complete a series of lessons and activities to help you construct elements of the DNP Project methodology. The goal is to develop, implement, and evaluate evidence-based solutions to the problem of interest. By the end of this chapter, you will be able to:

- Construct a plan and draft components of DNP Project methodology.
- Determine the best approach for evaluation of outcomes and processes.
- Review criteria for DNP Project quality and rigor.

INTRODUCTION

Organizing the DNP Project methodology is a milestone in the DNP Project process. You have invested significant time and effort at this point to fully understand the problem in its local context. You have explored and appraised literature. You have met with your DNP team to determine what is needed to achieve the project outcomes. The methodology is simply a road map that explains in detail how this goal of improving health outcomes will be achieved. This chapter gets you started pulling the elements of the map together.

The chapter begins with a review of the American Association of Colleges of Nursing (AACN, 2015) recommendations for the DNP Project methodology. Before you begin the methodology development, ensure that you are in compliance with the rules and regulations at your school and partnering agency. What types of DNP Projects are allowed? Is there a preferred outline or way of writing the methodology? What are the requirements of the institutional review board (IRB)? At some schools, DNP Projects qualify for IRB exemption status. At others, the DNP Project must be reviewed by the IRB or undergo full review if vulnerable populations are involved. You must also know whether the agency has its own process for IRB or project approval. Gather all of that information before you begin work on this section.

Later, as you begin to formally write the methodology section of your paper, you may notice a shift in the tone of the writing compared to the beginning of the proposal. Writing the methodology is specific and prescriptive. It must be very clear and precise so that those reading your proposal can understand exactly what you plan to do and how you plan to evaluate it. It would be extremely helpful to re-read examples of DNP Project methodologies from your school prior to starting your own. You may also consult a textbook dedicated to writing proposals (see Related Textbooks sections).

In essence, developing a methodology is making a plan. As Dwight Eisenhower said, "Plans are nothing; planning is everything" (White, Dudley-Brown, & Terhaar, 2020, p. 199). It is important to consider and troubleshoot potential challenges. When this project is implemented, it is unlikely that everything will go 100% according to the plan. That is why it is important to evaluate both outcomes and process. Evaluating the process will help you know more about what to change and how to make better plans the next time.

Plans also help you lead a team more effectively. You will not accomplish this project alone. Others will be involved. You have support from your DNP team. The method, the plan, will help your DNP team, participants, and stakeholders have clear expectations and instructions. Let's begin.

REFERENCES AND RESOURCES

American Association of Colleges of Nursing. (2015). *The doctor of nursing practice: Current issues and clarifying recommendations* [White paper]. Retrieved from https://www.aacnnursing.org/Portals/42/News/White-Papers/DNP-Implementation-TF-Report-8-15.pdf

White, K. M., Dudley-Brown, S., & Terhaar, M. F. (Eds.). (2020). *Translation of evidence into nursing and healthcare* (3rd ed.). New York, NY: Springer Publishing Company.

MY GOALS FOR PROJECT METHODOLOGY ARE TO:

Lesson 7.1

PERSPECTIVES ON DNP PROJECT METHODS

BACKGROUND

The AACN does not give specific recommendations for the methodology used in the DNP Project; it asserts that faculty should support innovation and evolve as the nature of practice evolves (AACN, 2015). Primarily, it emphasizes the importance of all DNP Projects having components of planning/development, implementation, and evaluation. Its position statement is intentionally broad. Key clarifying points include:

- Integrative and systematic review *alone* does not meet the requirements for the DNP Project because it lacks the components of implementation into practice (p. 4).
- Portfolios are tools to document and evaluate students rather than satisfy DNP Project requirements (p. 4).
- Group projects must demonstrate individual evaluation of each student (pp. 4–5).
- Those who aspire to be nurse educators will need additional training beyond the DNP in the role of nursing education (p. 7).

The methodology of DNP Projects may borrow concepts from research. But the purpose of the DNP Project is unique. The goal is to translate and implement evidence into practice (AACN, 2015). In other words, to close the 17-year gap between the two.

Quality improvement has emerged as the dominant model of the DNP Project. As a reminder, the Institute for Healthcare Improvement (IHI) offers a free training program on how to improve based on the Model for Improvement. Melnyk and Morrison-Beedy (2018) point out that there is a difference between quality improvement and evidence-based quality improvement. The DNP Project is about leading evidence-based projects to create practice changes that improve health outcomes.

Methodology is often categorized and described based on the process of data collection. For example, will the data points be quantitative, qualitative, or mixed? Will the data points be collected one time or at intervals over a period of time? Does the project evaluate a program? Please review the requirements of the institutional review board (IRB) as part of your planning process.

LEARNING OBJECTIVES

- Examine the required content for the methodology of the DNP Project.
- Gather perspectives and outline your approach.

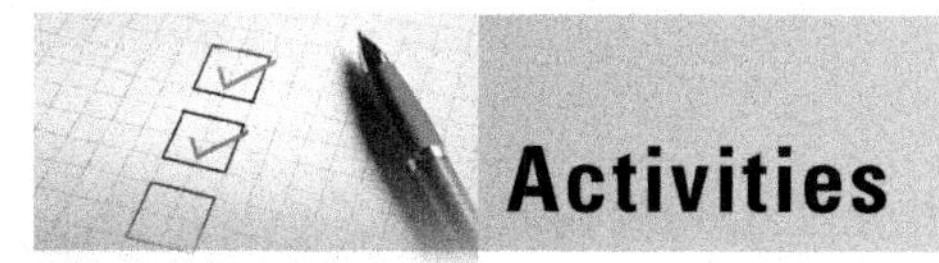

Activities

Review the DNP Project and IRB requirements for your school regarding methodology. Make a list of the required elements and key concepts.

Review of your project aims and objectives, make a list of the outcomes that need to be measured. Describe your plan to measure the outcome.

Outcome: ____

Measurement Plan:

Outcome: ____

Measurement Plan:

Outcome: ____

Measurement Plan:

*Add or subtract more outcomes as determined by your aims and objectives.

Evaluate the process for implementing the intervention. Consult with faculty and/or agency representatives to determine whether there is a standardized form used for the evaluation process.

Describe your plan to evaluate the project process:

____

____

____

____

____

NEXT STEPS

- Talk with your DNP chair and DNP team.
- Gather their perspective on the best method to use for your DNP Project.

REFERENCES AND RESOURCES

American Association of Colleges of Nursing. (2015). *The doctor of nursing practice: Current issues and clarifying recommendations* [White paper]. Retrieved from https://www.aacnnursing.org/Portals/42/News/White-Papers/DNP-Implementation-TF-Report-8-15.pdf

Institute for Healthcare Improvement. (2019). How to improve. Retrieved from http://www.ihi.org/resources/Pages/HowtoImprove/default.aspx

Melnyk, B. M., & Morrison-Beedy, D. (2018). *Intervention research and evidence-based quality improvement: Designing, conducting, analyzing, and funding* (2nd ed.). New York, NY: Springer Publishing Company.

RELATED TEXTBOOKS

Sylvia, M. L., & Tehaar, M. F. (2018). *Clinical analytics and data management for the DNP*. New York, NY: Springer Publishing Company.

White, K. M., Dudley-Brown, S., & Terhaar, M. F. (Eds.). (2020). *Translation of evidence into nursing and healthcare* (3rd ed.). New York, NY: Springer Publishing Company.

Chapter 2: The Science of Translation and Major Frameworks

Chapter 8: Methods for Translation

Chapter 9: Project Management for Translation

Chapter 14: Information Technology: A Foundation for Translation

Lesson 7.2

A LOOK AT IMPLEMENTATION SCIENCE

BACKGROUND

Nurses are responsible for providing evidence-based care (Christenbery, 2018). There are several models that outline the steps:

EBP model examples:

- Evidence-based process (Melnyk, Fineout-Overholt, Stillwell, & Williamson, 2010)
- The Iowa Model (Titler et al., 2001)
- The Johns Hopkins Nursing Evidence-Based Practice (EBP) Model, PET (Practice, Evidence, Transfer) process (Dearholt & Dang, 2017)

DNP-prepared nurses are needed to help close the 17-year research-to-practice gap (Vincent, Johnson, Velasquez, & Rigney, 2010). There are no data to indicate that this gap has been closed. There are many reasons why the translation of research into practice takes so long, including lack of knowledge, skills, and resources, as well as a mismatch between research and organizational priorities (Bauer, Damschroder, Hagedorn, Smith, & Kilborune, 2015). E. Rogers (1962) began studying the diffusion of innovations over 50 years ago. He defined an "innovation" as anything that is new to a particular group or individual. Rogers indicated that some innovations would diffuse more rapidly than others, but his work did not focus on the implementation stage (White et al., 2020). Since then, the field of implementation science has emerged.

By definition, implementation science is research that seeks to understand why and how implementation of evidence or projects succeed or fail (Nilsen, 2015). "It is the scientific study of methods to promote systematic uptake of research findings and other evidence-based practices (EBPs) into routine practice, and hence to promote the quality and effectiveness of health services" (Eccles & Mittman, 2006, p. 1). Just as DNP Projects borrow concepts from traditional research, applying concepts from implementation science may also guide and inform DNP Projects.

All DNP Projects are context specific. This means that the project leader needs to be able to tailor the implementation strategies and tactics based on the specific context of each DNP Project. DNP students must draw from the body of human subjects research evidence to decide what to implement and then draw from the body of evidence from implementation science to determine how to best implement the DNP Project plan.

The theories, frameworks, and models of implementation science can be categorized as:

1. Describing and/or guiding the process of translation of research to practice (Nilsen, 2015)
2. Understanding and explaining what influences implementation outcomes (Nilsen, 2015)
3. Evaluating implementation (Nilsen, 2015)
   a. Process evaluation (Bauer, Damschroder, Hagedorn, Smith, & Kilbourne, 2015)
   b. Formative evaluation (Bauer et al., 2015)
   c. Summative evaluation (Bauer et al., 2015)

LEARNING OBJECTIVES

- Review the comparison of EBP models.
- Read about implementation science.
- Consider the relationships in the context of Bingham's (n.d.) *Evidence-Based Practice, Quality Improvement, Research, and Improvement Science Flowchart.*

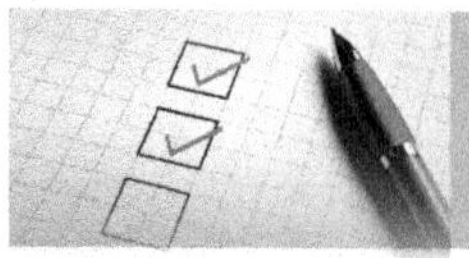

Activities

Refer to the PDF comparing evidence-based practice models (www.va.gov/nursing/ebp/docs/EBP_Process ComparisonStepsCurriculumHandout_www.pdf).

Read about implementation science using these open-access articles:

1. Bauer, M. S., Damschroder, L., Hagedorn, H., Smith, J., & Kilbourne, A. M. (2015). Implementation science for the non-specialist. *BMC Psychology, 3,* 32. doi:10.1186/s40359-015-0089-9
2. Nilsen, P. (2015). Making sense of implementation theories, models and frameworks. Retrieved from https://implementationscience.biomedcentral.com/track/pdf/10.1186/s13012-015-0242-0
3. Riner, M. E. (2014). Using implementation science as the core of the DNP Project. Retrieved from https://www.sciencedirect.com/science/article/pii/S8755722314001926?via%3Dihub

Bingham (n.d.) has developed a flowchart to illustrate how EBP, human subjects research, and implementation and improvement science interact with and inform each step in the DNP Project process (Figure 7.1). The steps to follow when using the flowchart are outlined with descriptive examples for DNP students.

Step 1: Evaluate and Grade the Research or Evidence for the Practice and Review Population Health Data and Clinical Outcomes is where the student summarizes the human subjects research literature to determine which evidence-based intervention they will implement.

> For example, there are many research studies that have outlined the benefits of flu vaccinations, especially among vulnerable populations. Yet, there are many populations of patients who are not receiving the benefits of vaccinations. The DNP Project should focus on figuring out how to increase utilization of flu vaccines, not study whether flu vaccines are efficacious. If the research has not determined that the intervention is evidence based, then the student needs to find a different project. DNP Projects should focus on the hard work of increasing utilization of an EBP.

As the flowchart illustrates, human subjects research is what will help the student sort through the research evidence to determine which interventions have enough evidence to justify being the focus of the DNP Project. In addition to evaluating the research evidence, Step 1 is also where the student assesses whether there is a gap in what the evidence says should be done and the actual practice at a specific clinic or hospital unit for a particular population.

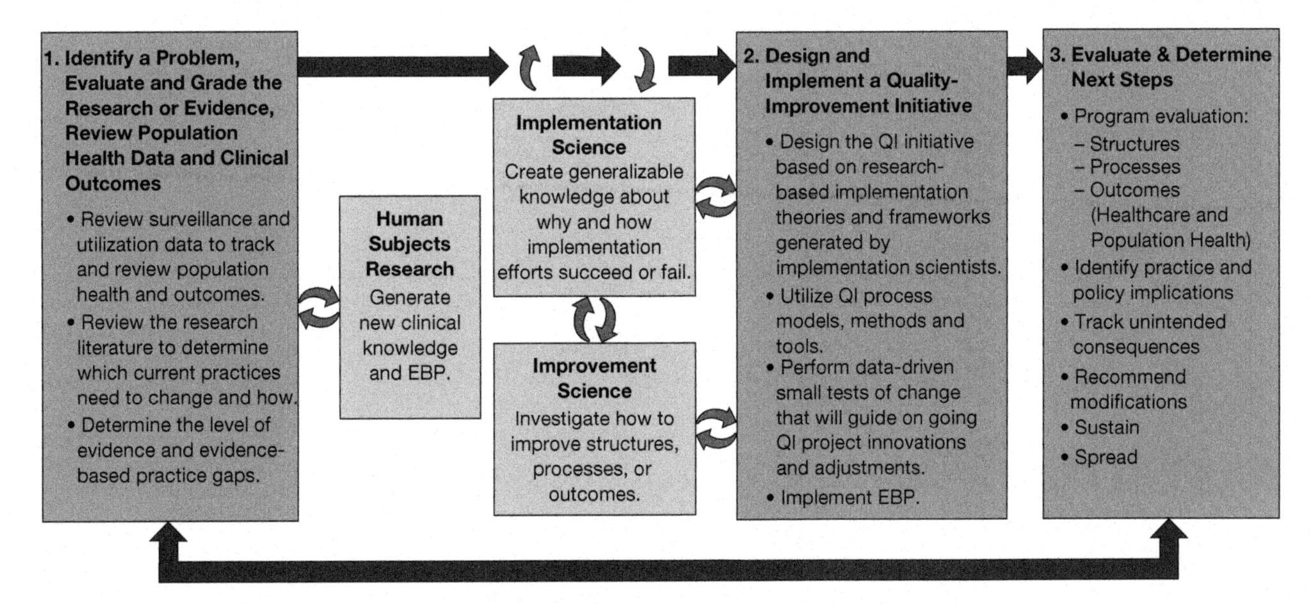

Figure 7.1 Bingham's evidence-based practice quality-improvement flowchart.

EBP, evidence-based practice; QI, quality improvement.
Source: Reprinted with permission from Bingham, D. (n.d.). Institute for Perinatal Quality Improvement. Retrieved from https://www.perinatalqi.org

For example, nearly 100% of patients cared for in one clinic may receive the flu vaccine, whereas less than 50% of patients cared for at another clinic may receive flu vaccines. Students should focus on ensuring that all patients, especially vulnerable populations of patients, receive EBPs. It is not a good use of resources for the student to focus on trying to implement an EBP in a setting that has already adopted that practice.

Step 2: Design and Implement a Quality-Improvement Initiative is the step that the student enters once they have has identified the efficacious evidence-based structure or process (practice) change that needs to be implemented within a particular population. Step 2 is primarily informed by the implementation science research that gives insight into how to more effectively implement the changes in structures and processes that have been identified to bring about the desired patient outcomes. Step 2 is informed by research-derived implementation theories, such as E. Rogers' (1962) classic Diffusion of Innovation theory or Klein and Sorra's (1996) implementation frameworks, which are a summation of implementation reports and studies; these are also useful for guiding how the student designs and implements the project.

For example, the following are some frameworks used in nursing:

- Knowledge-to-Action
- Plan-Do-Study-Act (PDSA)
- Mobilize-Assess-Plan-Implement-Track (MAP-IT)
- Define-Measure-Assess-Improve-Control (DMAIC)

Students should thoughtfully tailor their implementation strategies and tactics to ensure their implementation efforts are as effective as possible (Bingham & Main, 2010).

Step 3: Evaluate and Determine Next Steps. There are facilitators and barriers to all implementation efforts. Some things go as planned, but most often, there are unexpected challenges and barriers that are identified. We need to more effectively learn from each other's implementation efforts if we are going to be able to reduce the 17-year research-to-practice gap. Implementation science research models, such as Harvey and Kitson's (2015) PARiHS (Promoting Action on Research Implementation) framework or Laura Damschroder and colleagues' (2009) use of Consolidated Framework for

Implementation Research outline key constructs that can inform the evaluation process. Sharing implementation insights with others also makes it possible for subsequent students or leaders to build on what the student learned that affected implementation effectiveness, for example, the implementation context or the characteristics of the intervention.

NEXT STEPS

- In reflection, how does implementation science impact your project?
- Discuss what you have learned in this lesson with your DNP team.

REFERENCES AND RESOURCES

Bauer, M. S., Damschroder L., Hagedorn H., Smith J., & Kilbourne A. M. (2015). An introduction to implementation science for the non-specialist. *BMC Psychology, 3*, 32. doi: 10.1186/s40359-015-0089-9

Bingham, D. (n.d.). Institute for Perinatal Quality Improvement. Retrieved from https://www.perinatalqi.org/

Bingham, D., & Main, E. K. (2010). Effective implementation strategies and tactics for leading change on maternity units. *The Journal of Perinatal & Neonatal Nursing, 24*(1), 32–42.

Christenbery, T. (Ed.). (2018). *Evidence-based practice in nursing*. New York, NY: Springer Publishing Company.

Eccles, M. P., & Mittman, B. S. (2006). Welcome to implementation science. *Implementation Science, 1*(1). doi: 10.1186/1748-5908-1-1

Damschroder, L. J., Aron, D. C., Keith, R. E., Kirsh, S. R., Alexander, J. A., & Lowery, J. C. (2009). Fostering implementation of health services research findings into practice: A consolidated framework for advancing implementation science. *Implementation Science, 4*(1), 50.

Dearholt, D. & Dang, S. L. (2017). *Johns Hopkins nursing evidence-based practice: Model and guidelines* (3rd ed.). Indianapolis, IN: Sigma Theta Tau International.

Harvey, G., & Kitson, A. (2015). PARIHS revisited: From heuristic to integrated framework for the successful implementation of knowledge into practice. *Implementation Science, 11*(1), 33.

Institute of Medicine. (1999). *Crossing the quality chasm: A new health system for the 21st century*. Washington, DC: National Academies Press.

Klein, K. J., & Sorra, J. S. (1996). The challenge of innovation implementation. *The Academy of Management Review, 21*(4), 1055–1080. doi:10.2307/259164

Melnyk, B. M., Fineout-Overholt, E., Stillwell, S. B., & Williamson, K. M. (2010). Evidence-based practice: Step by step: the seven steps of evidence-based practice. *AJN The American Journal of Nursing, 110*(1), 51–53.

Nilsen, P. (2015). Making sense of implementation theories, models, and frameworks. *Implementation Science, 10*,53. doi: 10.1186/s13012-015-0242-0

Office of Nursing Service. (2015). Comparison of EBP process steps. Retrieved from https://www.va.gov/nursing/ebp/docs/EBP_ProcessComparisonStepsCurriculumHandout_www.pdf

Riner, M. E. (2014). Using implementation science as the core of the doctor of nursing practice inquiry project. *Journal of Professional Nursing, 31*(3), 200–207. doi: 10.1016/j.profnurs.2014.11.002

Rogers, E. M. (1962). *Diffusion of innovations*. New York, NY: Free Press of Glencoe.

Titler, M. G., Kleiber, C., Steelman, V. J., Rakel, B. A., Budreau, G., Everett, L. Q., ... Goode, C. J. (2001). The Iowa model of evidence-based practice to promote quality care. *Critical Care Nursing Clinics of North America, 13*(4), 497–509.

Vincent, D., Johnson, C., Velasquez, D., & Rigney, T. (2010). DNP-prepared nurses as practitioner-researchers: Closing the gap between research and practice. *The American Journal for Nurse Practitioners, 14*(11/14), 28–34.

White, K. M., Dudley-Brown, S., & Terhaar, M. F. (Eds.). (2020). *Translation of evidence into nursing and healthcare* (3rd ed.). New York, NY: Springer Publishing Company.

RELATED TEXTBOOK

Melnyk, B. M., & Morrison-Beedy, D. (2018). *Intervention research and evidence-based quality improvement: Designing, conducting, analyzing, and funding* (2nd ed.). New York, NY: Springer Publishing Company.

Chapter 29: Factors Influencing Successful Uptake of Evidence-Based Interventions in Clinical Practice

Table 29.1: Evidence for Implementation Strategies

Lesson 7.3

THINK BEYOND EDUCATION

BACKGROUND

We believe that nurses are born with a heart for teaching. There is something in our nursing DNA that tells us that education is always the right answer. Our instinct to teach others is rooted in good intentions. But the evidence says that education alone does not change behavior. In fact, when an educational intervention is delivered, it will only result in change 4% of the time (Institute of Medicine, 2011). To make a bigger impact on practice, we have to think beyond education. How can we get people to apply the information?

Almost every DNP Project involves delivery of information: an in-service training event, a simulated activity, or delivery of information to patients. We support the importance of this concept. However, best practices are necessary. You need to develop learning objectives and establish an evaluation plan for the educational session(s). We further recommend that there has to be some type of follow-up. How do you know the information is getting used and making an impact?

To make a bold statement, we believe the DNP Project must include an intervention that is more than just education alone. Measure something more than knowledge. Increasing awareness is great, but what is next? What tools are offered? What changes will be made? How will the outcomes be benchmarked over time?

LEARNING OBJECTIVES

- Determine what education is needed in your project.
- Plan the education event.
- Outline strategies to ensure the application and impact of knowledge.

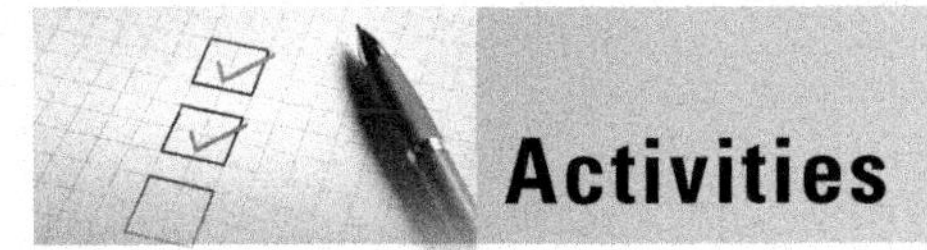

Activities

Answer the following questions:

- Will your DNP Project deliver information directly to patients or families?
  Explain Your Vision:

- Will your DNP Project deliver information to healthcare workers?
  Explain Your Vision:

When information is delivered directly to patients, here are some important considerations:

- Is the information based on evidence and is the source cited?
- Is the information written at the appropriate level of health literacy?
- Is the information culturally appropriate?
- How will the session take place? Individually? In a group?
- How long will each session last?
- What resources are needed?
- What are the intended learning outcomes and how are the outcomes evaluated?

The approach to education for healthcare workers may differ. When continuing-education credits are offered, there is generally a planning form required from the organization endorsing the content. Here are some important considerations:

- Does the organization/agency you are working with have a form for educational events? (To view a sample educational planning form, refer to the editable forms supplement available at springerpub.com/dpw. This supplement is also available at connect.springerpub.com/content/book/978-0-8261-7433-8.)
- Have you outlined the learning objectives?
- How will the knowledge be applied in practice?
- Does the evaluation of your educational session match up to the learning objectives?

After information and knowledge is delivered, regardless of the audience, how will the information be reinforced? Are there tools that you can offer to help remind the audience (e.g., handouts, pocket card, magnet, badge information card)?

Now, think beyond education. What else needs to happen to ensure that there is a change in practice that impacts outcomes (directly or indirectly) for patients?

NEXT STEPS

- Talk to your DNP team about interventions beyond education alone.
- Ensure that your DNP Project requires application of knowledge in practice.

REFERENCES AND RESOURCES

Bluestone, J., Johnson, P., Fullerton, J., Carr, C., Alderman, J., & BonTempo, J. (2013). Effective in-service training design and delivery: Evidence from an integrative literature review. *Human Resources for Health, 11*, 51. doi: 10.1186/1478-4491-11-51

Institute of Medicine. (2011). *Clinical practice guidelines we can trust.* Washington, DC: National Academies Press. Retrieved from https://www.nap.edu/read/13058/chapter/8#149

Medline Plus. (n.d.). Choosing effective patient education materials. Retrieved from https://medlineplus.gov/ency/patientinstructions/000455.htm

Strodtman, L. K. (1984). A decision-making process for planning patient education. *Patient Education and Counseling, 5*(4), 189–200. doi: 10.1016/0738-3991(84)90179-4

White, K. M., Dudley-Brown, S., & Terhaar, M. F. (Eds.). (2020). *Translation of evidence into nursing and healthcare* (3rd ed.). New York, NY: Springer Publishing Company.

RELATED TEXTBOOKS

Sylvia, M. L., & Tehaar, M. F. (2018). *Clinical analytics and data management for the DNP.* New York, NY: Springer Publishing Company.

White, K. M., Dudley-Brown, S., & Terhaar, M. F. (Eds.). (2020). *Translation of evidence into nursing and healthcare* (3rd ed.). New York, NY: Springer Publishing Company.

Chapter 13: Education: An Enabler of Translation

Lesson 7.4

IMPLEMENTATION FRAMEWORKS AND DNP PROJECT DESIGN

BACKGROUND

In the previous lessons, you reviewed perspectives on DNP Project methods, looked at implementation science, and spent time thinking about interventions beyond education. Now, it is time to describe your project methodology by selecting an implementation framework. The implementation framework helps you design the project. This is an important step to consider because you want to use a framework that will fit with your aim.

LEARNING OBJECTIVES

- Explore implementation frameworks.
- Sketch the DNP Project methodology.

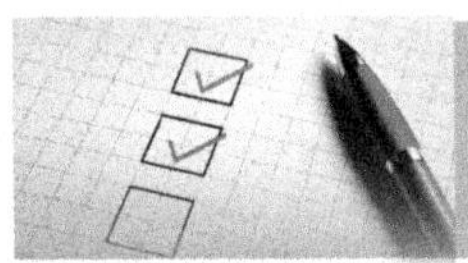

Activities

Implementation frameworks will help you think through the elements of the DNP Project and operationalize the components. Explore each model and others if needed. Determine the best fit for your project.

- Institute for Healthcare Improvement (IHI) Model for Improvement (Plan-Do-Study-Act [PDSA])
- Iowa Model for Evidence-Based Practice (EBP)
- Knowledge-to-Action Model
- Agency for Healthcare Research and Quality (AHRQ) Knowledge Transfer Framework
- Ottawa Model of Research
- RE-AIM (reach, effectiveness, adoption, implementation, maintenance) Model

Notes:

Selected theory: ______________________________

Selected framework: ______________________________

Why is this framework a "fit" for your DNP Project methodology? List three reasons.

1.

2.

3.

Sketch the framework. Next to the elements, describe the components of your DNP Project. You may need to revise your sketch after completing other lessons in this chapter.

NEXT STEP

- Discuss your plan with your DNP team.

RELATED TEXTBOOKS

Bonnel, W., & Smith, K. (2018). *Proposal writing for clinical nursing and DNP Projects*. New York, NY: Springer Publishing Company.

Chapter 10: Mapping It Out From Problem to Advanced Clinical Project Plan

Chapter 11: Writing the Methods Section: Organizing the Advanced Clinical Project

Melnyk, B. M., & Morrison-Beedy, D. (2018). *Intervention research and evidence-based quality improvement: Designing, conducting, analyzing, and funding* (2nd ed.). New York, NY: Springer Publishing Company.

Chapter 4: Using Theory to Guide Intervention Research

Sylvia, M. L., & Tehaar, M. F. (2018). *Clinical analytics and data management for the DNP*. New York, NY: Springer Publishing Company.

White, K. M., Dudley-Brown, S., & Terhaar, M. F. (Eds.). (2020). *Translation of evidence into nursing and healthcare* (3rd ed.). New York, NY: Springer Publishing Company.

Chapter 8: Methods for Translation

Chapter 9: Project Management for Translation

Lesson 7.5

INTERVENTION POPULATION, INCLUSION/ EXCLUSION CRITERIA, AND RECRUITMENT

BACKGROUND

The DNP Project is designed to impact patients and populations (American Association of Colleges of Nursing [AACN], 2015). To achieve this goal, the DNP Project intervention may or may not directly involve the targeted patient population. Often, the intervention population is not the same group. For example, if you are implementing a new protocol, the healthcare team will be the intervention population. In the methodology section, we need to identify the population participating in the intervention.

There may be reasons that you especially want to include or exclude project participants. You need to establish the rules for including or excluding people ahead of time. After the intervention population is identified, we will develop a recruitment strategy. How will the intervention population be made aware of your DNP Project? How, and by what means, will they be recruited to participate?

LEARNING OBJECTIVES

- Identify the intervention population.
- Outline inclusion/exclusion criteria of potential participants.
- Identify/develop plans for recruitment.

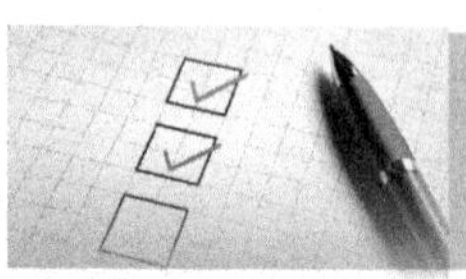

Activities

What patient population is the DNP Project designed to impact? ______________________________
—

What population(s) will participate in the project intervention? ______________________________

Are there certain circumstances or rules by which you would include or exclude participants? List your inclusion/exclusion criteria.

INCLUSION	EXCLUSION

Recruitment Strategies

In our experience, most DNP Projects require a letter of introduction to the intervention population and a recruitment flyer at minimum. Please refer to the rules at your school and involve the institutional review board (IRB) as needed. A letter of introduction is a one-page, single-spaced letter that describes the context of the DNP Project. You should introduce yourself as a DNP student, state the full title of the project, and mention that this is a required component of your doctoral education. In the second paragraph, you should describe the intervention and the inclusion/exclusion criteria, and outline what will happen. Describe the data-collection process and explain that the identity of the participant is protected. If the participant is being compensated for participation, describe the nature of the compensation. The letter should end by providing your contact information so that interested parties can follow up. The letter may also include the information of your DNP chair (faculty).

A recruitment flyer is simply a more concise, visual representation of the information included in the letter. It should contain the title of the DNP Project, provide a bulleted overview of the same elements described in the letter, and end with your contact information.

Both the letter and the recruitment flyer can be circulated in a number of ways: personal communication, email, traditional mailing, social media (if appropriate). There are often rules about proper ways to obtain contact information of participants and how this information is stored. Depending on your DNP Project approach, these may vary; consult with your DNP Project team and IRB.

Describe your strategies to spread the word about securing participants for your DNP Project:

____

____

____

____

Then, write a first draft of your recruitment letter.

To create the recruitment flyer, use templates in Word, Google Forms, or other sources. Also, refer to the following resources.

- Free templates: www.designcap.com/create/recruitment.html
- Community Tool Box: https://ctb.ku.edu/en/table-of-contents/participation/promoting-interest/posters-flyers/main

NEXT STEPS

- Consult with your DNP team.
- Revise your strategy as necessary.

REFERENCE AND RESOURCE

American Association of Colleges of Nursing. (2015). *The doctor of nursing practice: Current issues and clarifying recommendations* [White paper]. Retrieved from https://www.aacnnursing.org/Portals/42/News/White-Papers/DNP-Implementation-TF-Report-8-15.pdf

RELATED TEXTBOOKS

Melnyk, B. M., & Morrison-Beedy, D. (2018). *Intervention research and evidence-based quality improvement: Designing, conducting, analyzing, and funding* (2nd ed.). New York, NY: Springer Publishing Company.

Chapter 14: Participant Recruitment and Retention

Sylvia, M. L., & Tehaar, M. F. (2018). *Clinical analytics and data management for the DNP*. New York, NY: Springer Publishing Company.

Lesson 7.6

IRB, CITI TRAINING, AND ETHICAL CONSIDERATIONS

BACKGROUND

The institutional review board (IRB) is an entity designed to ensure humane and ethical conduction of research. The DNP Project is not research; however, the DNP Project must still be designed in a way that protects the project participants from harm. Human subjects research training is often required for any student, faculty, or essential staff looking to have a role in your DNP Project. Each school will have its own requirements for human subjects research training.

Although DNP Projects vary from school to school, a common debate revolves around the need for approval by an IRB. Quality-improvement (QI) projects are geared toward improving the quality of programs, existing services, or a process flow. Depending on the nature of the project and the data being collected, it may result in the project being categorized under the federal definition of human subject research.

The CITI (Collaborative Institutional Training Initiative) Program is designed to ensure basic understanding of research-related ethics. Most schools require DNP students to complete this training, which is transferable to other universities. If the student remains involved in research and evidence-based practice beyond DNP graduation, it is necessary to periodically update one's training. Ask your DNP faculty about which modules are required for your school. To learn more, visit the CITI website (https://about.citiprogram.org/en/homepage).

In an effort to protect human subjects, there are some considerations to be made when including "vulnerable populations" in your project. This is specifically outlined in the U.S. Department of Health and Human Services Part 46 of Protection of Human Subjects. Examples of vulnerable populations include children, prisoners, pregnant women, victims of traumatic experiences, economically/educationally disadvantaged persons, and mentally disabled persons.

DNP Projects that include vulnerable populations often undergo full IRB review regardless of the methodology of the project. Again, the purpose is to ensure humane treatment and protection for these populations. This type of information is included in the CITI Training.

When developing the DNP Project methodology, it is advisable to include a paragraph about relevant ethical concepts and the connection to the DNP Project. The American Nurses Association (n.d.) offers foundational content on ethical practice for all nurses (www.nursingworld.org/practice-policy/nursing-excellence/ethics).

LEARNING OBJECTIVES

- Review the IRB requirements for your school.
- Ensure completion of required CITI Training.
- Identify vulnerable populations involved in the DNP Project.
- Articulate concepts of ethics applicable to the DNP Project.

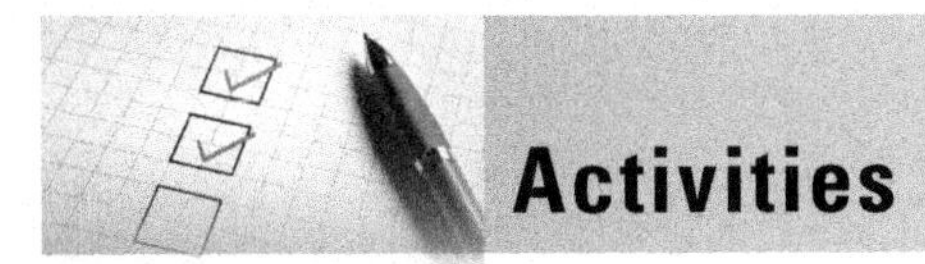

Activities

Review the IRB requirements for your school and partnering organization. Then discuss CITI Training requirements with faculty and complete the required training. Ensure you get a copy of your completed CITI Training certificate in the event the IRB asks to see it.

Questions for Consideration: Is there a vulnerable population involved in your DNP Project? If so, how will the risk to this group be mitigated in your DNP Project process?

Define the following ethical terms. Then write a paragraph about two terms and their relevance to your DNP Project. Use the National Institutes of Health (NIH) glossary to help you (www.niehs.nih.gov/research/resources/bioethics/glossary/index.cfm).

Autonomy: Be accountable for & make ones own decisions.

Justice: to treat everyone equally & s̄ bias

Beneficence: to do or promote good

Nonmaleficence: to do no harm, to remove from harm &/or to prevent harm

Fidelity: Do what you say; be honest to your word.

Veracity: to tell the truth

Other term of your choosing:

Other term of your choosing:

Selected Ethical Term #1: ____________________

Write one paragraph on this term and its relationship to your DNP Project.

____

____

____

____

____

____

____

____

____

Selected Ethical Term #2: ____________________

Write one paragraph on this term and its relationship to your DNP Project.

____

____

____

____

____

____

____

____

____

IRB Planning Checklist

Project Site Name	West Coast Family Practice
Research Personnel Contact	
Required Process at Site	Site Approval Letter Only Yes ☒ No ☐ Nursing Research Council Yes ☐ No ☒ Research Council Yes ☐ No ☒ IRB Yes ☐ No ☒
Expected Time for Review	Nursing Research Council How often does it meet? ____________ When are materials due? ______ How do I get on the agenda? ____________ Research Council How often does it meet? ______ When are materials due? ________ How do I get on the agenda? ____________ IRB How often does it meet? ____________ When are materials due? ________ How do I get on the agenda? ____________
Anticipated Type of Review	Exempt ☐ Expedited ☐ Full Review ☐
Required Supporting Documents	Human Subject Certification Yes ☐ No ☐ Informed Consent Yes ☐ No ☐ Recruitment Flyer Yes ☐ No ☐ Data-Collection Tool(s) Yes ☐ No ☐ IRB Application Yes ☐ No ☐
Review Before Submission	Review of Application by Chair Yes ☐ No ☐ Consistency Throughout Yes ☐ No ☐ Written in Simple Terminology Yes ☐ No ☐ Attachments of Supporting Documentation Yes ☐ No ☐ Previous Approvals Yes ☐ No ☐

IRB, institutional review board.

Expert Commentary: Tips for the IRB and Method Section: Gina Purdue, DNP, RN, CNE

One of the most common mistakes that I see students make in regard to the research procedures, IRB application, and the Methods section in the DNP Project report is missing information and a lack of detail. Both the IRB application and the DNP Project Proposal should discuss the steps of project implementation in enough detail that outsiders (those other than the DNP team) can fully and clearly understand the project. To assist students in outlining the project in detail, I encourage students to make a bulleted or numbered list consisting of each step of project implementation from recruitment of participants to evaluation of the project outcomes. In some cases, it may help to answer the IRB application questions first. Then the student can take the lists developed in the IRB application and turn the content into a written format for the methodology.

NEXT STEPS

- Discuss your work with your DNP team.
- Plan to mention ethical considerations in your DNP Project proposal.

REFERENCES AND RESOURCES

American Nurses Association. (n.d.). Ethics & human rights. Retrieved from https://www.nursingworld.org/practice-policy/nursing-excellence/ethics

CITI Training. (n.d.). Research ethics and compliance training. Retrieved from https://about.citiprogram.org/en/homepage

U.S. Department of Health and Human Services. (n.d.). Part 46. Common Rule. Retrieved from http://www.healthinfolaw.org/sites/default/files/Common%20Rule%20Subpart%20A.pdf

RELATED TEXTBOOKS

Melnyk, B. M., & Morrison-Beedy, D. (2018). *Intervention research and evidence-based quality improvement: Designing, conducting, analyzing, and funding* (2nd ed.). New York, NY: Springer Publishing Company.

Chapter 7: Ethical Considerations in Designing Intervention Studies

Chapter 13: Navigating the IRB for Investigators

White, K. M., Dudley-Brown, S., & Terhaar, M. F. (Eds.). (2020). *Translation of evidence into nursing and healthcare* (3rd ed.). New York, NY: Springer Publishing Company.

Chapter 16: Legal Issues in Translation

Lesson 7.7

PARTICIPATION CONSENT

BACKGROUND

Consent is a process, not just a form. Consent allows the potential participant to make an informed decision about whether to participate in a project/research study. This is "a fundamental mechanism to ensure respect for persons through provision of thoughtful consent for a voluntary act" (U.S. Department of Health and Human Services [USDHHS], 1993, para. 1). When you obtain informed consent, specific tasks and objectives must be met. These include having consent that provides information in a manner participants can understand. This includes all aspects of the project/study, including the project's purpose, the time commitment involved, what will occur during the project/study, alternatives, as well as any risks or benefits of participating (USDHHS, 1993).

Inclusion of participants, or their personal data, in the project requires some form of consent. Depending on the method, either a waiver of informed consent or informed consent is needed. It is necessary to consider the details of obtaining that consent. You need to describe the details and circumstances of how the consent will be obtained. The IRB has standards and requirements. It will be necessary to familiarize yourself with any templates your project site or institution requires for consent. Consider that your institution may have templates for different types of consents depending on the nature of the project. Various consent types include written informed consent, parental permission form, paper or online survey/questionnaire consent, and waiver of informed consent. The type of consent that is required depends on the nature of the project you are conducting, the data you will be collecting, and the manner in which you collect the data.

LEARNING OBJECTIVES

- Describe the elements involved in informed consent.
- Determine the type of consent that may be required for your project.
- Identify special situations that may require additional consent considerations.

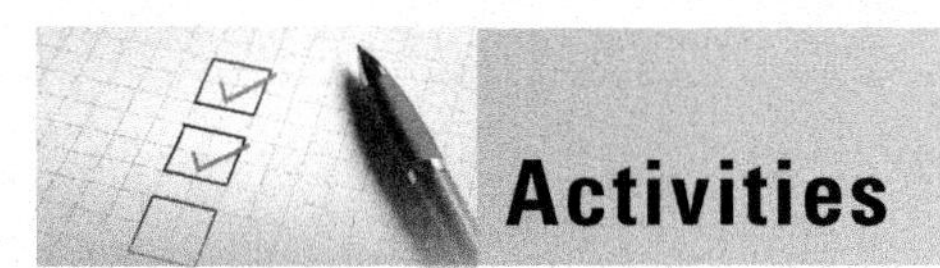

Activities

Next to each prompt, answer the question in one to two sentences. Use the information as a foundation to construct your informed consent form for your DNP Project. Write as if you are speaking to the project participants. Use plain language.

Who is conducting the project? (Introduce yourself)	
What is the project about? (Problem and purpose statements)	
What is being done? (Overview of project intervention)	
What does the participant have to do? (Describe the participant role)	
Will there be compensation? (Describe the benefits of participating)	
Will there be consequences for not participating? (Describe what could happen by not participating? Could the person suffer harm?)	
How will confidentiality be maintained? (Explain the process of de-identification or securing of personal information)	
How much time will this take and over what period of time will the project occur? (Include intervention time and period of data collection)	
Who can the individual contact if they have questions? (IRB contact information for participant)	
Other:	

NEXT STEPS

- Discuss the plan with your DNP team.
- Retrieve your organization's requirements for when consent is required.
- Review available consent templates from your organization to review specific requirements.

REFERENCE AND RESOURCE

U.S. Department of Health and Human Services. (1993). Office for Protection from Research Risks. Informed consent tips. Tips on informed consent. Retrieved from https://www.hhs.gov/ohrp/regulations-and-policy/guidance/informed-consent-tips/index.html

RELATED TEXTBOOK

Melnyk, B. M., & Morrison-Beedy, D. (2018). *Intervention research and evidence-based quality improvement: Designing, conducting, analyzing, and funding* (2nd ed.). New York, NY: Springer Publishing Company.

Chapter 7: Ethical Considerations in Designing Intervention Studies

Lesson 7.8

EVALUATION OF OUTCOMES AND PROCESS

BACKGROUND

The American Association of Colleges of Nursing (AACN) recommends that DNP Projects include evaluation of both outcomes and process (AACN, 2015). Reflect back on your project aim and objectives. What outcomes were targeted? How will these outcomes be measured? DNP Project outcomes are often based on quality indicators, clinical measures, and other data. The process of making a practice change must also be evaluated.

Descriptive information, such as demographics, is helpful to articulate the composition of the population. It is also sometimes helpful to ask questions that confirm or deny findings in the literature. Do you need to formally complete a needs assessment? What was the opinion of stakeholders involved in the project? What went well? What could be improved?

The project evaluation plan will be individualized and should be planned with your DNP team. Since the DNP Project is a learning experience, you will benefit from interacting with multiple types of evaluations. You should incorporate different techniques.

LEARNING OBJECTIVES

- Explore validated instruments.
- Devise a plan for benchmarking outcomes data.
- Review strategies for survey development for the purpose of collecting feedback.

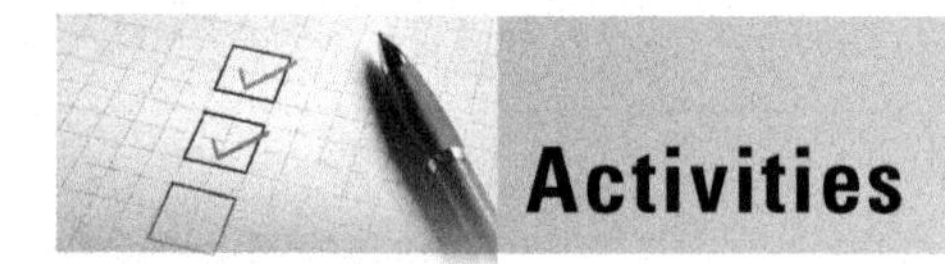

Activities

Finding a data-collection instrument(s) that is right for your project is challenging. The instrument must measure the targeted outcome. The instrument must meet acceptable levels of *validity* and *reliability*. Some instruments may be used free of charge, whereas others may not. The DNP student may need permission from the developer to use the instrument. Developing a new, validated instrument is beyond the scope of a DNP Project. It is often more practical to use an instrument that has already been developed.

Expert Commentary: Tips for Finding Validated Instruments: Nancy Owens, DNP, APRN, FNP-C

Search the literature. Retrieve instruments that assess the practice-based problem in question. Databases may help you find out the name of an appropriate instrument, but it can still be difficult finding the instrument itself.
Assess each potential instrument. Identify those with established results, good indicators of validity and reliability. Has the instrument been extensively used by the scientific community?
Instrument sensitivity and specificity. Select an instrument that measures what you want to measure. For what purpose was this instrument developed? How was the instrument validated?
Contact the author or publisher for permission to use the instrument. You may be required to purchase the instrument. Consider the project or agency budget and time constraints.
Logistics. Consider the length of time required for completion of the instrument and complexity. Could your intervention population complete the instrument?

List your DNP Project outcomes and potential validated instruments to measure the outcome. Discuss your findings with your DNP team.

Outcome #1:

Potential Instruments:

Outcome #2:

Potential Instruments:

Outcome #3:

Potential Instruments:

Benchmarking Outcomes Data

In the quality-improvement process, benchmarking is a process of tracking an outcome over a period of time. This information can later be displayed as a run chart. For example, data may be collected from a patient chart by conducting a chart audit before the intervention and then at designated intervals after the intervention. It may be necessary to develop a chart-audit tool or data-extraction form. If you are looking at multiple outcomes, it can be helpful to have the information centrally organized.

Tips for Developing Chart-Audit Tools

1. **Determine number of audits needed.** For most rapid-cycle quality improvement, 30 to 60 audits or 10% of the total population are rules of thumb (Agency for Healthcare Research and Quality, 2013). The number and approach should be discussed by the DNP team.
2. **Plan to collect data multiple times.** We recommend a minimum of three collection points for a DNP Project: baseline (preintervention) and two points postintervention. Three data points can help determine trends. If available, trending data from the previous year(s) could be used to establish a baseline and/or comparisons.
3. **Privacy and data security.** *Never* take patient information from a chart without going through the proper channels. This process should not start until after the DNP Project proposal is fully approved and cleared by the given IRBs (if applicable).
4. **Use guidelines, protocols, and standards of care.** These help to outline what information needs to be included in the tool.

Will your project benchmark certain clinical data points or performance measures? Develop a sketch of a chart-audit tool or data-extraction form. Present the sketch to your DNP team.

Survey Development

Surveys are developed for different purposes. DNP-prepared nurses require basic skills in survey development. The survey should collect information that is of value to the DNP team. Examples of feedback include demographics of the intervention population, validation of findings in the literature, documentation of needs, perspectives of stakeholders on current problems, and advice for improving the process for the next improvement cycle. Resources for survey development: Survey Monkey. (2019). Survey 101. Retrieved from https://www.surveymonkey.com/mp/survey-guidelines; Vannette, D. (2010). 10 Tips for building effective surveys. Retrieved from https://www.qualtrics.com/blog/10-tips-for-building-effective-surveys

Consider the questions you will need to ask as part of your DNP Project. What will you need feedback on during this process? Draft the survey questions for review by your DNP team.

Remember that when you are evaluating the process anticipated for your DNP Project, you will most likely need to develop your own tool or survey so that you can capture the data that are relevant to your project. The goal is to get feedback on what to improve during the next project or improvement cycle.

NEXT STEPS

- Review your evaluation plan with your DNP team.
- Ensure that both outcomes and process are included.
- Revise your approach as necessary.

REFERENCES AND RESOURCES

American Academy of Family Physicians. (n.d.). Eight steps to a chart audit for quality. Retrieved from https://www.aafp.org/fpm/2008/0700/pa3.html

American Association of Colleges of Nursing. (2015). *The doctor of nursing practice: Current issues and clarifying recommendations* [White paper]. Retrieved from https://www.aacnnursing.org/Portals/42/News/White-Papers/DNP-Implementation-TF-Report-8-15.pdf

Agency for Healthcare Research and Quality. (2013). Practice facilitation handbook: Chapter 8, Collecting data with chart audits. Retrieved from https://www.ahrq.gov/professionals/prevention-chronic-care/improve/system/pf-handbook/mod8.html

RELATED TEXTBOOK

Sylvia, M. L., & Tehaar, M. F. (2018). *Clinical analytics and data management for the DNP.* New York, NY: Springer Publishing Company.

Lesson 7.9

PROJECT DATA AND PLANS FOR DATA ANALYSIS

BACKGROUND

We would venture to say that when it comes to data and data analysis, there is a polar effect . . . you either love it, or it makes you cringe. We must recognize our limitations, and if you require help with part of the project, you should ask for assistance from data experts. Why must we even consider data analysis and statistics? Conducting data and statistical analyses allows us to interpret the results into useful, meaningful information. With the diversity of projects and designs, it is challenging to address all possible types of data analysis here, but we give you a jump start and explore common themes. Several important reminders:

- Make sure your measures match what you outlined in the aim(s) and objectives.
- Collect the exact same data at different points in time to benchmark appropriately. Analysis cannot be conducted if measurements are inconsistent.
- Don't forget to capitalize on collecting qualitative data via focus groups or open-ended responses on feedback surveys. There may be a unique perspective that quantitative measures fail to capture.

LEARNING OBJECTIVES

- Identify the dependent and independent variables of the project.
- Select the appropriate statistical test based on the type of data collected.
- Outline an initial data analysis plan.

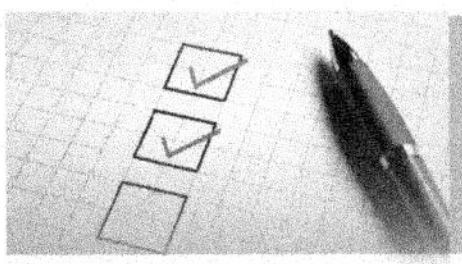

Activities

Simply put, the dependent variable is the outcome you are measuring.

Q: In this PICO question, what is the dependent variable? "Among diabetics (P), what is the impact of a 5-minute counseling session (I) on fasting a.m. glucose (O) and A1c (O)?"

A: Fasting a.m. glucose AND A1c

The independent variable is the factor that you are planning to influence (intervention). The outcome that will be measured is the dependent variable. In this example, the independent variable is the 5-minute counseling session.

Write your PICO question: ______________________________

Based on your DNP Project, fill in the blanks:

INDEPENDENT VARIABLE (HINT: YOUR PLANNED INTERVENTION(S)	DEPENDENT VARIABLE (HINT: YOUR OUTCOMES THAT WILL BE MEASURED)

Before you select an appropriate statistical test, you must label the variable by category: nominal, ordinal, or scale (interval/ratio). Here are some definitions to help you:

TYPE OF VARIABLE	EXAMPLE
Nominal: Used to label or classify into groups or categories	Race, gender, hair color
Ordinal: Used to rank or order variables	Agree, neutral, disagree
Scale: Used when variables have a set standard of space	Temperature, blood pressure

All of these variables can often be analyzed using descriptive statistics (statistics used to describe a group of variables), including, mean, median, mode, range, frequencies, percentages, and so on. You are trying to describe the variables. You are not really comparing them to anything at this point, just reporting them for what they are.

DNP Projects compare outcomes between two or more groups to draw conclusions (inferential statistics). To select the appropriate test, you must know the independent and dependent variables and know the type of variable (nominal, ordinal, scale). Common inferential statistics used in DNP Projects include a *t*-test, paired *t*-test, or analysis of variance (ANOVA). Here are some definitions to help you:

TEST	DEFINITION
t-test	Used to test the difference between two groups
Paired *t*-test	Used to test the difference between two groups at different points in time
ANOVA	Used to test the difference among three or more groups

Qualitative data are often collected in interviews, focus groups, or via open-ended questions on surveys. When the data are collected, they are reviewed, ideally by two reviewers. The reviewers each identify common themes. After they compare notes, they outline themes and derive the main point. The main point is sometimes translated into a synthesis statement—one single statement that captures the main point/idea. With this information in mind, outline your data analysis plan:

- Write your PICO question.
- Be clear on your independent and dependent variable(s).
- Pull each instrument used in the project.
- Determine whether it is quantitative or qualitative.
- Next to the quantitative measures, label the variable as nominal, ordinal, or scale.
- Mark your qualitative measures.

When this is complete, talk to your faculty about the best approach to use for data analysis.

NEXT STEPS

- Review your data analysis with your DNP team.
- Confirm that each of the data points you plan to collect is necessary and helps answer your clinical question.

RELATED TEXTBOOKS

Holly, C. (2019). *Scholarly inquiry and the DNP capstone*. New York, NY: Springer Publishing Company.
Chapter 5: Qualitative Descriptive Research

Sylvia, M. L., & Tehaar, M. F. (2018). *Clinical analytics and data management for the DNP*. New York, NY: Springer Publishing Company.
Chapter 1: Introduction to Clinical Data Management
Chapter 2: Statistical Concepts and Power Analysis

Lesson 7.10

TIMELINE, BUDGET, AND RESOURCES

BACKGROUND

As a team leader, you are responsible for establishing the timeline and budget and identifying additional resources that may be required for your project. Appreciating the time and resources necessary for your project is just as important as the project itself. Establishing a timeline will allow you to keep yourself on track in an effort to meet the objectives of your project and ensure forward progress. Just as we have helped you bring a very broad, grandiose plan to a manageable size, we do the same in terms of setting a realistic timeline. Specific to the timeline, you may have an idea of when you expect milestones to be reached, but it is also important to consider the tasks that may be outside your control. This includes external and internal site institutional review board (IRB) approvals.

LEARNING OBJECTIVES

- Develop a project timeline.
- Organize a project budget and list necessary resources.

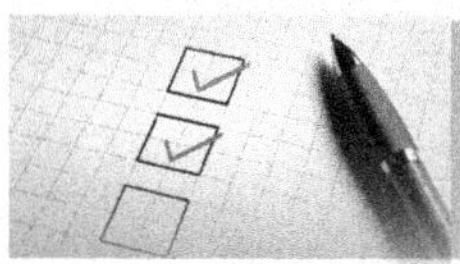

Activities

Consider the time requirements of your academic program and how these align with your DNP Project. Establish a project timeline and consider the following milestones (at a minimum) and how long each will take:

TASK	START	DURATION
Project planning/proposal development		
Proposal approval (by DNP team)		
IRB submission/approval (site)		
IRB submission/approval (school)		

TASK	START	DURATION
Implementation		
Data collection		
Data analysis		
Writing results, discussion, implications		
Final presentation/dissemination		

Displays of your timeline should be easy to read and follow. You can develop a Gantt chart or create your own. Using the tools shown in Figures 7.2 and 7.3, create a timeline for the major milestones of your project:

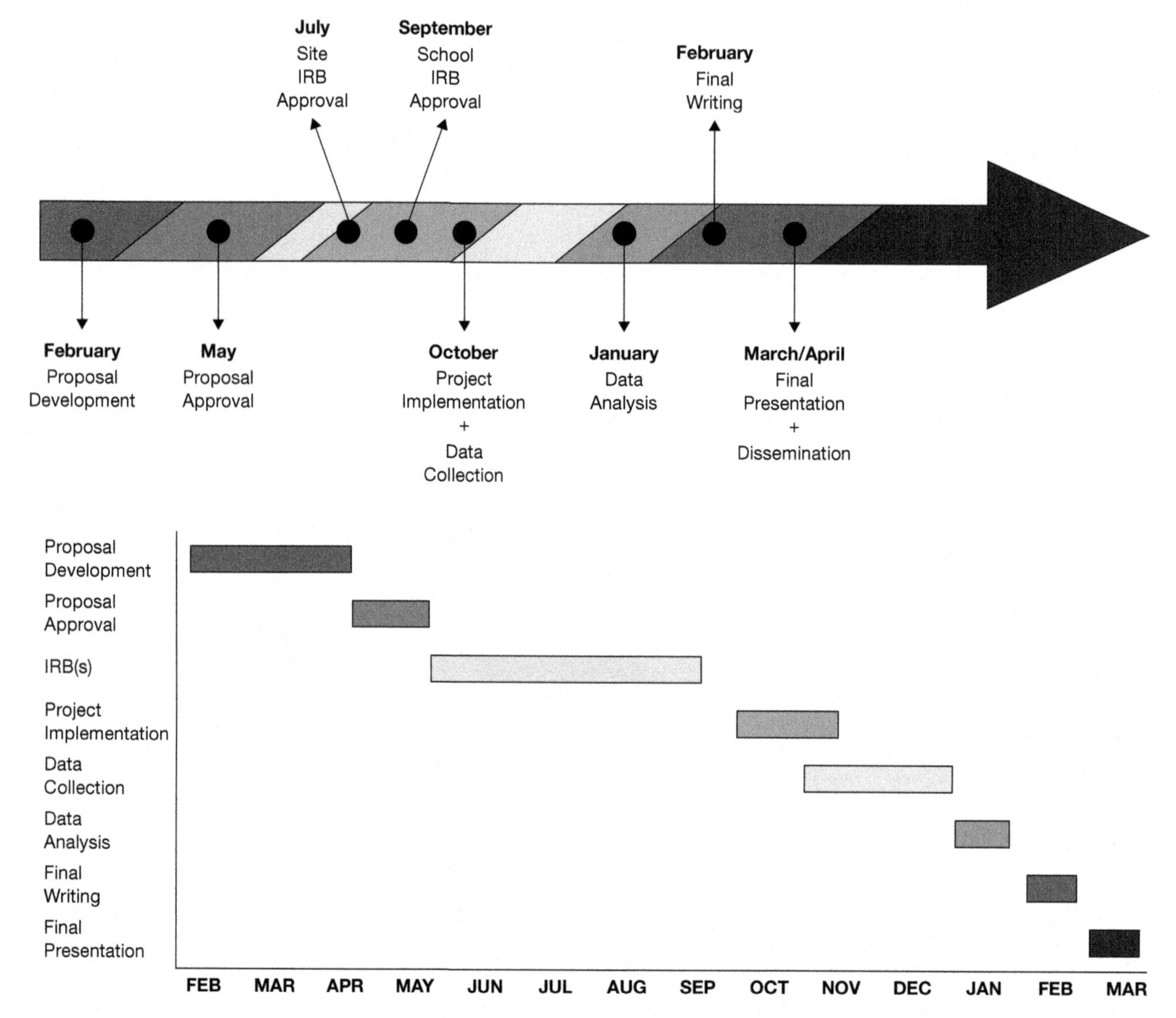

Figure 7.2 Sample Gantt chart.

AIM 1										
Activity	1	2	3	4	5	6	7	8	9	10
AIM 2										
Activity	**1**	**2**	**3**	**4**	**5**	**6**	**7**	**8**	**9**	**10**

Figure 7.3 Gantt chart template.
Source: Reproduced from White, K. M., Dudley-Brown, S., & Terhaar, M. F. (Eds.). (2020). *Translation of evidence into nursing and healthcare* (3rd ed.). New York, NY: Springer Publishing Company.

Project Budget and Resources

As with any project, it is important to consider any costs associated with your DNP Project. Most times, the costs associated with a project are nominal, but you want to be mindful so you do not end up surprised by out-of-pocket expenses. In general, budgets consider both expenses and revenue related to the project. They also include both direct (equipment/supplies) and indirect (day-to-day costs like electricity) costs. Consider the following types of expenses and resources that may be necessary specific to your project and establish an anticipated budget:

PROGRAM EXPENSE	PROJECTED COST	ACTUAL COST (ADD LATER)
Salaries/wages (Admin support, practitioners, statistics consultant)		
Start-up costs (copies, charts, displays, etc.)		
Capital costs (hardware, equipment)		
Operational costs (heat/ electricity)		
Other:		
Total Project Expenses	**$**	**$**

NEXT STEPS

- Discuss your timeline and budget with your DNP team.
- Discuss feasibility of timeline in terms of providing enough time for each task.
- Consider how the timeline aligns with program requirements and your other academic responsibilities.
- Consider the required budget and resources. Are there opportunities for grant funding or donation of services?

REFERENCES AND RESOURCES

Smartsheet. (2019). How to create a simple Gantt chart in any version of excel. Retrieved from https://www.smartsheet.com/blog/gantt-chart-excel

Teamgantt. (2019). Free Google sheets Gantt chart template. Retrieved from https://www.teamgantt.com/google-sheets-gantt-chart-template

RELATED TEXTBOOK

White, K. M., Dudley-Brown, S., & Terhaar, M. F. (Eds.). (2020). *Translation of evidence into nursing and healthcare* (3rd ed.). New York, NY: Springer Publishing Company.

Chapter 9: Project Management for Translation

Lesson 7.11

ANTICIPATED FINDINGS

BACKGROUND

What is it that you are trying to achieve by conducting your project? What are the data expected to show you? Consider the original aim of the project and the objectives you created in order to get there. Because you developed SMART (specific, measurable, achievable, relevant, time-bound) objectives, you will be able to evaluate whether you successfully achieved them. In consideration of why you are doing your project, what do you anticipate your results to be? You need to consider the potential implications of your findings.

What are the potential facilitators and barriers to the project? How are you working to either remove them or use them to your advantage in the project?

LEARNING OBJECTIVES

- Describe anticipated project findings.
- Outline potential barriers to success.
- List potential strategies to mitigate barriers.

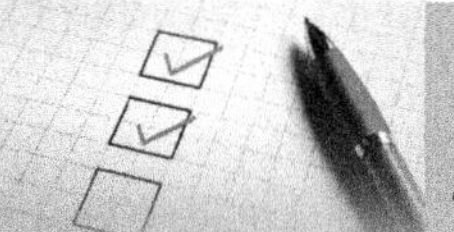

Activities

Answer these reflective questions. Then translate your thoughts into a formal paragraph for your DNP Project proposal.

1. When you conduct this project, what do you think will happen? Will it be welcomed? Do you think the outcomes will be met? Explain.

2. What barriers to the successful implementation of your project exist? List them and then write a strategy to mitigate the barrier.

NEXT STEPS

- Translate your thoughts on anticipated findings and facilitators and barriers into two formal paragraphs for the DNP Project proposal.
- Discuss your concerns with the DNP team.

RELATED TEXTBOOK

Bonnel, W., & Smith, K. (2018). *Proposal writing for clinical nursing and DNP Projects*. New York, NY: Springer Publishing Company.

Lesson 7.12

PREPLANNING FOR SUSTAINABILITY AND DISSEMINATION

BACKGROUND

The DNP Project should be designed with sustainability in mind (American Association of Colleges of Nursing [AACN], 2015). The AACN (2015) states the DNP Project should "Include a plan for sustainability (e.g. financial, system or political realities, not only theoretical abstraction)" (p. 4). Essentially, this means that the project should be designed in a way that it makes meaningful change in practice and has potential to continue beyond the DNP Project.

Likewise, the AACN (2015) states that dissemination of the DNP Project should "Include a product that describes the purpose, planning, implementation, and evaluation components of the project, and should be required for each project . . . and may include a variety of forms depending upon the focus" (p. 5). Appendix A of the same document outlines examples of dissemination (AACN, 2015). At minimum, we endorse White, Dudley-Brown, and Terhaar's (2020) recommendation for the 3 P's of dissemination: paper, poster, and presentation.

LEARNING OBJECTIVES

- Review the AACN requirements.
- Determine your plans for sustainability and dissemination of the DNP Project.

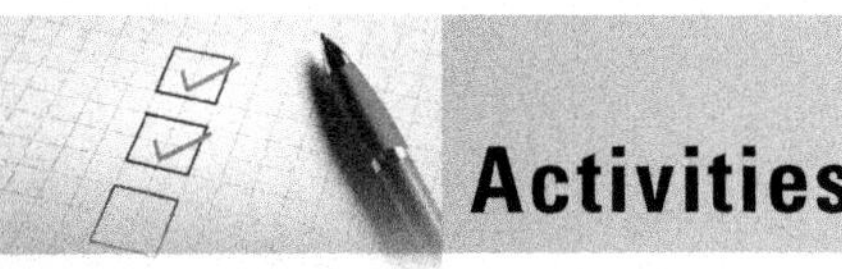

Activities

Review the DNP Project requirements at your school. In addition to the AACN requirements, take notes on other specifics:

____

____

____

____

____

____

Sustainability: Answer the following questions as you plan for DNP Project sustainability.

1. How will the practice change (intervention) be reinforced over time?

   ____

   ____

2. Are there resources in place to support the project in the future?

   ____

   ____

3. After this project is completed, when will the next quality cycle begin?

   ____

   ____

4. Can the practice change (intervention) carry on without you?

____

____

5. Is there a mechanism in place to continue to collect and monitor data on patient outcomes?

____

____

As a leader, it is important to diversify. Ensure that multiple people can execute given tasks. Leave tools, protocols, or guidelines with an organization to ensure that a practice change is sustained.

Dissemination: We recommend White et al.'s (2020) approach to dissemination:

Poster, paper, and presentation. These are discussed in the next chapter.

- Review the suggested list adapted from the AACN (2015) examples of dissemination.
- Select one additional dissemination technique that would be appropriate for the population your project is targeting.
- Describe your plan to include this dissemination in addition to the 3 P's.

Dissemination Suggestions to Target Populations:

- Webinar or online modules
- Video (YouTube)
- Submission of written summary to a lay publication
- Oral presentation to public at large
- Digital posters, grand rounds, or PowerPoint presentations
- Blog, Infographic, or Listicle
- Social media release: Facebook, Instagram, SnapChat, LinkedIn, and so on.
- Other: ______________________________

Write your plan for dissemination.

____

____

____

____

NEXT STEPS

- Discuss your strategies with your DNP team.
- Revise your approach as necessary.

REFERENCES AND RESOURCES

American Association of Colleges of Nursing. (2015). *The doctor of nursing practice: Current issues and clarifying recommendations* [White paper]. Retrieved from https://www.aacnnursing.org/Portals/42/News/White-Papers/DNP-Implementation-TF-Report-8-15.pdf.

White, K. M., Dudley-Brown, S., & Terhaar, M. F. (Eds.). (2020). *Translation of evidence into nursing and healthcare* (3rd ed.). New York, NY: Springer Publishing Company.

RELATED TEXTBOOKS

Smith-Stoner, M. (2018). *A guide to disseminating your DNP Project*. New York, NY: Springer Publishing Company.

Chapter 1: Why Take the Time to Disseminate Your Work?
Chapter 3: Choosing Your Method of Sharing Your Project
Chapter 4: Determining the Unique Contribution to Health Care
Chapter 5: Setting Up the Project
Chapter 6: Group Dissemination Projects

White, K. M., Dudley-Brown, S., & Terhaar, M. F. (Eds.). (2020). *Translation of evidence into nursing and healthcare* (3rd ed.). New York, NY: Springer Publishing Company.

Lesson 7.13

ASSESSING DNP PROJECT QUALITY AND RIGOR

BACKGROUND

Across the country, there is much debate about the quality and rigor of DNP Projects. This is because there is a high rate of variation among projects. Ultimately, our goal as faculty is to create equity. The American Association of Colleges of Nursing (2015) published a white paper to establish minimum expectations for DNP Projects. The recommendation of the white paper was a first step toward equity among DNP Projects.

Quality, by definition, may refer to the degree of excellence with which a project is executed (Merriam-Webster.com, 2019). The measure of the quality and the indicators of quality are determined by each school. We believe these standards should be in alignment with the AACN recommendations in order to create national equity of DNP Projects. Each DNP program should have a grading rubric to evaluate the DNP Project. The rubric is the school's measure of DNP Project quality. It is always the faculty's responsibility to evaluate student performance, although others may give additional feedback.

Rigor is a different concept. Technically, "rigor" refers to the strict, precise adherence to procedure. We believe that rigor is a term more appropriately applied to research, which does require strict adherence to procedure. Eventually, standards may be developed for DNP Project "rigor," but it may be unreasonable to demand "rigor" before establishing project quality indicators. If the term "rigor" is used in the context of DNP Projects, the definition offered by Roush and Tesoro (2018) sounds clear. They define "DNP Project rigor" as "a systematic, logical, and thorough approach to the design and implementation of a project that addresses a significant problem and includes an evaluation process based on appropriate metrics, collected and analyzed using methods that provide a valid and reliable determination of project outcomes" (Roush & Tesoro, 2018, p. 438).

LEARNING OBJECTIVES

- Review the DNP Project requirements and grading rubrics at your school.
- Read the recommended articles.
- List potential quality indicators for your DNP Project.

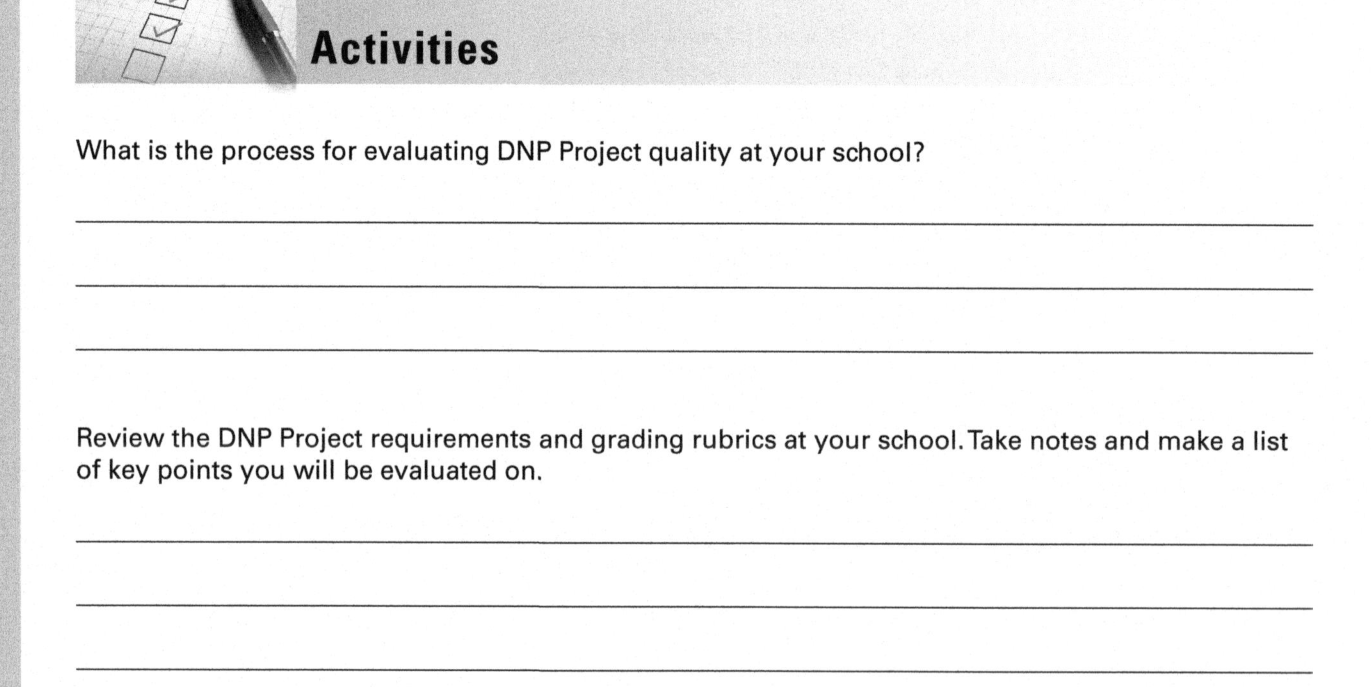

Activities

What is the process for evaluating DNP Project quality at your school?

Review the DNP Project requirements and grading rubrics at your school. Take notes and make a list of key points you will be evaluated on.

Review the content of each article listed in the resource list. Focus on the article by Roush and Tesoro (2018). Based on their study and examples of problems in DNP Projects, list three elements of your DNP Project method that may need revisions.

1.

2.

3.

NEXT STEPS

- Review your list with your DNP team.
- Revise your proposed DNP methodology to improve quality and rigor of the project.

REFERENCES AND RESOURCES

American Association of Colleges of Nursing. (2015). *The doctor of nursing practice: Current issues and clarifying recommendations* [White paper]. Retrieved from https://www.aacnnursing.org/Portals/42/News/White-Papers/DNP-Implementation-TF-Report-8-15.pdf

Doles, J., Hernández, C., & Miles, H. (2017). The DNP Project: Quandaries for nursing scholars. *Nursing Outlook, 65*(1), 84–93. doi: 10.1016/j.outlook.2016.07.009

Merriam-Webster.com. (2019). Quality. Retrieved from https://www.merriam-webster.com/dictionary/quality

Roush, K., & Tesoro, M. (2018). An examination of the rigor and value of final scholarly projects completed by DNP nursing students. *Journal of Professional Nursing, 34*(6), 437–443. doi: 10.1016/j.profnurs.2018.03.003

Waldrop, J., Curaso, D., Fuchs, M., & Hypes, K. (2014). EC as PIE: Five criteria for executing a successful DNP Project. *Journal of Professional Nursing, 30*(4), 300–306. doi: 10.1016/j.profnurs.2014.01.003

CHAPTER SUMMARY

To review, the methodology of the project describes the processes followed by the intended intervention and includes an evaluation plan. This chapter engaged you in the prework and planning required to develop a successful DNP Project. Your DNP team should be involved in this process. Use this methodology planning checklist as you prepare your DNP Project proposal.

☐ Select Implementation Framework.

____

☐ Visual Representation of Method Step

Use Framework to Guide You.

- Develop
- Implement
- Evaluate
- Sustain
- Disseminate

☐ Poster
☐ Paper
☐ Presentation
☐ Other:

☐ Intervention Population:

☐ Recruitment Plan:
- ☐ Letter
- ☐ Flyer

☐ Consent:
- ☐ IRB
- ☐ CITI Training Complete

☐ Evaluation: Objectives are evaluated? Y/N

Outcomes ☐ Tools
☐ Instrument
☐ Benchmarks

Process ☐ ______________
☐ ______________
____
____

☐ Data Analysis Plan
☐ Storage
☐ Ethics Mentioned
☐ Timeline
☐ Budget

Anticipated Findings:

Barriers:

Solutions:

8

Strategies to Organize, Disseminate, and Sustain DNP Project Findings

Molly J. Bradshaw, Tracy R. Vitale, Thomas Christenbery, and David G. Campbell-O'Dell

Lessons

OBJECTIVES

Organizations play a key role in successful DNP Project management. After the implementation of the DNP Project, the student must analyze data, interpret the findings, and finalize a strategy for sustainability. Students are required to present the final academic products of the DNP Project, which should include at minimum a paper, presentation, and poster. Beyond the academic setting, it is also important to communicate the project findings to stakeholders, colleagues, and the community. Storing and sharing DNP Projects in electronic repositories is considered best practice. In this chapter, students will examine skills for project management, composing final academic products, and plan dissemination of information in appropriate formats to others. By the end of this chapter, you will be able to:

- Consider best practices of project management.
- Finalize plans for sustainability after data collection.
- Develop a plan to finish the academic products.
- Utilize multiple formats for dissemination of project findings.

INTRODUCTION

The DNP Project proposal must be approved by the DNP team, the institutional review board (IRB), and other appropriate entities before project implementation begins. As the project gets underway, you must stay organized and utilize your leadership skills for successful project management.

Detailed data-management strategies and clinical analytics are beyond the scope of this workbook. However, we advise you to consult with your faculty and other experts with skill sets to help you set up code books, use data-analysis software, and accurately interpret your findings. For additional support, we recommend the textbook by Sylvia and Terhaar (2018), *Clinical Analytics and Data Management for the DNP*.

You will need to consider the impact of the intervention on identified outcomes for the targeted population. What contribution did your project make to the organization, education, practice, policy, and health systems? You will make final plans for project sustainability. Likewise, you will examine the process itself and make recommendations about what could be improved.

All of this information must be communicated. In the academic setting you will most likely be asked to present a final academic paper with an oral presentation. The paper generally builds on the DNP Project proposal. The proposal is changed to past tense. Instead of saying what will happen, the tone shifts to what was done. Then additional sections are added beyond the methodology such as results, discussion, and implications. The oral presentation is just an alternate format of the academic paper content. DNP students should have skills to present information in multiple ways. Again, we support the concept of the 3P's of academic products: paper, presentation, and scholarly poster (White, Dudley-Brown, & Terhaar, 2020).

Remember to check the requirements at your school. We discuss the differences between digital repositories and peer-reviewed publications. Social media considerations are outlined.

Presenting information to stakeholders, the community, and patient populations may require a different approach and you may need to revise your original plans depending on your project findings. Let's begin.

REFERENCES AND RESOURCES

Sylvia, M. L., & Terhaar, M. F. (2018). *Clinical analytics and data management for the DNP*. New York, NY: Springer Publishing Company.

White, K. M., Dudley-Brown, S., & Terhaar, M. F. (Eds.). (2020). *Translation of evidence into nursing and healthcare* (3rd ed.). New York, NY: Springer Publishing Company.

MY GOALS FOR STRATEGIES TO ORGANIZE, DISSEMINATE, AND SUSTAIN DNP PROJECT FINDINGS ARE TO:

Lesson 8.1

PROJECT MANAGEMENT AND EMOTIONAL INTELLIGENCE

BACKGROUND

In addition to leadership skills, the DNP student must demonstrate an ability to manage the implementation of the DNP Project. Effective project management often translates to project success and includes emotional intelligence.

LEARNING OBJECTIVES

- Correlate the elements of the critical success factors for project management with the context of your DNP Project.
- Identify one key factor to carefully manage your project implementation.
- Determine the role of emotional intelligence in project management.

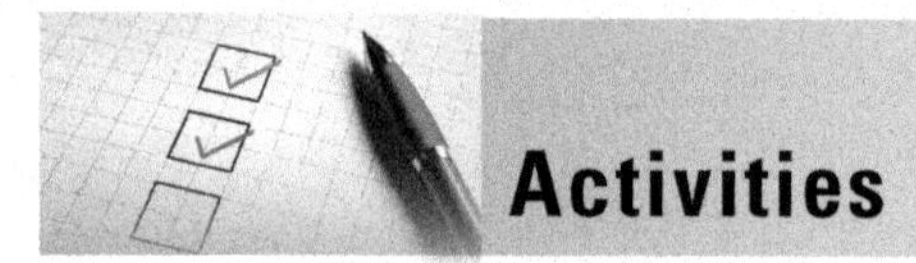

Activities

Successful project management incorporates the following elements. Highlight one key area of concern that may need careful management.

- Communication
- Planning effort
- Organization
- Attention to safety and quality
- Management of project participants

Project Procedures

- Obtaining resources
- Developing an appropriate method and rollout plan

Human Factors

- Experience of participants
- Nature of the participants
- Size of organization and number of participants
- Mission/values of the organization
- Mission/values of participants

Project Factors

- Project type
- Complexity of the project
- Project timing

External Factors

- Fiscal/resource components
- Social issues
- Political issues
- System/technology issues

List three strategies to ensure success.

1.

2.

3.

Emotional intelligence is an emotional awareness about yourself and others (Goleman, 1995). The five domains of emotional intelligence include:

The five domains of emotional intelligence include self-awareness, self-regulation, social skills, empathy, and motivation.

1. Assess your emotional intelligence with this free web-based resource (Mind Tools, 2019).
2. Based on your results, list two components for improvement. Describe the potential impact on the successful management of your DNP Project.

Emotional Intelligence Component #1:

Strategy to Improve:

Potential Impact on DNP Project Success:

Emotional Intelligence Component #2

Strategy to Improve:

Potential Impact on DNP Project Success:

Tips for DNP Project Management

- Have a clear rollout plan and follow the methodology you described.
- Take notes of observations and incidental comments.
- After completion of the intervention, reflect on what could be improved.
- Resolve conflicts and issues in a timely manner.
- Communicate regularly with the DNP team.
- Do not change the project method without consulting the DNP team/IRB.

NEXT STEPS

- Communicate regularly with your DNP team.
- Utilize the suggested tips for DNP Project management.

REFERENCES AND RESOURCES

Alias, Z., Zawawi, E. M. A., Yusof, K., & Aris, N. M. (2014). Determining critical success factors of project management practice: A conceptual framework. *Social and Behavioral Sciences, 153*, 61–69. doi: 10.1016/j.sbspro.2014.10.041

Ellis, P. (2017). Learning emotional intelligence and what it can do for you. *Wounds UK, 13*(4), 66–69. Retrieved from https://www.wounds-uk.com

Goleman, D. (1995). *Emotional intelligence*. New York, NY: Bantam Books.

Mind Tools. (2019). How emotionally intelligent are you? Retrieved from https://www.mindtools.com/pages/article/ei-quiz.htm

RELATED TEXTBOOK

Marshall, E. S., & Broome, M. E. (2018). *Transformational leadership in nursing* (2nd ed.). New York, NY: Springer Publishing Company.

Chapter 1: Expert Clinician to Transformational Leader in a Complex Health Care Organization: Foundations

Lesson 8.2

FINALIZING PLANS FOR SUSTAINABILITY AFTER DATA COLLECTION

BACKGROUND

According to the American Association of Colleges of Nursing (2015), the DNP Project should include a plan for sustainability. The plan you conceptualized in the DNP Project proposal may shift as a result of findings recognized after data collection and analysis.

LEARNING OBJECTIVES

- Revisit your sustainability plan described in the DNP Project proposal.
- Revise your plan according to project findings.

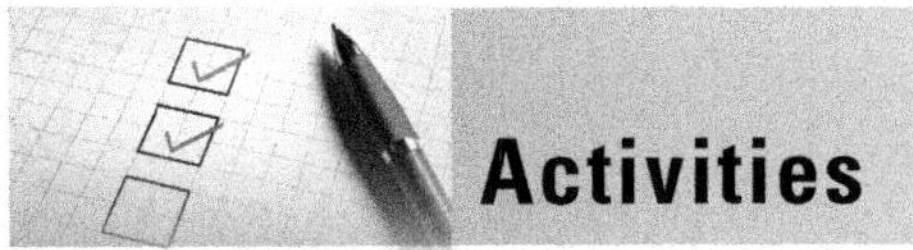

Activities

1. List the key components of your original plan for DNP Project sustainability.

2. Based on the analysis of your project data, answer the following questions:
   a. Did the evaluation of process identify any changes that should be made in the future?

   b. Was the outcome of the project favorable?

   c. Are there any practices that should be abandoned?

3. Revise your DNP Project sustainability plan by outlining key changes here:

NEXT STEPS

- Discuss the revisions with your DNP team.

REFERENCE AND RESOURCE

American Association of Colleges of Nursing. (2015). *The doctor of nursing practice: Current issues and clarifying recommendations* [White paper]. Retrieved from https://www.aacnnursing.org/Portals/42/News/White-Papers/DNP-Implementation-TF-Report-8-15.pdf

RELATED TEXTBOOK

Christenbery, T. (Ed.). (2018). *Evidence-based practice in nursing*. New York, NY: Springer Publishing Company.

Lesson 8.3

WRITING THE RESULTS AND DISCUSSION SECTIONS

BACKGROUND

After data collection and data analysis, you are ready to begin writing the next components of your final academic paper for the DNP Project. In most cases, you will take the DNP Project proposal, change it to past tense, and then make other small revisions. Then you will begin to add additional sections to follow the methodology section:

- Results
- Discussion
- Limitations
- Implications
- Plan for Sustainability
- Plan for Dissemination
- Conclusion

Results of the DNP Project must first be reported. Generally, the approach for reporting follows the logical or sometimes chronological order of data collection. It includes data on project outcomes and process. The key to the Results section is to be unbiased and simply report the information. Avoid the temptation to discuss the meaning of the information. That part comes later under Discussion. Tables and text are both utilized to convey the information. Read the Results section of several studies or other DNP Projects to better understand how findings are reported in text and graphically.

Discussion of the results offers the opportunity to interpret and convey meaning. In the Discussion section, start by briefly reminding the reader of the project aim(s) and objectives. Move the discussion through the order in which it is presented in the Results section. Make meaning out of the information. Does it support the findings of the literature or is it different? Were there any outliers? Now discuss limitations. Limitations are handicaps of the project. Is there a reason the sample size was small? Was there a sentinel event during the project? Try to explain why the results turned out the way they did.

LEARNING OBJECTIVES

- Organize the approach to writing the Results section.
- Organize the approach to the Discussion section and address any limitations.

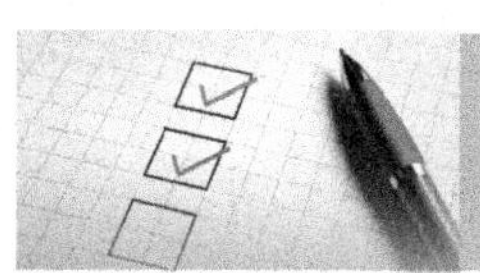

Activities

Use this outline to organize your approach to writing the DNP Project results (Sacred Heart University Library, n.d.; University of Southern California, 2019).

Structure and Approach

- Provide a short statement of context.
- Present information with a brief description.

Content

- Summarize key findings.
- Write in the past tense.
- Keep information in logical sequence.
- Use tables, charts, and figures to illustrate your findings.
- Focus on findings that are important.

Problems to Avoid

- Be factual and concise.
- Avoid presenting the same information more than once.
- Do not interpret the meaning in this section.

Outline your approach to writing your Results section.

Use this outline to organize your approach to writing your Discussion section.

Structure and Approach

- Use the past tense.
- Follow a logical approach.
- Use subheadings if appropriate to organize themes.

Content

- Reiterate the project problem.
- Explain key results and explain why they are important.
- Make connections between your findings and findings in the literature.
- Discuss limitations, lessons learned, and the evaluation of the DNP Project process.
- Make recommendations for future quality improvement, practice change, or research.

Problems to Avoid

- Do not introduce new results.
- Do not waste sentences restating your results.
- Do not omit negative information; present it in an objective way.

Outline your approach to writing your Discussion section.

NEXT STEPS

- Draft your DNP Project Results and Discussion sections.
- Review the draft with your DNP team.

REFERENCES AND RESOURCES

Quinn, C. T., & Rush, A. J. (2009, June). Writing and publishing your research findings. *Journal of Investigative Medicine, 57*(5), 634–639. doi: 10.231/JIM.0b013e3181aa089f

Sacred Heart University Library. (n.d.). Organizing academic research papers: 7. The results. Retrieved from https://library.sacredheart.edu/c.php?g=29803&p=185931

University of Southern California. (2019). Research guides. Organizing your social sciences research paper: 7. The results. Retrieved from https://libguides.usc.edu/writingguide/results

Lesson 8.4

WRITING ABOUT IMPACT ON PATIENTS, FAMILIES, AND POPULATIONS

BACKGROUND

The complexity of the healthcare system has put patients, families, and populations at risk (Institute of Medicine, 1999). The DNP degree involves a skill set to equip you to make practice changes that improve the quality and safety of healthcare for the target population. The project should improve health outcomes. The work of this project must culminate in your description of the impact you have made on the selected outcomes. What are the implications of your work for the population?

LEARNING OBJECTIVES

- Inventory the impact your DNP Project has made for patients, families, and populations.
- Draft a paragraph(s) summarizing your points.

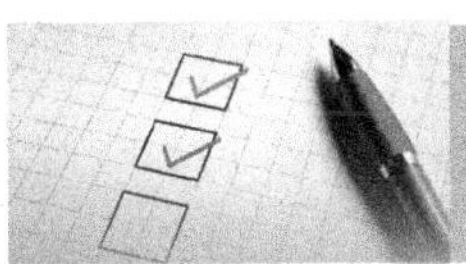

Activities

Reflect on the outcomes of your DNP Project. Describe the impact it has made for patients, families, and populations. Do you have direct quotes from your data that are significant? Did you make observations during the intervention that were meaningful? After your reflection, draft a paragraph summarizing your points.

____

____

____

____

NEXT STEP

- Translate your draft into the final DNP Project write-up.

REFERENCE

Institute of Medicine. (1999). To err is human: Building a safer healthcare system, summary. Retrieved from https://www.nap.edu/read/9728/chapter/1

Lesson 8.5

WRITING ABOUT THE IMPACT ON PRACTICE, EDUCATION, POLICY, AND SYSTEMS

BACKGROUND

The DNP Project should be designed to make an impact, direct or indirect, on health outcomes of the targeted population (American Association of Colleges of Nursing [AACN], 2015). The DNP Project could also make an impact on other related components of the healthcare environment. In the final academic write-up, it is important to address the project implications beyond those of the target population. The DNP Project offers an opportunity for the DNP student to demonstrate a skill set based on the DNP Essentials (AACN, 2015).

LEARNING OBJECTIVES

- Explain the impact of the DNP Project on practice, education, policy, and health systems.
- Incorporate this information into the final academic write-up.

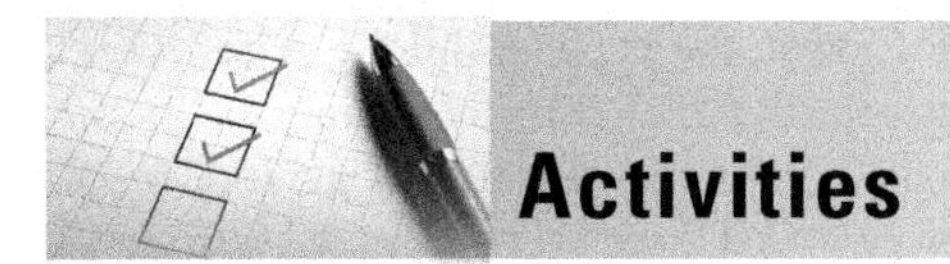

Activities

For each category, explain the impact on your DNP Project.

Impact on Practice	**Impact on Education**
Impact on Policy	**Impact on Health Systems**

NEXT STEP

- Based on your notes here, translate the information into a dedicated section of the final DNP Project write-up.

REFERENCE

American Association of Colleges of Nursing. (2015). *The doctor of nursing practice: Current issues and clarifying recommendations* [White paper]. Retrieved from https://www.aacnnursing.org/Portals/42/News/White-Papers/DNP-Implementation-TF-Report-8-15.pdf

Lesson 8.6

STRATEGIES FOR FINAL ACADEMIC PAPER

BACKGROUND

The final academic paper of the DNP Project will vary depending on the requirements of the given program. In most cases, the document evolves from the proposal to a completed report describing the findings and implications. Because it is written in sections over a period of time, it typically builds until one final academic paper is completed. The intended audience for this paper is the DNP faculty and other academic stakeholders. It is an academic product and may include components required to demonstrate DNP program outcomes.

Later, as you prepare to publish the findings of your DNP Project, the paper will need to be revised. Findings of quality-improvement projects are often written using the SQUIRE (Standards for QUality Improvement Reporting Excellence) 2.0 Guidelines (Ogrinc, Davies, Goodman, Batalden, Davidoff, & Stevens, 2016). Key information may need to be de-identified and removed. Some components of the paper that are necessary for academia are not necessary for a journal. It is important to streamline the content.

LEARNING OBJECTIVES

- Compare the SQUIRE 2.0 Guidelines to the requirements for the final academic paper at your school.
- Dissect the differences in writing for academic purposes versus for a journal audience.

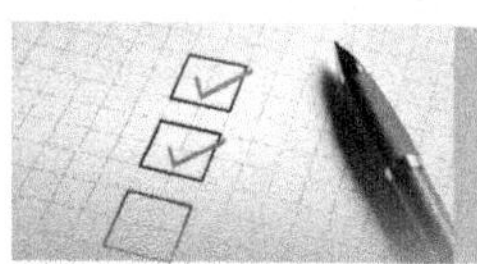

Activities

Review the requirements for the final academic paper at your school. Compare the requirements to the SQUIRE 2.0 Guidelines.

REQUIREMENTS AT YOUR SCHOOL: FINAL ACADEMIC PAPER	SQUIRE 2.0 GUIDELINES
	Title
	Abstract
	Problem description
	Available knowledge
	Rationale
	Specific aims
	Context
	Intervention
	Study of the intervention
	Measures
	Analysis
	Ethical considerations
	Results
	Summary
	Interpretation
	Limitations
	Conclusion
	Funding

NEXT STEP

- Discuss the strategy for your final academic paper with your DNP team.

REFERENCE AND RESOURCE

Ogrinc, G., Davies, L., Goodman, D., Batalden, P., Davidoff, F., & Stevens, D. (2016). SQUIRE 2.0 (Standards for Quality Improvement Reporting Excellence): Revised publication guidelines from a detailed consensus process. *BMJ Quality & Safety*, *25*(12), 986–992. doi: 10.1136/bmjqs-2015-004411

RELATED TEXTBOOK

White, K. M., Dudley-Brown, S., & Terhaar, M. F. (Eds.). (2020). *Translation of evidence into nursing and healthcare* (3rd ed.). New York, NY: Springer Publishing Company.

Lesson 8.7

STRATEGIES FOR ORAL PRESENTATIONS

BACKGROUND

DNP students are required to disseminate the findings of their project in multiple ways. Making oral presentations to various groups is a typical requirement. Therefore, DNP students benefit from practicing and honing public speaking skills. In preparing for oral presentations, give consideration to the target audience and the environment (Federal Emergency Management Agency, 2014). The oral presentation delivers the same content as the written paper in a more concise way.

LEARNING OBJECTIVE

- Outline strategies for effective oral presentations.

Reflection

- In the past, what have been your strengths when giving oral presentations?
- In the past, what have been your biggest challenges or weaknesses when giving oral presentations?

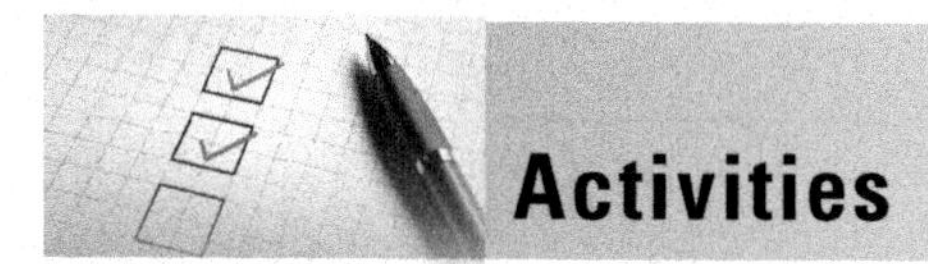

Activities

Complete the prompts to organize a strategy for an effective oral presentation based on your DNP Project.

	Notes
Planning • Who is the audience? • What is the purpose of the presentation? • How much time do you have? • What is the environment like?	

Outline and Visual Materials
• Create an outline of your oral presentation.
  • Most often, the outline follows the headings in your paper.
  • Do not use large paragraphs and complete sentences; keep the text focused and present using bullets.
  • List key points.	

Practice • Practice your presentation. • Prepare a transcript if you cannot stay focused. • Time yourself.	
Feedback • Videotape yourself for self-evaluation. • Have a colleague observe you give the presentation.	
Final Strategies for the Presentation Day • Arrive early. • Check audio/visual equipment. • Have backup access to your files.	

NEXT STEP

- Discuss your plan with your DNP team.

REFERENCE AND RESOURCE

Federal Emergency Management Agency. (2014). Lesson 4.0: Preparing for oral presentations. Retrieved from https://training.fema.gov/emiweb/is/is242b/student%20manual/sm_04.pdf

RELATED TEXTBOOK

White, K. M., Dudley-Brown, S., & Terhaar, M. F. (Eds.). (2020). *Translation of evidence into nursing and healthcare* (3rd ed.). New York, NY: Springer Publishing Company.

Lesson 8.8

STRATEGIES FOR CREATING SCHOLARLY POSTERS

BACKGROUND

A poster is a concise, visual summary of your DNP Project. Scholarly posters empower DNP students to kindle important *networking* connections and *communicate* critical translation of science into practice initiatives. To promote productive networking alliances, a poster must be visually interesting to capture a conference attendees' curiosity. Conference attendees are seldom interested in posters that serve as a storehouse for massive amounts of technical verbiage and data analyses. Wise DNP students carefully select poster information and visuals that entice attendees to stop and view their posters. Once an attendee is attracted to a DNP student's project, the poster must serve as a conversation starter. As attendees begin to view a poster, the DNP student should mention the project's most important outcome, which enables the attendee to place the DNP Project into a meaningful context. This is the point at which you succinctly state your project's take-home message. For example: *From the literature, we learned that grit and social interaction are the biggest predictors for completing DNP programs and subsequently designed an intervention that helps DNP students maximize grit and social capacity.* At this point, you have provided just enough information to encourage the attendee to talk and ask questions.

LEARNING OBJECTIVES

- Design an effective scholarly poster based on your DNP Project.

Reflection

When developing a poster, who is the intended audience? Where will the poster be displayed? Are there specific requirements from the conference/event on the size or poster design?

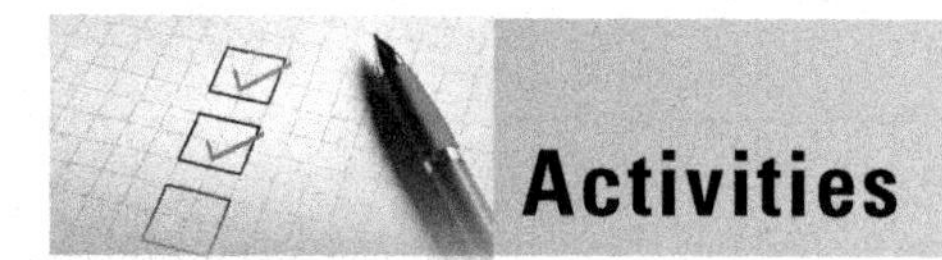

Activities

Because the purpose of a poster is to encourage networking and stimulate professional conversation, it is counterproductive when posters are burdened with an abundance of words impossible to pronounce, let alone define; passive tense; and convoluted structure. These drawbacks are easily avoidable by following a few simple tips about poster sections and *design*.

Sections

Organize your poster into seven sections (Figure 8.1):

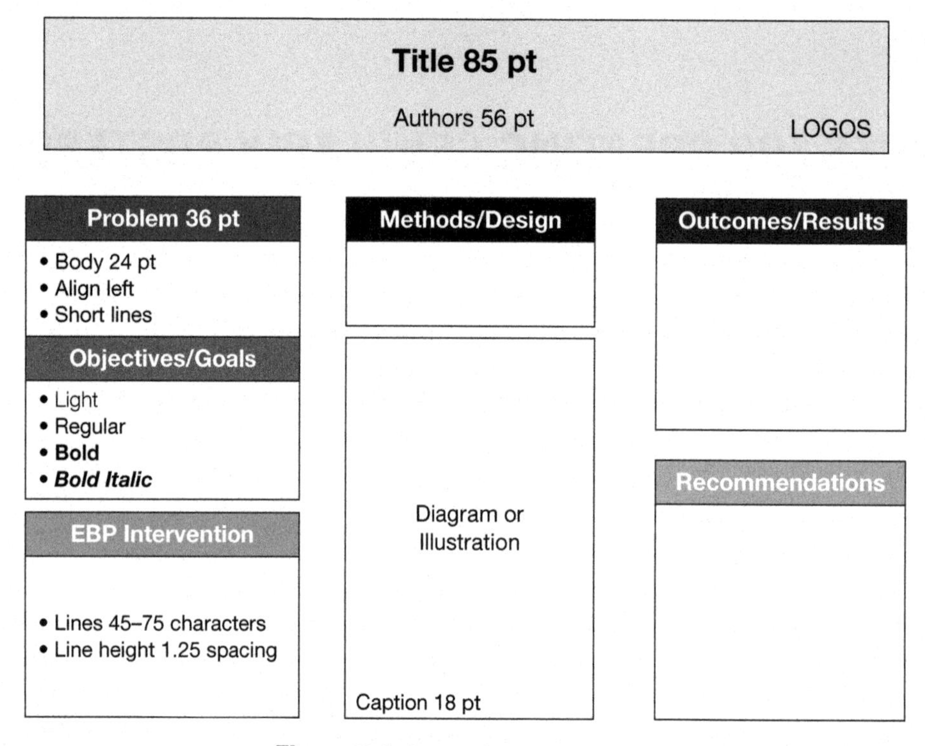

Figure 8.1 Poster design template.

Source: Reproduced from Christenbery, T. (Ed.). (2018). *Evidence-based practice in nursing* (Figure 11.3). New York, NY: Springer Publishing Company.

Section I: Title

- A title is often the first feature of the poster an attendee sees. The title needs to be large, bold, and easy to read.
- Aim for a likable title. For example: "Comfort vs. Fear: The ICU Experience" instead of "Experiences of Critically Ill Cardiac Patients: Focus Group Findings About Fear and Quality of Life."
- A title rule of thumb: *Less is more.* That is, be judicious in your selection of words for the title.
- Title header should include your name, credentials, and name of school or organization.

Section II: Clinical Problem and Key Objectives

- Must be brief and convey the project's importance.
- Limit to two or three key objectives and relate them directly to the problem statement.
- State key objectives unambiguously and write them in bullet form.

Section III: Description of Patients, Setting, and Project

- Include important clinical and demographic data for patients.
- Briefly describe the sample selection.
- List major steps taken to implement the project and *brief* rationalizations for taking those steps.
- Describe measurement tools in this section and how data were collected.

Section IV: Outcomes and Clinical Relevance

- This is the section most attendees find of maximum interest—the so what!
- Display data analysis in this section with judicious use of charts, graphs, and pictures.
- Do not overwhelm with visuals. Generally, two graphs or charts are sufficient to display analyses.

Section V: Primary Conclusions

- State the importance of your work as a whole.
- Emphasize nursing implications and direction for future collaborative work.

Section VI: References

- Reference all sources, including images and graphs.

Section VII: Acknowledgments

- Thank those who contributed to your project. DNP work is not accomplished in a vacuum. This might include faculty advisor, institution, or funding sponsors.

Design

- **Organization:** Adhere to conference guidelines for layout (e.g., vertical, horizontal) and size. Leave space at the edges, this will help the poster to seem less cluttered. Remember, 40% of the poster should be blank or negative space. Viewers need to rest their eyes and the negative space helps fulfill that purpose.

- **Flow:** Readers appreciate the logical flow of content. Avoid visual confusion. Use numbered headers and/or arrows to help the reader follow the intended flow. In Western countries, people generally read left to right and top to bottom. Use large, easy-to-read, and numbered sections for each of the content areas.

- **Visuals:** Use recognizable images that draw the viewer toward the poster. A recognizable image prevents your poster from looking like a wall of text. People are not interested in reading large amounts of text. If you have placed over 250 words in any section, you are way over your word count. Remember, 40% of the poster needs to be clear space.
- **Color:** Use a limited number of colors, no more than three to five, and use those colors throughout the poster, including the graphs. Use two or three primary colors and an accent color that is noticeable. The accent color should draw the viewer's eye to what you want the viewer to see.
- **Background:** No matter how amazing the photo—do not blow it up and use it for the background. Photo backgrounds are very distracting and eliminate all negative space.
- **Fonts:** Much like colors, the fewer used the better. Only use one or two different fonts. A boldface title and headers should be 150 to 250 points, and body text uses a minimum of 48 points. The goal is to read the poster content from a distance of 3 to 4 feet. Avoid ornate lettering. A sans serif typeface, such as Arial or Helvetica, is more legible from a distance. Dark lettering on soft backgrounds is easiest to read.
- **Bullets:** Avoid making your poster look like a scholarly paper. Even a 200-word narrative placed on a poster is mind-numbing. Use bullets liberally to emphasize the salient points—they provide an easier and friendlier read for your viewer. Remember, the poster is a visual message and it is counterproductive to insert a lengthy 200-word narrative into it.

NEXT STEP

- Design a scholarly poster based on your DNP Project.

REFERENCE AND RESOURCE

Christenbery, T. (Ed.). (2018). *Evidence-based practice in nursing*. New York, NY: Springer Publishing Company.

RELATED TEXTBOOK

Christenbery, T. (Ed.). (2018). *Evidence-based practice in nursing*. New York, NY: Springer Publishing Company.

Chapter 11: Organizing and Evidence-Based Implementation Plan

Lesson 8.9

DNP PROJECT REPOSITORIES

BACKGROUND

The American Association of Colleges of Nursing (2015) recommends that a summary of DNP Project findings be shared beyond the academic setting. To facilitate that goal, DNP students and faculty should encourage use of digital DNP Project repositories (AACN, 2015). A repository is basically an electronic warehouse where intellectual property can be stored. "A digital repository for DNP final projects should be used to advance nursing practice by archiving and sharing of this work and outcomes" (AACN, 2015, p. 5).

There are different types of repositories. Determine whether a repository is available and/or required by your school. If your school does not have a repository available, some are available via professional nursing organizations. As you explore the best choice for your situation, remember to include your DNP team in the conversation. It may be necessary to de-identify agency information. You may also need to consider your plans for future publication. In most cases, use of a repository is considered a "pre publication" and does not interfere with publication in academic journals. However, read the details carefully. We recommend that an abstract of the DNP Project be uploaded to a repository at minimum.

LEARNING OBJECTIVES

- Compare options for digital repositories.
- Determine the best fit for your situation based on your school requirements.

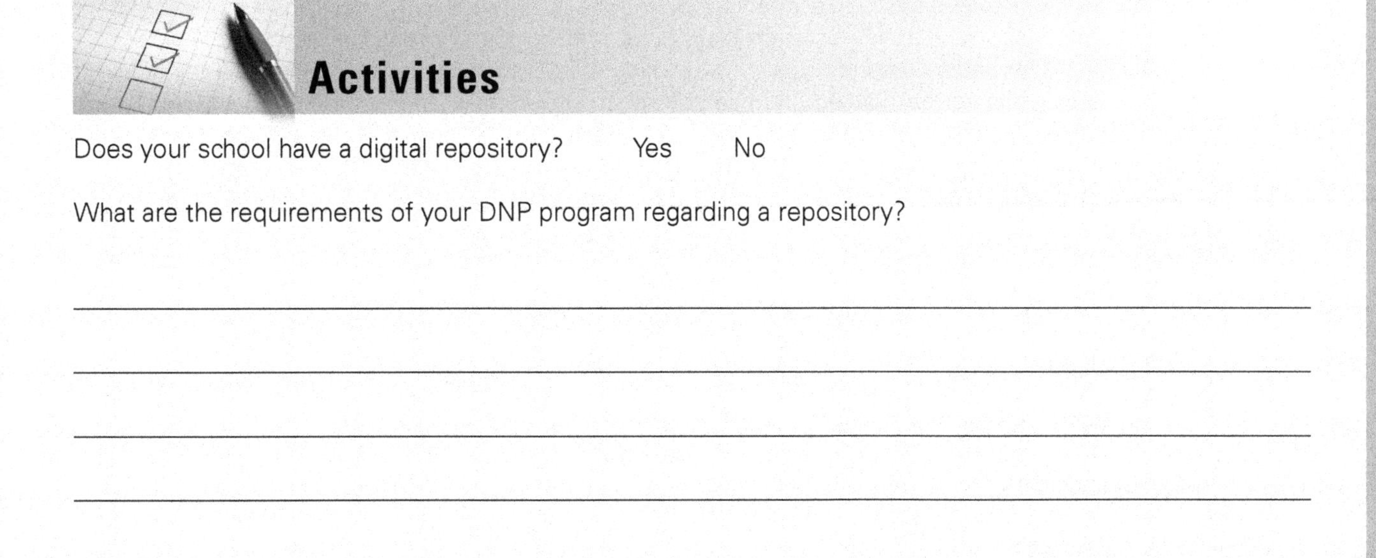

Activities

Does your school have a digital repository? Yes No

What are the requirements of your DNP program regarding a repository?

____

____

____

____

____

Explore two additional DNP Project repositories.

Virginia Henderson Global Nursing e-Repository:

- About Us: www.nursingrepository.org/about/
- Policies and Guidelines: www.nursingrepository.org/helpfulguides/

Doctors of Nursing Practice:

- About Us: www.doctorsofnursingpractice.org/about-us/
- Doctoral Project Repository: www.doctorsofnursingpractice.org/doctoral-project-repository/

Notes

Expert Commentary: DNP Project Repositories: David G. Campbell-O'Dell, DNP, APRN, FNP-BC, FAANP

The Doctoral project repository sponsored by Doctors of Nursing Practice, Inc. is an archive of curated documents. This repository is proud to accept completed projects and displays both abstracts and full projects to all site visitors. Submission of projects does not replace or presume any publication efforts. Each listing is owned by the individual who uploads the completed academic scholarly practice project. This service allows the nursing practice scholar to share ideas and work products with the scholarly practice and general public community.

Once uploaded and posted, the owner of the documents may share the URL web page address with any individual or organization desired. Each listing helps to educate patients, employers, organizations, and other stakeholders about DNP capabilities and competencies. Your posted scholarly practice doctoral project will:

- Support a collaborative engagement with practice partners and employers.
- Showcase a DNP-prepared professional's impact on improving outcomes.
- Disseminate DNP-generated content for all interested in the theme, environment, and process of impacting the complex processes of healthcare delivery.
- Build a foundation for sustainable change, future practice, and the research of practice scholarship.
- Support the growth and development of DNP students in the process of developing their projects.

Based on the findings of this lesson, my tentative plan for using a repository is to:

____

____

____

____

____

NEXT STEP

- Discuss your plan with your DNP team.

REFERENCE

American Association of Colleges of Nursing. (2015). *The doctor of nursing practice: Current issues and clarifying recommendations* [White paper]. Retrieved from https://www.aacnnursing.org/Portals/42/News/White-Papers/DNP-Implementation-TF-Report-8-15.pdf

Lesson 8.10

SOCIAL MEDIA AND ALTERNATIVE DISSEMINATION

BACKGROUND

From an academic perspective, White, Dudley-Brown, and Terhaar (2020) describe the 3P's of dissemination: (a) paper, (b) poster, and (c) presentation. The American Association of Colleges of Nursing (2015) recommends that some form of DNP Project dissemination occur beyond the academic setting.

LEARNING OBJECTIVES

- Describe the target users of given social media platforms.
- Consider alternative strategies for dissemination of DNP Project findings.

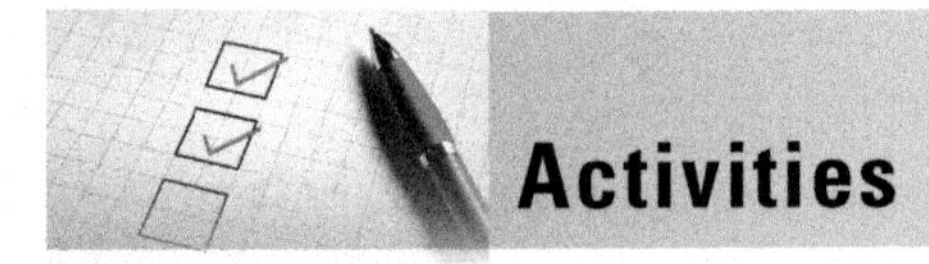

Activities

Read the Pew Research Center (2019) report and the Smith and Anderson (2018) report on social media use. Consider the descriptions of each social media platform. Highlight one social media platform for potential dissemination of DNP Project findings.

Facebook	Twitter	Pinterest
SnapChat	YouTube	Instagram

Other:

Selected Social Media Platform: ______________________________

Rationale for Selection: ______________________________

Tentative Dissemination Plan:

____

____

____

Review the following types of dissemination of DNP work and highlight three strategies you would like to use to disseminate your findings.

PRINT	PRESENTATION
Peer-reviewed journal Review of the literature for an article, project or practice or policy change	Scholarly presentation at professional meetings
Publications in professional publications such as newsletters and special reports	Continuing-education presentations for professionals Innovative instructional methods for students
Organizational policies and procedures Website content Budgetary analysis, review of systems processes and outcomes	Continuing education for staff, benefactors, and volunteers Bulletin boards in public locations

(continued)

PRINT	PRESENTATION
Health education material for the public	Presentations at support groups for specific conditions, wellness presentations for community groups
Letters to the editor, elected representatives on health issues	Testimony at public meetings
Digital media	
Blogs, websites maintained	Videos—YouTube, Vimeo Maintain a board on Pinterest Facebook page Twitter feed
Social media: Facebook, Twitter, Instagram, Tumblr, Reddit, etc.	SlideShare Infographic
eBooks and other electronic media	Public domain photos in repositories
Broadcast	
Social media streaming Periscope Blab Facebook streaming Google Hangouts	Television interviews Radio interviews Podcast interviews Podcasts
Performances	
Poetry Fiction Drawing Photographic exhibit	Theater performances Song
Reflective and Process Oriented	
Description of process of preparing, completing DNP Return on investment Return on expectations	Lessons learned regarding: Working, getting an education, having a family What happened after the degree? Was it worth it?
Other	
Grant applications Quality reports	Travel project to apply principles in the field

Source: From Smith-Stoner, M. (2018). *A guide to disseminating your DNP Project.* New York, NY: Springer Publishing Company.

NEXT STEP

- Discuss your plan with your DNP team.

REFERENCES AND RESOURCES

American Association of Colleges of Nursing. (2015). *The doctor of nursing practice: Current issues and clarifying recommendations* [White paper]. Retrieved from https://www.aacnnursing.org/Portals/42/News/White-Papers/DNP-Implementation-TF-Report-8-15.pdf

Pew Research Center. (2019). Social media fact sheets. Retrieved from https://www.pewresearch.org/internet/fact-sheet/social-media/

Smith, A., & Anderson, M. (2018). Social media use in 2018. Retrieved from https://www.pewinternet.org/2018/03/01/social-media-use-in-2018

White, K. M., Dudley-Brown, S., & Terhaar, M. F. (Eds.). (2020). *Translation of evidence into nursing and healthcare* (3rd ed.). New York, NY: Springer Publishing Company.

RELATED TEXTBOOK

Smith-Stoner, M. (2018). *A guide to disseminating your DNP Project.* New York, NY: Springer Publishing Company.

Unit 1: Planning Your Dissemination Strategy
Unit 2: Introducing Types of Dissemination Methods
Unit 3: Disseminating Your Work via Print Methods
Unit 4: Disseminating Your Work via Oral Presentation Methods
Unit 5: Disseminating Work via Art and Performance Methods
Unit 6: This Is the Beginning

CHAPTER SUMMARY

Completing the work in this chapter is a major achievement! As you take these lessons and apply them to your DNP work, utilize these lessons to stay organized.

NOTES

9

The DNP Experience

Molly J. Bradshaw, Tracy R. Vitale, and Irina Benenson

Lessons

OBJECTIVES

The purpose of this chapter is to suggest potential activities for the DNP experience and beyond. The lessons related to the activities may be relevant at different points of the DNP Project process depending on the nature of the project and trajectory of the DNP curriculum. They may also contain ideas that extend beyond graduation. Consult with your faculty for further clarification on the DNP practice experience at your school. By the end of this chapter, you will be able to:

- Understand the requirements for the DNP experience at their school.
- Incorporate the lessons and suggested activities into the DNP Practice Experience.
- Refer to these resources post-DNP graduation.

INTRODUCTION

According to the American Association of Colleges of Nursing (AACN; 2006, 2015), the nurse completing the DNP degree must complete a minimum of 1,000 practice hours beyond the BSN degree in order to achieve the desired outcomes. These DNP experience hours must be part of a supervised academic program. If a student has a master's degree in nursing that required clinical hours, they will often get credit for those hours upon admission to a post-master's DNP program. For students completing BSN–DNP programs, the hours are often collective, yet spent on both learning your new nursing role and completion of DNP-related work. Discuss your situation with your DNP academic advisors and refer to Lesson 1.10, The DNP Practice Experience and Practice Hours.

The hours spent toward application of the DNP Essentials and/or the DNP Project should be referred to as the "DNP practice experience" or "practice hours" (AACN, 2015). The faculty are responsible for assessing the needs of the students and determining the nature of the experience. The AACN (2015) notes that the immersion experience should allow for application and integration of the DNP Essentials into practice and not focus entirely on Essential VIII, Advance Nursing Practice (meaning patient contact or traditional nursing "clinicals"). The DNP practice experience should provide unique perspectives of the healthcare system, be nontraditional, interprofessional, and expand the skill set of the DNP student. Work hours do not count and students should not receive "credit" for years of experience (AACN, 2015). The goal is to expand horizons. Both faculty and students should carefully read the content of the AACN (2015) white paper regarding the practice experience, practice hours, and collaborative partnerships.

Because the DNP experience is widely interpreted, it begs the question, "What can I do to complete the required DNP experience hours?" The work of completing the DNP Project accounts for a good majority of the hours. However, the purpose of this chapter is to offer a series of lessons that guide you through potential activities that may contribute to your DNP experience. It is important to track all of the time spent on activities that related to both your DNP Project and the DNP Essentials. We are often asked if reading, writing, or spending time at the library counts. It may be reasonable to include a small, predetermined number of hours toward these activities. *This is up to your faculty and the policies at your school.*

We kick off this chapter by making a bold statement. Remember, you are completing a *doctoral* degree in nursing. Devoting numerous hours of reading, writing, and investigation of literature is a natural expectation. *Move* beyond *these activities.* Get out and engage in some aspect of healthcare, learning or the community that you have not explored. Several suggestions are offered. Short descriptions in the words of DNP students regarding their DNP practice experiences are found in the Chapter Summary. A log to help you track your DNP experience hours is found in the Appendix. Let's begin.

REFERENCES

American Association of Colleges of Nursing. (2006). *The essentials of doctoral education for advanced nursing practice.* Retrieved from https://www.aacnnursing.org/Portals/42/Publications/DNPEssentials.pdf

American Association of Colleges of Nursing. (2015). *The doctor of nursing practice: Current issues and clarifying recommendations* [White paper]. Retrieved from https://www.aacnnursing.org/Portals/42/News/White-Papers/DNP-Implementation-TF-Report-8-15.pdf

MY GOALS FOR THE DNP EXPERIENCE ARE TO:

Lesson 9.1

REVIEWING POLICIES ON THE DNP EXPERIENCE AT YOUR SCHOOL

BACKGROUND

As part of your program, you will complete a minimum of 1,000 clinical or "DNP experience" hours. These include clinical hours and the time put toward your DNP Project. As you consider your DNP practice experience, it is important to recognize what your school will allow. Some are very prescriptive, whereas others allow you to individualize your hours and have more leeway as long as your project aligns with the DNP Essentials.

Chamberlain University (2017) has identified some common practice experiences that align with the DNP Essentials. Consider some of the following activities and whether they align with your school's policy:

I. Scientific Underpinnings for Practice
- Attend a conference/workshop related to the project focus or EBP.
- Appraise literature for inclusion.
- Review EBP materials.
- Construct a PICO(T) (patient/population, intervention, comparison, outcome, time) question.
- Synthesize your literature review.

II. Organizational and Systems Leadership for Quality Improvement (QI) and Systems Thinking
- Attend/participate in QI meetings.
- Implement a rapid-cycle improvement project.
- Meet stakeholders.
- Conduct needs assessment of practice setting.
- Perform a SWOT (strengths, weaknesses, opportunities, threats) analysis.
- Develop a business plan.

III. Clinical Scholarship and Analytical Methods for Evidence-Based Practice
- Construct an institutional review board (IRB) proposal.
- Create tools for sustainability.
- Develop a professional portfolio.
- Prepare a final DNP Project paper or manuscript.
- Collect/analyze data.
- Disseminate DNP Project findings.
- Implement your DNP Project.

IV. Information Systems/Technology and Patient Care Technology for the Improvement and Transformation of Healthcare
- Use large data sets for data extraction activities.
- Evaluate web-based training/education.
- Design a mobile application for healthcare.
- Participate in health information technology as an evaluator.

V. Healthcare Policy for Advocacy in Healthcare
- Meet with an elected official for review of health policy.
- Participate on the committee at an institutional, local, state, and national level.

VI. Interprofessional Collaboration for Improving Patient and Population Health Outcomes
- Consult with mentor/preceptor.
- Consult with content experts.
- Participate in an interprofessional team.

VII. Clinical Prevention and Population Health for Improving the Nation's Health
- Collect/analyze epidemiological data.
- Identify gaps in care for individuals, communities, and/or populations.
- Implement and evaluate health promotion/disease prevention.

VIII. Advanced Nursing Practice
- Assess clients, populations, or organizations in the practice setting.
- Implement therapeutic interventions in the practice/community/non direct care setting.
- Disseminate knowledge to other healthcare providers and community members.
- Consult with experts regarding nursing practice.
- Mentor other healthcare providers.

LEARNING OBJECTIVES

- Describe acceptable DNP hours based on the policies of your DNP Project.
- Create a form to log your DNP hours.

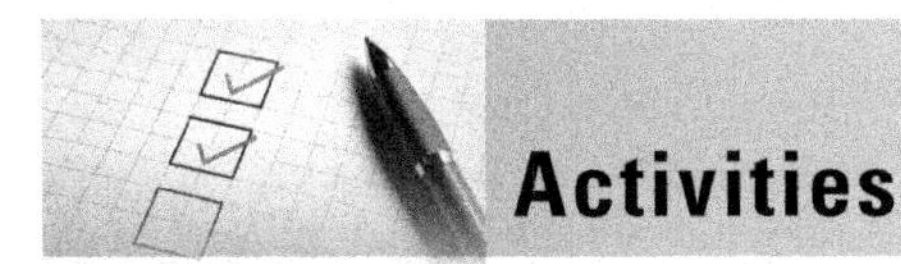

Activities

Develop a log of hours completed and align your hours with a DNP Essential.

DATE	DESCRIPTION OF EXPERIENCE HOURS	DNP ESSENTIAL	# OF HOURS ANTICIPATED	# HOURS COMPLETED	CUMULATIVE HOURS
01/02/2019	Meeting with CNO to discuss DNP Project needs	II, VI	1	1.5	1.5

NEXT STEPS

- Review the log with your chair to confirm the appropriateness of your DNP hours.
- List any questions you have for your DNP chair.

REFERENCES

American Association of Colleges of Nursing. (2006). *The essentials of doctoral education for advanced nursing practice.* Retrieved from https://www.aacnnursing.org/Portals/42/Publications/DNPEssentials.pdf

American Association of Colleges of Nursing. (2015). *The doctor of nursing practice: Current issues and clarifying recommendations* [White paper]. Retrieved from https://www.aacnnursing.org/Portals/42/News/White-Papers/DNP-Implementation-TF-Report-8-15.pdf

Chamberlain University. (2017). Doctorate of nursing practice (DNP) practicum activities. Retrieved from https://www.chamberlain.edu/docs/default-source/academics-admissions/dnp/practicum-activities_form_073015.pdf?status=Temp&sfvrsn=0.42956183198839426

Lesson 9.2

PLANNING A PRECEPTED DNP EXPERIENCE

BACKGROUND

The American Association of Colleges of Nursing (AACN; 2015) suggests that DNP experiences extend beyond direct patient care. This may include indirect care practices, including larger organizations (i.e., Red Cross, organizational information technology departments, community health organizations, long-term care facilities, urgent care facilities, prisons, school systems, public health, non government agencies, or private corporations). In addition to having a precepted experience, it is possible that one of these locations may also be able to translate to the site for the DNP Project (AACN, 2015).

When considering practice experiences, learning objectives should align with the DNP Essentials and application of theory and evidence to practice (AACN, 2015). DNP practice experiences are a great opportunity for the student to interact and collaborate both intraprofessionally and interprofessionally in order to facilitate leadership and communication. The AACN (2015) outlines that the DNP program practice experiences should provide:

- Systematic opportunities for feedback and reflection
- In-depth work/mentorship with experts in nursing, as well as other disciplines
- Opportunities for meaningful student engagement within practice environments
- Opportunities for building and assimilating knowledge for advanced nursing practice at a high level of complexity
- Opportunities for further application, synthesis, and expansion of learning
- Experience in the context of advanced nursing practice within which the final DNP Project is completed
- Opportunities for integrating and synthesizing all of the DNP Essentials and role requirements necessary to demonstrate achievement of defined outcomes in an area of advanced nursing practice

The purpose of this lesson is to ensure that you are adequately prepared for planning a precepted DNP experience.

LEARNING OBJECTIVES

- Outline the DNP Project requirements at your school.
- Identify potential precepted DNP experiences.
- List questions to clarify with faculty.

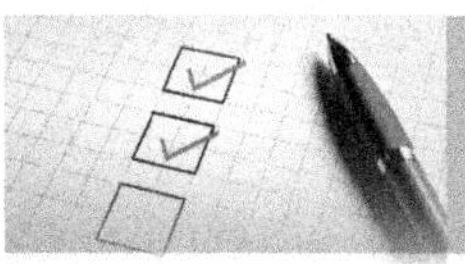

Activities

Using the information from Lesson 9.1 and Lesson 9.3, consider potential precepted experiences that will help meet your needs related to your program track and DNP Project.

Are there any limitations on the requirements of a precepted DNP experience set forth by your academic institution?

____

____

____

What are your experiential needs:

____

____

____

What experiential needs will help you develop, implement, and evaluate your DNP Project?

____

____

____

Who in your professional network may be able to work with you on a precepted DNP experience?

____

____

____

NEXT STEPS

- Organize a plan with your faculty to facilitate these experiences.
- Review requirements of a precepted experience and the necessary documentation of its occurrence.

REFERENCES

American Association of Colleges of Nursing. (2006). *The essentials of doctoral education for advanced nursing practice.* Retrieved from https://www.aacnnursing.org/Portals/42/Publications/DNPEssentials.pdf

American Association of Colleges of Nursing. (2015). *The doctor of nursing practice: Current issues and clarifying recommendations* [White paper]. Retrieved from https://www.aacnnursing.org/Portals/42/News/White-Papers/DNP-Implementation-TF-Report-8-15.pdf

Lesson 9.3

MAPPING THE DNP ESSENTIALS TO YOUR PROJECT

BACKGROUND

The American Association of Colleges of Nursing's (AACN; 2006) DNP Essentials "outline the curricular elements and competencies that are required for schools conferring the Doctor of Nursing Practice degree" (p. 8). All DNP Essentials should be met by the end of the DNP program. The DNP Project provides the student with an opportunity to operationalize skills and demonstrate competency in the DNP Essentials. Students are responsible for accruing hours that have contributed to their DNP experience.

The Essentials are:

1. Scientific Underpinnings
2. Organizational and Systems Leadership for Quality Improvement
3. Clinical Scholarship and Analytical Methods for Evidence-Based Practice
4. Information Systems and Patient Care Technology
5. Healthcare Policy for Advocacy in Healthcare
6. Interprofessional Collaboration for Improving Patient and Population Health
7. Clinical Prevention and Population Health for Improving the Nation's Health
8. Advanced Nursing Practice

LEARNING OBJECTIVE

- The learner is able to list potential activities that help meet the objectives of the DNP Project while also meeting the DNP Essentials.

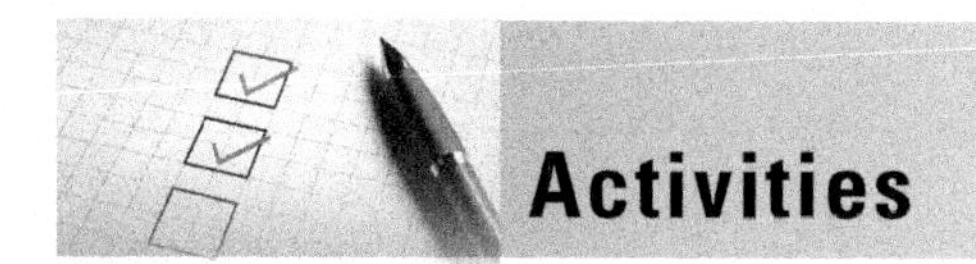

Activities

Complete the following mapping activity to plan for anticipated activities related to the DNP Project.

DNP ESSENTIAL	PLANNED DNP EXPERIENCE	EVIDENCE ASSIGNMENT/ EXPERIENCE HAS BEEN MET
i. Scientific Underpinnings for Practice		
ii. Organizational and Systems Leadership for Quality Improvement and Systems Thinking		
iii. Clinical Scholarship and Analytical Methods for Evidence-Based Practice		
iv. Information Systems/ Technology and Patient Care Technology for the Improvement and Transformation of Healthcare		
v. Healthcare Policy for Advocacy in Healthcare		
vi. Interprofessional Collaboration for Improving Patient and Population Health Outcomes		
vii. Clinical Prevention and Population Health for Improving the Nation's Health		
viii. Advanced Nursing Practice		

NEXT STEP

Questions from faculty/DNP chair regarding DNP Project Experience Log:

____

____

____

REFERENCE

American Association of Colleges of Nursing. (2006). *The essentials of doctoral education for advanced nursing practice.* Retrieved from https://www.aacnnursing.org/Portals/42/Publications/DNPEssentials.pdf

Lesson 9.4

CREATING A DNP PORTFOLIO

BACKGROUND

A DNP portfolio is a collection of your work that showcases different assignments or elements of your doctoral scholarship. It could be used to demonstrate learning outcomes (DNP Essentials) presented during a job interview or included as a part of your current promotion/tenure procedure. The DNP portfolio is not a substitution for a DNP Project (American Association of Colleges of Nursing, 2015).

Before you develop a DNP portfolio, consider its purpose and intended audience. Determine whether the DNP portfolio will be organized in hard copy or electronically. If it is electronic, consider whether you will be able to access it beyond graduation. Remember that certain information or assignments may need to be de-identified if it is accessible by the public.

LEARNING OBJECTIVES

- Determine the purpose and intended audience.
- Identify the components of the portfolio.
- Ensure safe-keeping of sensitive information.
- Explore the options for creating a dedicated website.

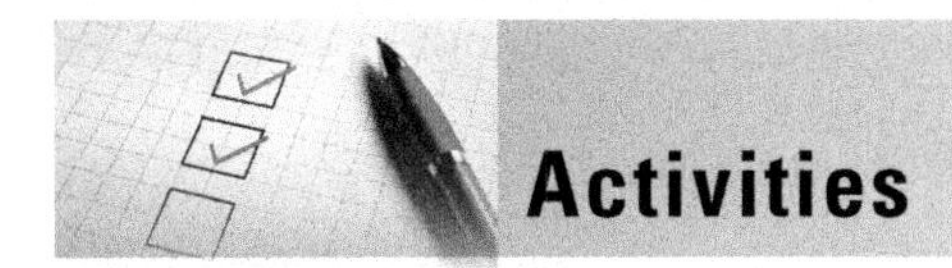

Activities

Complete these prompts.

DNP portfolio:

- Purpose:
- Intended audience:
- List potential items to include:
  - Assignments?
  - Unique or creative work?
  - DNP Project executive summary?
  - Other
  - Consider mapping content to the DNP Essentials

Maintaining a website-based DNP portfolio is an excellent way to ensure that your portfolio is easily accessible. There are several companies that offer free capabilities for creating websites. One of our favorites is WIX.com. Explore their services (www.wix.com).

Review these examples of DNP portfolios:

- https://npmollyb.wixsite.com/who4nprx
- https://tracyvitalednp.wixsite.com/mysite
- https://rampages.us/peggiepowellfnp
- https://depaul.digication.com/linda_a_graf_dnp_portfolio/Welcome/published

NEXT STEPS

- Discuss your plan with your DNP team and DNP faculty.
- Develop a DNP portfolio.

REFERENCES AND RESOURCES

American Association of Colleges of Nursing. (2015). *The doctor of nursing practice: Current issues and clarifying recommendations* [White paper]. Retrieved from https://www.aacnnursing.org/Portals/42/News/White-Papers/DNP-Implementation-TF-Report-8-15.pdf

Havercamp, J., & Vogt, M. (2015). Beyond academic evidence: Uses of technology within e-portfolio for the doctor of nursing practice program. *Journal of Professional Nursing, 31*(4), 284–289. doi: 10.1016/j.profnurs.2015.03.007

Melander, S., Hardin-Pierce, M., & Ossage, J. (2018). Development of a rubric for evaluation of the DNP portfolio. *Nursing Education Perspectives, 39*(5), 312–314. doi: 10.1097/01.NEP.0000000000000381

University of Arizona. (2019). DNP portfolio. Retrieved from https://www.nursing.arizona.edu/resources/dnp-portfolio

RELATED TEXTBOOK

Smith-Stoner, M. (2018). *A guide to disseminating your DNP Project*. New York, NY: Springer Publishing Company.

Lesson 9.5

HONING SKILLS IN HEALTH LITERACY

BACKGROUND

In a report titled "Health Literacy: A Prescription to End Confusion," the Institute of Medicine (2004) outlined the current state of health literacy by presenting a cultural context, described needed skills, and talked about strategies to improve patient communication. Health literacy is defined in the report as the degree to which someone can understand and use health information to make decisions. The literature suggests that assessing the level of health literacy among patients may be time-consuming and ineffective. Rather, it suggests using a "universal precaution," which assumes a basic level of health literacy among all patients (Agency for Healthcare Research and Quality [AHRQ], 2015).

Honing health literacy skills can be time well spent for DNP students. To learn more about health literacy, consider completing the free modules available from the Centers for Disease Control and Prevention (CDC) (www.cdc.gov/healthliteracy/gettraining.html).

It may also be beneficial to spend time reviewing materials used to communicate with patients. For example, if you are developing a patient tool kit as part of your DNP Project, you need to ensure that it meets health literacy standards. Explore this resource:

Agency for Healthcare Research and Quality. (2015). *Health literacy universal precautions toolkit* (2nd ed.). Rockville, MD: Author. Retrieved from https://www.ahrq.gov/health-literacy/quality-resources/tools/literacy-toolkit/healthlittoolkit2.html

LEARNING OBJECTIVES

- Complete the free health literacy training and examine the AHRQ Tool kit.
- Assess the understandability of patient materials in your nursing practice.

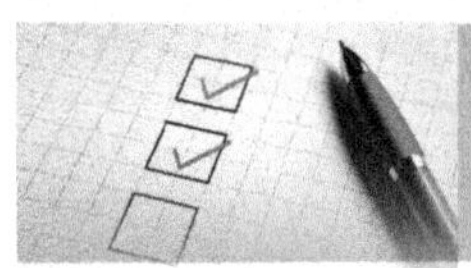

Activities

1. Use the tools from the CDC Clear Communication Index to assess whether materials for patients are understandable.

2. Select a written or audiovisual piece of patient educational material.

   Item selected: ______________________________

   Link: CDC Modified Clear Communication Index

   Final score: ______________________________

3. Reflect on what you have learned:

____

____

____

____

____

____

____

____

NEXT STEPS

- Continue honing skills in health literacy.
- Use universal precautions and resources in your nursing practice.

REFERENCE AND RESOURCE

Institute of Medicine. (2004). *Health literacy: A prescription to end confusion.* Washington, DC: The National Academies Press. Retrieved from https://www.nap.edu/catalog/10883/health-literacy-a-prescription-to-end-confusion

RELATED TEXTBOOK

Marshall, E. S., & Broome, M. E. (2020). *Transformational leadership in nursing* (3rd ed.). New York, NY: Springer Publishing Company.

Chapter 3: Current Challenges in Complex Health Organizations and the Quadruple Aim

Improving Health Literacy to Increase Safety and Patient Engagement in Healthcare (p. 73)

Lesson 9.6

INCREASING YOUR POLITICAL AWARENESS AND ENGAGEMENT

BACKGROUND

Awareness and engagement in policy development are key to changing health outcomes. DNP-prepared nurses should have skill sets to become influential in policy conversation, otherwise nursing influence on policy is lost. Without influence, our ability to transform care is limited (Dreher & Smith Glasgow, 2017). Many nursing organizations also have policy/advocacy information available on their website. The American Nurses Association (n.d.) has an Advocacy Toolkit Policy; National League for Nursing (n.d.) has an Advocacy Action Center where you can sign up for alerts, identify/contact legislators, and follow current legislation.

Expert Commentary: Understanding the Role of the DNP in Health Policy:
Tracy R. Vitale, DNP, RNC-OB, C-EFM, NE-BC

During our doctoral education, we were challenged as students to identify key policy makers. What was originally perceived to be a civic lesson quickly turned into a reality check. When the class was presented with the headshots of some obviously recognizable figures like the President of the United States and the state governor, overall confidence quickly decreased as the images of our state senators, local representatives, and other key players, including the U.S. Secretary of Health and Human Services and chair of the Institute of Medicine committee on the Future of Nursing, Donna Shalala, were presented and we did not know who they were.

As nurses, especially those with a DNP, it is our obligation not only to be aware but also to be active in health policy. This may include working within an organization at the local, state, or national level. Regardless of our intended roles, our lawmakers are guiding the way we practice. On a state level, legislators are currently making decisions on topics, including a joint protocol with physicians, a multistate nurse licensure compact, nurse staffing ratios, requiring newly licensed RNs to attain a BSN within 10 years of initial licensure as a condition of license renewal, minimal staffing, and other legislation impacting nurses and overall healthcare delivered. We would be remiss if we didn't also acknowledge the historic passing of The Patient Protection and Affordable Care Act (shortened to Affordable Care Act and nicknamed "Obamacare"), which was signed into law in March 2010 and has been challenged in recent years. You can review the Affordable Care Act at www.hhs.gov/healthcare/about-the-aca/index.html (HHS.gov, n.d.).

LEARNING OBJECTIVES

- The learner will be able to identify key policy makers in her or his geographic area.
- The learner will be able to identify current state legislation impacting nurses/ the nursing profession.
- The learner will be able to develop a letter to a local/state representative on a healthcare topic of interest.

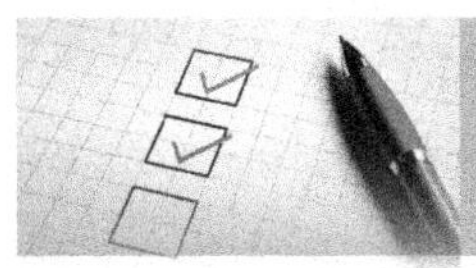

Activities

1. Using the website links, identify your representative and his or her contact information:

   State governor: www.usa.gov/state-governor

   U.S. senators: www.senate.gov/general/contact_information/senators_cfm.cfm

   U.S. representative: www.house.gov/representatives/find-your-representative

   Federal, state, and local representatives: www.usa.gov/elected-officials

2. Identify the names of the people in the following positions in your state/area:

   State governor

   U.S. senator:

   U.S. senator:

   National representative:

   National representative:

   Local representative (state senator/assembly/etc.):

   Local representative (state senator/assembly/etc.):

3. Using the information collected, navigate your state's legislative website and identify a bill currently being considered. Review the bill, identify any groups that are supporting/opposing the bill, and determine your stance. Once you have done this, draft a letter to the appropriate representative supporting/opposing the bill using the following sites as samples for templates:

   https://www.ncsbn.org/APRN_formletter_Legislator_web.pdf

   http://www.nea.org/home/19657.htm

   http://advocacy.aone.org/legislative-basics/how-communicate-and-build-relationship-your-legislators

NEXT STEPS

- Identify political/advocacy efforts being done by any of your professional organizations.
- Discuss with your mentors/leaders any advocacy they have been involved in.

REFERENCES AND RESOURCES

American Association of Nurse Practitioners. (n.d.). Championing the NP role and amplifying the NP voice. Retrieved from https://www.aanp.org/advocacy

American Nurses Association. (n.d.). ANA advocacy toolkit. Retrieved from https://www.nursingworld.org/practice-policy/advocacy/ana-advocacy-toolbox/

American Organization for Nursing Leadership. (2019). How to communicate with your legislators. Retrieved from http://advocacy.aone.org/legislative-basics/how-communicate-and-build-relationship-your-legislators

Dreher, H. M., & Smith Glasgow, M. E. (2017). *DNP role development for doctoral advanced nursing practice* (2nd ed.). New York, NY: Springer Publishing Company.

HHS.gov. (n.d.). About the Affordable Care Act. Retrieved from https://www.hhs.gov/healthcare/about-the-aca/index.html

National Council of State Boards of Nursing. (n.d.). Template letter to a legislator. Retrieved from https://www.ncsbn.org/APRN_formletter_Legislator_web.pdf

National Education Association. (n.d.). Writing to your legislators. Retrieved from http://www.nea.org/home/19657.htm

National League for Nursing. (n.d.). Advocacy action center. Retrieved from http://www.nln.org/advocacy-public-policy/legislative-issues

RELATED TEXTBOOK

Dreher, H. M., & Smith Glasgow, M. E. (2017). *DNP role development for doctoral advanced nursing practice* (2nd ed.). New York, NY: Springer Publishing Company.

Lesson 9.7

CREATING BUSINESS PLANS

BACKGROUND

Doctorally prepared nurses should develop an ability to engage in fiscal conversations. Managing department budgets and participating in conversations related to reimbursements are natural expectations. In fact, as a DNP experience, spending time with the organization's chief financial officer may provide some unique insight.

Beyond engagement in pre established business, some DNP students may consider an entrepreneurial approach to the work of the DNP Project. Is there a product that you want to sell to improve health outcomes? Is there a service you want to provide? There are time limits to DNP Projects. However, developing a business plan to later launch a business could be a beneficial learning experience.

LEARNING OBJECTIVES

- Review some practical tips for getting started.
- Explore further reading and resources for writing business plans.
- Get inspired by DNP student ideas.

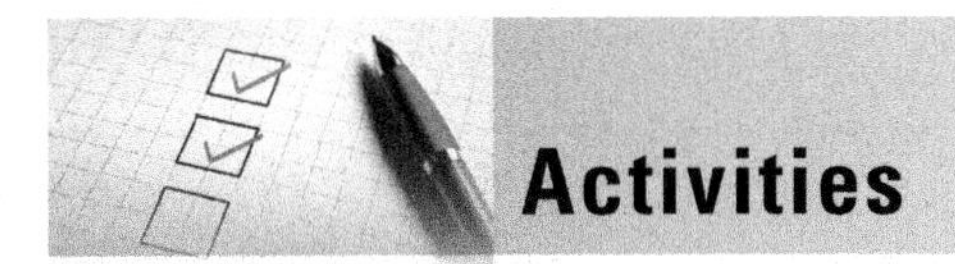

Activities

Business plans start with a product or service that you want to sell to a consumer. Ramsey Solutions (2019) offers some basic tips to get started. Answer the questions using their prompts:

Why do you want to start this business?

Logistics:

Product/service offered:

Schedule:

Budget:

What will you charge?

What will your policies be?

Make it official:

Will there be incorporation, licensing, and so on?

How will income and expenses be tracked?

Will you need start-up funding?

Ensure proper tax withholding.

Put yourself out there:

How will you advertise your services/product?

Examples of DNP student projects turned to businesses:

- Development of a mobile app
- Development of a mobile health clinic
- Development of an online business

As this lesson concludes, remember that you do not have to go into debt or start a large-scale business at first. Make plans to scale business at a reasonable pace.

NEXT STEPS

- To learn more, visit www.daveramsey.com/blog/the-basics-of-starting-a-business
- Draft a plan for discussion with your DNP team.

REFERENCES AND RESOURCES

Ramsey Solutions. (2019). Basics of starting a business. Retrieved from https://www.daveramsey.com/blog/the-basics-of-starting-a-business

Wright, C. (2017). *Business boutique: A woman's guide to making money doing what she loves*. Brentwood, TN: Ramsey Press. Retrieved from https://academy.businessboutique.com/store/?_ga=2.83802838.1978302816.1558024788-1595694451.1558024788

Lesson 9.8

DEVELOPING MARKETING PLANS AND STORYTELLING

BACKGROUND

"Marketing" is a term used to describe a series of activities designed to create buy-in among consumers. The consumer may be seeking information, services, or a product. However, there is definite skill and science involved in the process. The DNP student and graduate must have a marketing strategy and skills. Effective marketing helps others understand the abilities of DNP-prepared nurses and engages our patients, staff, stakeholders, and other "consumers" in our products and services. Creating a clear marketing message is the first step.

Donald Miller (2017) is the author of the best-selling book, *Building a StoryBrand: Clarify Your Message So Customers Will Listen*. He has developed a marketing framework that he calls the "SB7 Framework." He bases this marketing strategy on the ancient art of storytelling. He believes that by telling a story well, you create effective marketing. According to Miller, a good story starts with a character (consumer) who encounters a problem. The consumer then meets a guide (DNP student) who understands his or her fear and gives the consumer a skill, solution, or product to solve his or her problem. Effective marketing should always present a call to action with a clear indication of the success or failure that could occur. In the end, the consumer is the hero of the story (consumer/patient).

As you work with organizations to improve health outcomes, consider the impact of marketing. Does the organization market its services well? Do you market yourself well as a professional? Use the DNP practice experience to improve your business-related marketing skills.

LEARNING OBJECTIVES

- Complete the 5-Minute Marketing Makeover.
- Identify one way to improve the marketing related to your DNP Project or practice.

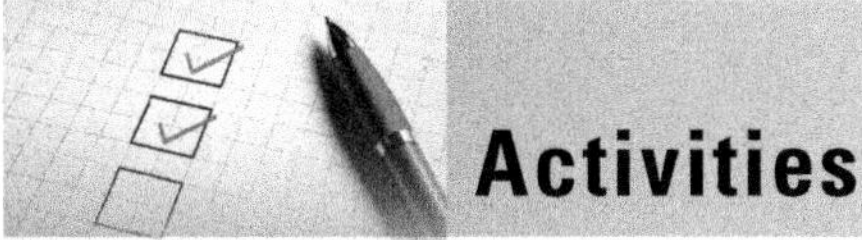

Activities

Go to https://storybrand.com to read more about Story Brand. Based on your DNP Project or DNP practice experience, identify an element that would benefit from effective marketing. List it here:

If you are having difficulty thinking of a practice application, consider how you will market your DNP career when you graduate.

On the website https://storybrand.com, scroll down and complete the free 5-Minute Marketing Makeover. Based on what you learned, list three things you will do to improve the marketing of your DNP Project or practice.

1.

2.

3.

NEXT STEPS

- Discuss your plans with your DNP team.
- Read the complete book by Donald Miller.

REFERENCE AND RESOURCE

Miller, D. (2017). *Building a story brand: Clarify your message so customers will listen.* Nashville, TN: Harper Collins Leadership. https://www.amazon.com/Building-StoryBrand-Clarify-Message-Customers/dp/0718033329

Lesson 9.9

DATA VISUALIZATION, INFOGRAPHICS, AND LISTICLES

BACKGROUND

Translating data into visual form makes it easier to understand. It is estimated that 65% of people are visual learners; the brain can process visual images 60,000 times faster than information written in words (Bradshaw & Porter, 2017). As part of the DNP practice experience, consider incorporating data visualization into your DNP Project dissemination plan.

Beyond data visualization, there are infographics and listicles. An infographic is composed of synthesized data that are visually translated, arranged in a way that tells a story, have a call to action, and are a verifiable source of information (Bradshaw & Porter, 2017). Infographics are often best suited for quantitative data. For qualitative information consider writing a listicle. A listicle is information, written in a way that combines the concepts of "article" and "lists." Listicles often have a cardinal number in the title, have an opening comment, and are supported by key information in list format. At the end, there should also be a closing remark, call to action, and a verifiable source of information.

LEARNING OBJECTIVES

- Gather data that need to be presented.
- Investigate resources for developing an infographic or listicle.

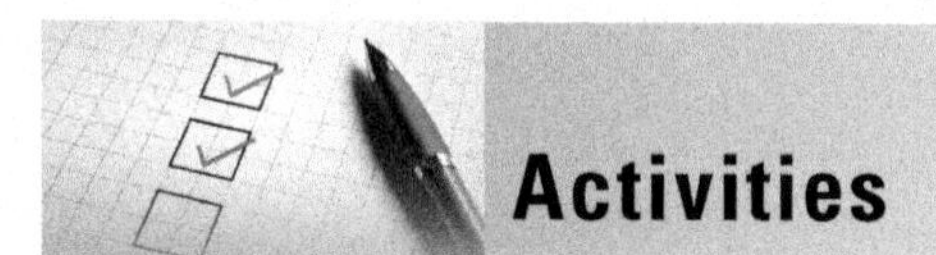

Activities

Data Visualization

Figure 9.1 features the coxcomb diagram by Florence Nightingale, an example of organizing large data content. In this figure, each month of the year is represented by a wedge with portions of the wedge representing the percentage of deaths resulting from certain causes. The outside of the wedge is light gray and represents the largest proportion of deaths from contagious diseases such as cholera and typhus. The middle section of the wedge is dark gray and represents deaths from other causes, whereas the inside of the wedge closest to the center represents deaths from wounds. Further information can be found on the YouTube video: "Lady with a Pie Chart" (https://youtu.be/lLzrYJ3OR7E).

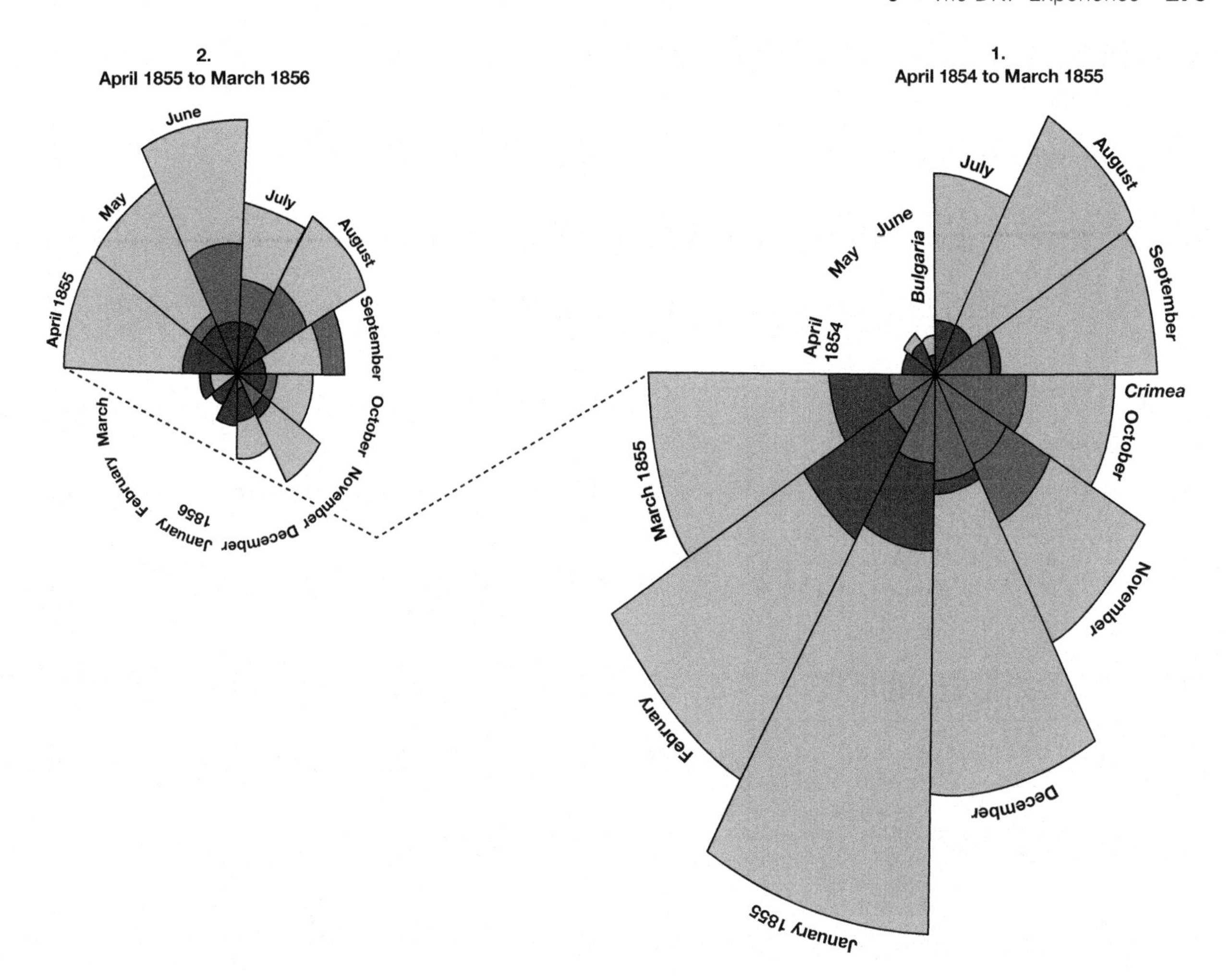

Figure 9.1 Florence Nightingale's coxcomb diagram.
Source: From Nightingale, F. (1858). *Notes on matters affecting the health, efficiency, and hospital administration of the British army.*

Infographics

1. Review the following article, noting the process for developing an infographic.

   Bradshaw, M., & Porter, S. (2017). Infographics: A new tool for the nursing classroom. *Nurse Educator, 42*(2), 57–59. doi:10.1097/nne.0000000000000316

2. After planning and sketching your infographics, explore the free version of Piktochart (https://piktochart.com). Select the free option for infographics and use their predesigned templates to create your infographic. Visit https://encompass.eku.edu/swps_facultygallery/42 for an infographic example.

Listicles

Explore these links to help you create listicles.

Mulholland, B. (2018). Writing a listicle: The 11 step guide and why they are awesome. Retrieved from https://www.process.st/listicle/

Shook, M. (2018). 5 simple tips for writing awesome listicles for medium. Retrieved from https://medium.com/publishous/5-simple-tips-for-writing-awesome-listicles-for-medium-d3e6e7112fa6

NEXT STEPS

- Discuss your plans with your DNP team.
- Work toward utilization of these concepts in practice beyond graduation.

REFERENCES AND RESOURCES

Bradshaw, M., & Porter, S. (2017). Infographics: A new tool for the nursing classroom. *Nurse Educator, 42* (2), 57–59. doi:10.1097/nne.0000000000000316

Mulholland, B. (2018). Writing a listicle: The 11 step guide and why they are awesome.

Nightingale, F. (1858). *Notes on matters affecting the health, efficiency, and hospital administration of the British army.*

Shook, M. (2018). 5 simple tips for writing awesome listicles for medium. Retrieved from https://medium.com/publishous/5-simple-tips-for-writing-awesome-listicles-for-medium-d3e6e7112fa6

Lesson 9.10

DNP ENGAGEMENT IN RESEARCH

> To him who devotes his life to science, nothing can give more happiness than increasing the number of discoveries, but his cup of joy is full when the results of his studies immediately find practical applications.
>
> —*Louis Pasteur*

BACKGROUND

The difference between PhD- and DNP-prepared nurses is well documented and was outlined in Chapter 1, Understanding the DNP Degree and DNP Project. Although the education and roles may have very different focuses, there is a wealth of opportunity for collaboration in which each can utilize his or her strengths in research. One such opportunity is the ability for DNPs to engage in research. The collaboration can allow for the dissemination of knowledge, scientific inquiry, and translational research (American Association of Colleges of Nursing [AACN], 2004, 2006, 2016).

In 2018, the AACN supported that PhDs and DNPs need to partner with each other in order to translate newly generated knowledge into practices. This can be achieved through implementation science, which is geared toward efforts to "identify barriers (personal, economic, and management) to effective evidence translation and examines the causal relationships of the interventions and the outcomes" (AACN, 2018, p. 4). How do we do this? Trautman, Idzik, Hammersla, and Rosseter (2018) suggest that DNP- and PhD-prepared nurses use their individual skill sets in an effort to advance each other's work. Consider a DNP-prepared nurse leader who recognizes a clinical problem that needs to be addressed based on available data from the organization. A PhD nurse scientist, in collaboration with the DNP nurse leader, can design a study to collect data to explore variations in the clinical problem. The DNP can explore current literature for potential implementation strategies while bringing organizational leadership expertise about potential financial implications and leadership to further improve the design of the research to answer this clinical question (Trautman et al., 2018). As the PhD-prepared nurse can design an interventional study, the DNP-prepared nurse can lead the shift of changing practice based on the results of the study.

LEARNING OBJECTIVES

- Recall and compare the differences between PhD and DNP areas of expertise related to research.
- Identify potential research collaborators who focus on a similar area of interest.

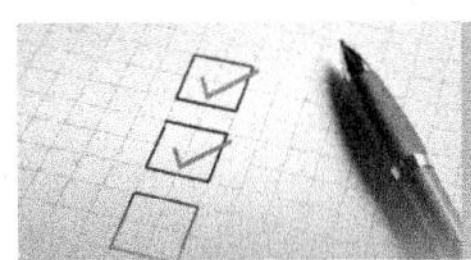

Activities

Identify nurse researchers at your facility who have a focus in your area of interest and review their publications on their work.

Are there recommendations that would warrant the work of a DNP in translating this evidence?

Are there recommendations for future scholarship/research that you could participate in?

How would you propose their evidence be used for translation into practice?

NEXT STEPS

- List any questions you have for your DNP team.
- Consider establishing a plan for future research.

REFERENCES AND RESOURCES

American Association of Colleges of Nursing. (2004). *AACN position statement on the practice Doctorate in nursing.* Washington, DC: Author.

American Association of Colleges of Nursing. (2006). *The essentials of doctoral education for advanced nursing practice.* Washington, DC: Author.

American Association of Colleges of Nursing. (2016). Advancing healthcare transformation: A new era for academic nursing. Retrieved from http://www.aacnnursing.org/Portals/42/Publications/AACN-New-Era-Report.pdf

American Association of Colleges of Nursing. (2018). Defining scholarship for academic nursing. Retrieved from http://www.aacnnursing.org/News-Information/Position-Statements-White-Papers/Defining-Scholarship-Nursing

Trautman, D. E., Idzik, S., Hammersla, M., & Rosseter, R. (2018). Advancing scholarship through translational research: The role of PhD and DNP prepared nurses. *The Online Journal of Issues in Nursing, 23*(2). doi: 10.3912/OJIN.Vol23No02Man02

RELATED TEXTBOOK

Melnyk, B. M., & Morrison-Beedy, D. (2018). *Intervention research and evidence-based quality improvement: Designing, conducting, analyzing, and funding* (2nd ed.). New York, NY: Springer Publishing Company.

Lesson 9.11

DNP ENGAGEMENT IN SYSTEMATIC REVIEW

BACKGROUND

A systematic review is often considered the basis for evidence-based practice (Holly, Salmond, & Saimbert, 2017). Systematic reviews can be helpful in interpreting knowledge from a large collection of studies about a particular topic or situation (Staffileno & Foreman, 2018). In a systematic review there is a focused question and specific protocol used to identify, critique, and eventually provide a collective summary of primary research (Baker & Weeks, 2014). There are several organizations that collect and publish systematic reviews, including Campbell Collaboration, Cochrane Collaboration, and Joanna Briggs Institute. These organizations provide guidance and training, as well as the necessary computer software to support evidence synthesis (Staffileno & Foreman, 2018).

The American Association of Colleges of Nursing (2015) states that systematic review as a DNP Project does not allow for integrating scholarship into practice. However, a systematic review can set the stage for evidence transfer/translation and provide a DNP with a skill set to change practice.

Expert Commentary: Use of Systematic Review in Nurse Practitioner Practice: Irina Benenson, DNP, FNP-C, CEN

A long time ago I read a study about what makes a good clinician. Some factors you might think were important, like grades achieved during your training, were irrelevant. What correlated the best was the number of medical journals a clinician read. I don't know whether that means good clinicians read more journals or reading more journals makes a better clinician. One thing I know is that reading and understanding medical literature requires critical analysis skills. However, it is not until I performed my first systematic review that I started to develop these skills.

Before knowing how to appraise literature, I really wasn't aware of all the things that can go wrong in a study, and I didn't know what to look for to decide whether the results were really credible. I thought the authors knew a lot more than I did, and I trusted them to a degree that was not warranted. The more I immersed myself in reviewing the literature and learned about fundamental bias of research (flaws in the process of participant selection, data collection and interpretation), the less I was willing to be a passive absorber of information. I learned to question the results and reach my own conclusions on what the best evidence is. Literature reading skills helped me to be a better consumer of medical journals and a better clinician. Understanding studies and making clinical decisions based on valid evidence became crucial to my everyday practice of diagnosing and treating patients—which of course is the ultimate purpose of medical research.

LEARNING OBJECTIVES

- Implement learned skills in using knowledge to integrate findings from a CSR into practice.
- Examine policies and clinical practice guidelines for integration of systematic reviews in their development.

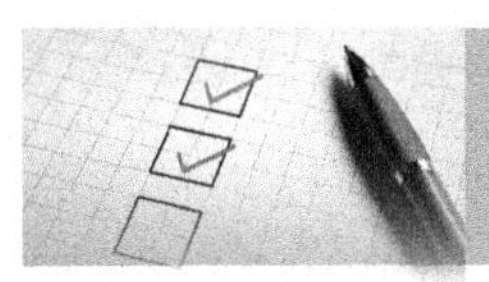

Activities

We have already discussed that DNPs are responsible for transferring knowledge into practice. With that said, if you find yourself able to participate in conducting a systematic review, you can bring the knowledge transfer component into play. Examples of knowledge transfer/translation options include using the results of the systematic review to:

- Develop an evidence-based teaching tool.
- Develop a pilot study to implement recommendations.
- Develop or update of an existing practice policy.
- Develop clinical audit criteria.

Identify a systematic review relevant to your DNP Project. Appraise the review using the Critical Appraisal Skills Programme Systematic Review (CASP SR) Checklist: (https://casp-uk.net/wp-content/uploads/2018/01/CASP-Systematic-Review-Checklist_2018.pdf).

List three ways the information can be applied in practice:

1.

2.

3.

NEXT STEP

- Consider additional training on the process of systematic review.

REFERENCES AND RESOURCES

American Association of Colleges of Nursing. (2015). *The doctorate of nursing practice: Current issues and clarifying recommendations*. Retrieved from https://www.aacnnursing.org/Portals/42/News/White-Papers/DNP-Implementation-TF-Report-8-15.pdf

Baker, K. A., & Weeks, S. M. (2014). An overview of systematic review. *Journal of PeriAnesthesia Nursing, 29*(6), 454–458. doi: 10.1016/j.jopan.2014.07.002

Holly, C., Salmond, S., & Saimbert, M. (Eds.). (2017). *Comprehensive systematic review for advanced practice nursing* (2nd ed.). New York, NY: Springer Publishing Company.

Staffileno, B. A., & Foreman, M. D. (2018). *Research for advanced practice nurses: From evidence to practice* (3rd ed.). New York, NY: Springer Publishing Company.

RELATED TEXTBOOKS

Holly, C., Salmond, S., & Saimbert, M. (Eds.). (2017). *Comprehensive systematic review for advanced practice nursing* (2nd ed.). New York, NY: Springer Publishing Company.

Staffileno, B. A., & Foreman, M. D. (2018). *Research for advanced practice nurses: From evidence to practice* (3rd ed.). New York, NY: Springer Publishing Company.

Lesson 9.12

DEVELOPING YOUR QUALIFICATIONS AS A NURSE EDUCATOR

BACKGROUND

The DNP degree is a practice-focused doctorate (American Association of Colleges of Nursing [AACN], 2015). "Practice" is defined by the AACN (2004) as "any form of nursing intervention that influences healthcare outcomes for individuals or populations, including the direct care of individual patients, management of care for individuals and populations, administration of nursing and healthcare organizations, and the development and implementation of health policy" (p. 2).

Many students enroll in DNP programs with the intention of becoming a nurse educator in the future. The DNP degree is designed to prepare you for the highest levels of nursing practice. To be an effective nurse educator, you must first be an expert in nursing practice. Obtaining a DNP degree does make you qualified to teach. However, it does not prepare you for the faculty role. Additional training will be needed. The AACN (2015) reaffirmed previous recommendations that nursing education requires a distinct body of knowledge and competencies that are not of the same scope as the DNP degree.

If you are interested in becoming a nurse educator, you can complete additional training and coursework within the DNP program (AACN, 2015). This is optional and may or may not be available as part of your school or DNP curriculum. You must discuss this endeavor with your DNP faculty and DNP program director. If it is an option, this additional study may help you further add to your qualification as a nurse educator. The purpose of this lesson is to explore options for professional development in the nurse educator role offered by the National League for Nursing.

LEARNING OBJECTIVES

- Review the mission statement of the National League for Nursing.
- Examine opportunities for further development in the role of nurse educator.

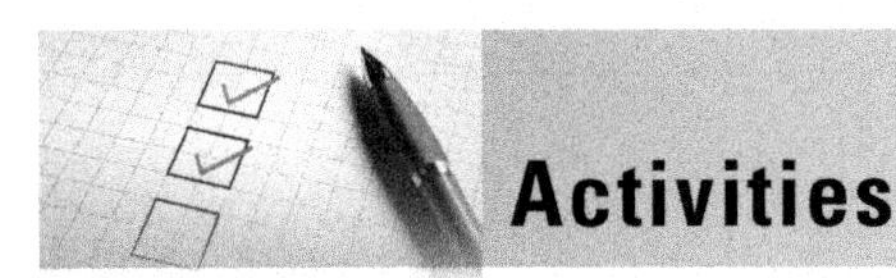

Activities

1. Visit the website of the National League for Nursing (www.nln.org). Review the NLN Vision for Doctoral Preparation of Nurse Educators (www.nln.org/docs/default-source/about/nln-vision-series-%28position-statements%29/nlnvision_6.pdf?sfvrsn=4).

Notes

2. Review the available professional development programs and teaching resources (www.nln.org/professional-development-programs).

Notes

3. Review the qualifications for certification in nursing education (CNE; www.nln.org/Certification-for-Nurse-Educators).

Notes

Identify nurse educator opportunities at your school.

Write a plan to develop your qualifications as a nurse educator.

NEXT STEPS

- Discuss your plans with your DNP team.
- Continue to develop your qualifications as a nurse educator beyond graduation.

REFERENCES AND RESOURCES

American Association of Colleges of Nursing. (2004). *AACN position statement on the practice doctorate in nursing* [White paper]. Retrieved from https://www.aacnnursing.org/Portals/42/News/Position-Statements/DNP.pdf

American Association of Colleges of Nursing. (2015). *The doctor of nursing practice: Current issues and clarifying recommendations* [White paper]. Retrieved from https://www.aacnnursing.org/Portals/42/News/White-Papers/DNP-Implementation-TF-Report-8-15.pdf

RELATED TEXTBOOK

Dreher, H. M., & Glasgow, M. (2018). *DNP role development for doctoral advanced practice nursing.* New York, NY: Springer Publishing Company.
Chapter 7: The Role of the Nurse Educator

Lesson 9.13

COMPLETING A STUDENT REFLECTION

BACKGROUND

Reflective journaling is an opportunity for students to look back on their experience and explore their thoughts (Stevens & Cooper, 2009). Reflective journaling may also allow you to think about how your thoughts have changed over time, recognize the impact of new experiences, and even recognize how you may have done things differently if given the opportunity (Stevens & Cooper, 2009). Use reflective journaling as a strategy for identifying professional growth and development throughout the DNP program.

LEARNING OBJECTIVES

- Use reflective journaling to explore feelings and thoughts about the DNP experience.

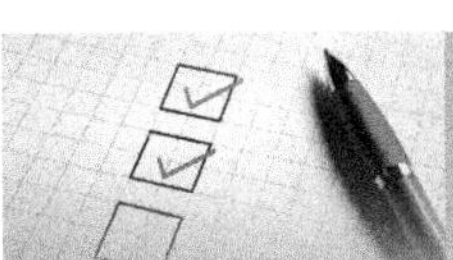

Activities

Using one of the following writing prompts, write a reflective piece related to your DNP experience.

- When I think about my DNP education, the "a-ha" moment that made me change the way I now think was …
- How will having a DNP change the way you practice?
- When you think about your DNP Project, how did your leadership skills allow you to ensure the successful implementation and execution of it?
- Recognizing you are at the end of your formal DNP journey, what would you tell yourself on the eve of the first day of the first class you took?
- How can you use what you have learned in the DNP program (either theoretically or clinically) to impact practice?

NEXT STEPS

- Consider creating a publication on your DNP Experience to encourage other students.
- Discuss your experience with your DNP classmates and faculty.

REFERENCE

Stevens, D., & Cooper, J. (2009). *Journal keeping: How to use reflective writing for effective learning, teaching, professional insight, and positive change.* Sterling, VA: Stylus Publications. Retrieved from http://mcgill.worldcat.org/oclc/646821096

CHAPTER SUMMARY

Here's what former DNP students have shared about their DNP practice experiences:

> "Besides my DNP Project (on a different topic), I spent time in an employer-owned, on-site primary care clinic. It provided care to employees and covered dependents. I led the evaluation of their health indicators (BP, A1c, lipid profile, etc.) for an entire year. The model was so successful the owner was invited to present the model at the Centers for Disease Control Prevention in Atlanta, Georgia. I had the opportunity to be a part of the presentation and the round-table discussion at the CDC."
>
> —*Margaret Zoellers, DNP*

> "My goal was to offer a support group to Jewish women who have experienced pregnancy loss. To learn more, I attended several support groups on pregnancy loss in other areas of the state. Some were focused to the general population and others were specifically for Jewish women of all levels of observance (my population of interest). Although that information was not in my DNP paper, attending those meetings helped me design my intervention."
>
> —*Martha DeCrise, DNP*

> "Besides implementing my project, I spent a lot of time talking with the staff about the project and getting their feedback. I had regular meetings, attended a tobacco cessation training course for providers, and attended other conferences/seminars to get up to date on changes in the healthcare field (related to tobacco abuse/misuse)."
>
> —*Michelle Santoro, DNP*

> "I spent quite a bit of time in a clinic for pregnant women with substance abuse issues ... and on a unit at another agency for infants with neonatal abstinence syndrome. I also shadowed a dean of nursing at another college of nursing who also specializes in perinatal research."
>
> —*Angela Clark, DNP*

> "The DNP experience was divided into three phases. In the planning phase, I completed the Institute for Healthcare Improvement (IHI) Open School courses to learn about the Model for Improvement. Then I hosted a kickoff party, which consisted of one-to-one education sessions on diabetes (my topic of interest), morning huddles, and use of white boards to improve communication. I developed tools, checklists, and a sticker system for providers to better identify diabetic patients. After other work, data collection, and analysis, the project work wrapped up with a SQUIRE (Standards for QUality Improvement Reporting Excellence) paper, storyboard preparation, and presentation to the facility and stakeholders."
>
> —*Tarnia Newton, DNP*

The American Association of Colleges of Nursing (AACN) asserts that a minimum of 1,000 hours of practice beyond the BSN must be performed as part of an academic program. The DNP practice experience hours should expand beyond direct patient care to embrace learning in contexts that align with the DNP Essentials. As you work with your faculty to determine your plan, draw on these student examples and the content of this chapter for inspiration.

10

Finishing Strong: Project Profiles and Empowerment

Molly J. Bradshaw and Tracy R. Vitale

Lessons

OBJECTIVES

In the final chapter, a series of student projects are profiled to illustrate key concepts of the workbook. The profiles summarize the key points of the selected DNP Projects, point out lessons learned, and engage other DNP students in case study. Strategies are offered to help DNP students manage common project-related problems. This chapter and the workbook conclude with a final lesson on the concept of nursing empowerment. By the end of this chapter, you will be able to:

- Review the DNP Project profiles and complete the case study questions.
- Apply the tips for success to your own DNP Project.
- Utilize strategies to address common DNP Project problems.
- Commit to a future of empowering your self and others.

INTRODUCTION

Envision completing your DNP Project. Abraham Lincoln said, "I do the very best I know how ... and I mean to keep doing so to the end (Wise Old Sayings, n.d.)." Ah, completing your DNP Project. Even better, the climax of the DNP program—graduation. What a moment, "Congratulations, Doctor ... (your last name)!" Your moment. This chapter offers final content to help get you to this moment, your moment, with a strong finish.

We believe in leadership by example. Therefore, we asked for the help of recent DNP graduates. We profile key features of their real-world projects to help illustrate major concepts of the workbook. These graduates were all completing their projects after publication of the American Association of Colleges of Nursing (AACN, 2015) white paper, which clarified the recommended content of the DNP Project. These students offer their experiences in overcoming the challenges of the project and present their advice for your success.

We use their projects as inspiration to challenge you. Based on what you have learned in this workbook, we ask you to apply your knowledge. There are no right or wrong answers. But if you were leading, or plan to lead a similar project, we gives you a chance to practice your DNP skills.

The DNP Project does not occur in a test tube. It occurs in the context of an organization, system, and population(s) with complexities. Because it is a first-hand, real-world experience, it is only natural that there you will experience complications, challenges, and problems. We reserve the final lessons of this workbook to help you think through strategies to manage common DNP Project-related problems.

The DNP degree should empower you to engage in the highest levels of nursing practice. As you are empowered, you should also empower others—your colleagues, your team, and, most important, your patients. Completing the DNP Project is only the beginning of the next chapter of your nursing journey. Oprah Winfrey makes a great point by saying, "Doing your best at this moment, puts you in the best spot for the next moment" (Wise Old Sayings, n.d.) Commit to a legacy of empowering self and others in the moments to come in the future. Let's begin.

REFERENCES

American Association of Colleges of Nursing. (2015). *The doctor of nursing practice: Current issues and clarifying recommendations* [White paper]. Retrieved from https://www.aacnnursing.org/Portals/42/News/White-Papers/DNP-Implementation-TF-Report-8-15.pdf

Wise Old Sayings. (n.d.) Finishing strong sayings and quotes. Retrieved from http://www.wiseoldsayings.com/finishing-strong-quotes/

Lesson 10.1

DNP PROJECT PROFILE: IMPLEMENTING EVIDENCE-BASED MESSAGES

Contributing DNP Student: Angela Wood

BACKGROUND

Motivational interviewing (MI) is a common technique utilized to improve communication in DNP Projects. This project was selected because it demonstrates the use of MI for a practice change to deliver an evidence-based message, the 5-2-1-0 message. The project adds value to the current delivery of care using evidence to address factors that contribute to pediatric obesity. In addition to validated instruments, there are clear health indicators for benchmarking patient outcomes.

PROJECT PROFILE

Student: Angela Wood
Project title: "Motivational Interviewing in Primary Care to Improve Lifestyle Choices for School-Age Children" (see Supplement 10.1 available at connect.springerpub.com/content/book/978-0-8261-7433-8/ch10).

Problem: Obesity is becoming an epidemic in the pediatric population. Primary care providers are in an ideal position to intervene; however, they may not approach counseling in an evidence-based way using a standardized message.

Purpose statement: The purpose of the DNP Project was to change practice to utilize MI and the 5-2-1-0 message to improve delivery of information during well-child examinations. The purpose of this lesson is to use this DNP Project as a case study in which to apply your project management and leadership skills.

Implementation framework: Model for Improvement ("Plan, Do, Study, Act" or PDSA)
Intervention population: Providers and parents/guardians of patients
Impact population: Obese children aged 4 to 12 years scheduled for well-child examinations

Methodology:

1. Develop = Train providers in use of 5-2-1-0, MI, and process for project
2. Implement = Evidence-based message (5-2-1-0) using MI
   a. Procedure:
      i. Consent
      ii. Well-child examination with MI and 5-2-1-0 message introduced at end of visit
      iii. 5-2-1-0 materials given, demographic survey, Family Nutrition & Physical Activity (FNPA) completed, Readiness Ruler completed, and information given to principal investigator (PI) in a sealed, numbered envelope; a 1-month follow-up was scheduled
      iv. Made a 2-week follow-up phone call to reinforce information and remind of appointment
      v. A 1-month follow-up appointment; FNPA and Readiness Ruler administered

3. Evaluate
   a. Describe the impact population
      i. Instrument: Self-developed demographic survey
   b. Outcome 1: Behavior modification related to nutrition and activity
      i. Instrument: The FNPA screening tool
   c. Outcome 2: Effectiveness of MI
      i. Instrument: Readiness Ruler from the *Keep Me Healthy Toolkit*

LEARNING OBJECTIVES

- Become inspired by other students.
- Apply project management and leadership skills.
- Transfer lessons learned and advice from DNP students to your DNP Project.

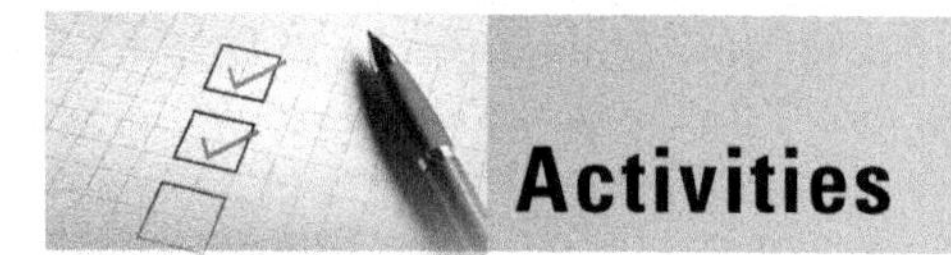

Activities

Part 1: There is clear evidence on the benefit of using both MI and the 5-2-1-0 message in clinical practice. The key is how to translate that information and actually get the providers to use it in practice. Student needs must align with agency needs.

"I identified the practice gap of this clinical agency with the help of the stakeholders (leadership, providers, and staff). It's important to assess and met the needs of the agency to improve patient outcomes. Personal interests may not align with the needs of the agency." —Angela Wood

In your project, how will you assess agency needs and align them with your needs?

____

____

____

____

"If I could change anything in hindsight, I wish I had involved the agency earlier. Their perspective of the problem may have influenced my work in the early DNP courses and prevented my project from changing focus to better align with their needs." —Angela Wood

Part 2: Obesity is an epidemic for all ages. Benchmarking is a quality-improvement technique used to help measure patient outcomes. In regard to benchmarking health outcomes of patients, list some indicators (direct and indirect) of obesity that are improving or being impacted?

"Since the intervention was performed at the well-child exam, we routinely document certain indicators such as height, weight, BMI (body mass index), and blood pressure. Those are certainly direct measures. We can also track the number of patients/families who return for follow-up visits using the electronic health record to show, in a more indirect way, that we are making an effort to impact obesity." —Angela Wood

List the potential indicators, or data points, that are related to your DNP Project outcomes.

____

____

____

____

NEXT STEPS

- Assess the needs of your partnering agency early to better align them with your needs.
- Determine what information is routinely collected that might measure the impact of your project outcomes, directly or indirectly.

REFERENCES AND RESOURCES

Wood, A. (2017, November). *Motivational interviewing in primary care to improve lifestyle choices for school aged children.* Paper presented for the degree of Doctor of Nursing Practice at Eastern Kentucky University, Richmond, Kentucky.

Wood, A. (2018, April). *Motivational interviewing in primary care to improve lifestyle choices for school aged children.* Poster session presented at the 3rd Annual College of Health Sciences Scholars Day, Eastern Kentucky University, Richmond, Kentucky.

RELATED TEXTBOOKS

Sylvia, M. L., & Terhaar, M. F. (2018). *Clinical analytics and data management for the DNP.* New York, NY: Springer Publishing Company.

Chapter 16: Ongoing Monitoring, Benchmarks, pages 291–307

White, K. M., Dudley-Brown, S., & Terhaar, M. F. (Eds.). (2020). *Translation of evidence into nursing and healthcare* (3rd ed.). New York, NY: Springer Publishing Company.

Chapter 1: Evidence-Based Practice

Chapter 4: Translation of Evidence to Improve Clinical Outcomes

Chapter 9: Project Planning and the Work of Translation

Chapter 13: Interprofessional Collaboration and Practice for Translation

Lesson 10.2

DNP PROJECT PROFILE: USE OF THE IHI MODEL FOR IMPROVEMENT

Contributing DNP Student: Tarnia Newton

BACKGROUND

The Institute for Healthcare Improvement (IHI, 2019a) Model for Improvement is more commonly known as the "Plan, Do, Study, Act" or "PDSA" cycle. The goal of this model is to accelerate improvement by making and testing small changes to allow for greater implementation over time. These rapid cycles foster more immediate results and can be adjusted to meet real-world time frames (IHI, 2019a). As mentioned in a previous lesson, we recommend completing the IHI Open School Online Courses and consider utilization of the free *tools* available.

In this lesson, we examine a DNP Project based on use of the Model for Improvement. The student completed the IHI training mentioned and then applied it to improve care for diabetic patients in the clinical setting. There were four rapid PDSA cycles completed in the context of one DNP Project. Keep in mind that many institutional review boards (IRBs) consider quality improvement (QI) an exempt activity.

LEARNING OBJECTIVES

- Appreciate that multiple tests of change can occur in the context of a DNP Project.
- Practice drafting plans for multiple tests of change.
- Envision the potential use of the Model for Improvement in your DNP Project and beyond in future practice.

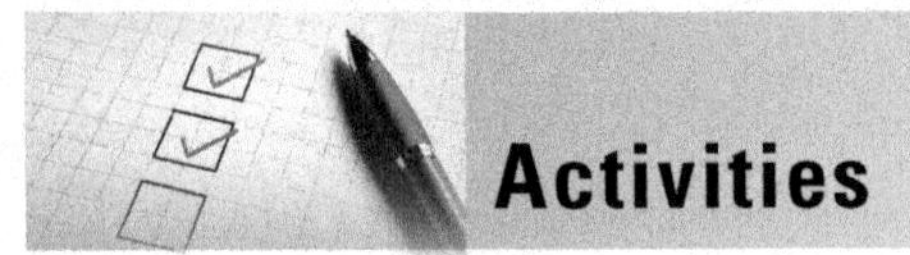

Activities

Use this DNP Project as an exemplar to draft a plan for multiple PDSA cycles.

Student: Tarnia Newton

Project title: "Implementing a Patient-Centered Approach to Standardization of Diabetes Care in a Nurse Practitioner-Led Clinic" (see Supplement 10.2 available at connect.springerpub.com/content/book/978-0-8261-7433-8/ch10).

"The purpose of this project was to improve patient outcomes with diabetes care utilizing the *American Diabetes Association Standards of Medical Care in Diabetes* as a map for creating a plan for improvement. An initial audit based on the key elements of the guideline was conducted to assess compliance. In this population, 75% of patients had HgA1c greater than 8 mg/dL and most patients were missing preventative care measures. My goal was to improve the percentage of diabetic patients receiving standardized, appropriate diabetic care according to the ADA guidelines to 90%." —Tarnia Newton

"I would say my initial predictions were naive and I did not understand the giant task in front of me. The QI project designed consisted of four rapid plan-do-study-act (PDSA) cycles over 90 days. Each PDSA cycle was approached with tests of change and categorized into team and patient engagement as well as two process changes: (1) Diabetic Care Measures Checklist (DCMC) and (2) a preventative care referral. Each cycle was modified and implemented every 2 weeks based on team, patient feedback, and data findings. Technically running four QI projects simultaneously" (see Figure 10.1 and Table 10.1). —Tarnia Newton

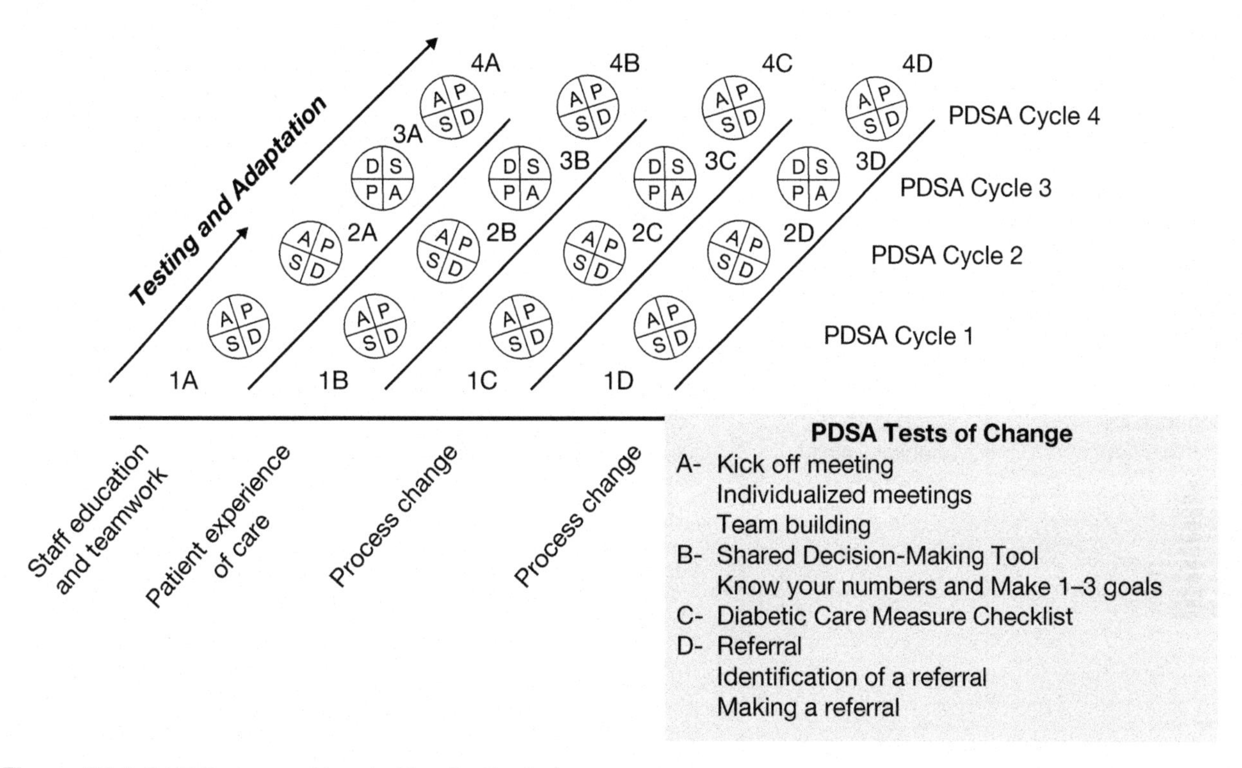

Figure 10.1 DNP Project rapid cycle Plan-Do-Study-Act ramps.
PDSA, Plan, Do, Study, Act.
Source: Reproduced with permission from Langley, G. J., Moen, R. D., Nolan, K. M., Nolan, T. W., Norman, C. L., & Provost, L. P. (2009). *The improvement guide: A practical approach to enhancing organizational performance* (2nd ed.). San Francisco, CA: Jossey-Bass.

Table 10.1 Plan-Do-Study-Act Cycles and Interventions

FOCUS	PDSA #1	PDSA #2	PDSA #3	PDSA #4
Team engagement	1. Weekly team meeting 2. Implement team on diabetes teaching confidence survey	1. Add end-of PDSA-cycle meetings 2. One-on-one educational sessions with team	Initiated 10-minute morning huddles to motivate and reinforce QI	Implement a huddle white board to assist the organic engagement for the team to discuss diabetic patients for the day
Patient engagement	Patient engagement forms placed on charts for use	Creation and placement of posters in patient areas to empower diabetic patients to complete engagement forms	Engagement form prefilled with patient lab numbers	Add additional information for patients to support diabetic goals
Diabetic care measure checklist	Implement using diabetic checklist and placed on chart	1. Placed checklist on the outside of chart 2. Reminder notes on laptops to complete form	Charts prepped the day prior with checklist filled with lab results	1. Create HPI template in EMR for checklist information 2. One-on-one educational session for providers to capture checklist in HPI template
Preventative Care Referral	Referring diabetic patient to ophthalmology, podiatry, and nutrition	Add referral focus area on checklist form	Referral cards created for patient to get at the front desk	Add provider profile in EMR for ophthalmology, podiatry, and nutrition

EMR, electronic medical record; HPI, history of the present illness; PDSA, Plan-Do-Study-Act; QI, quality improvement.

Use the example of this DNP Project as inspiration. In the context of your DNP Project, if the Model for Improvement is used, how might multiple cycles fit together and build on one another? Start with the four prompts given in Figure 10.2.

Cycle on Team Engagement:

Cycle on Patient Engagement:

Cycle on Process Change 1:

Cycle on Process Change 2:

"The DNP skill set is different than anything else you might have experienced. But this process will give you the skill set required to be a change agent. Be ready to put on a new pair of glasses because you won't see healthcare the same way." —Tarnia Newton

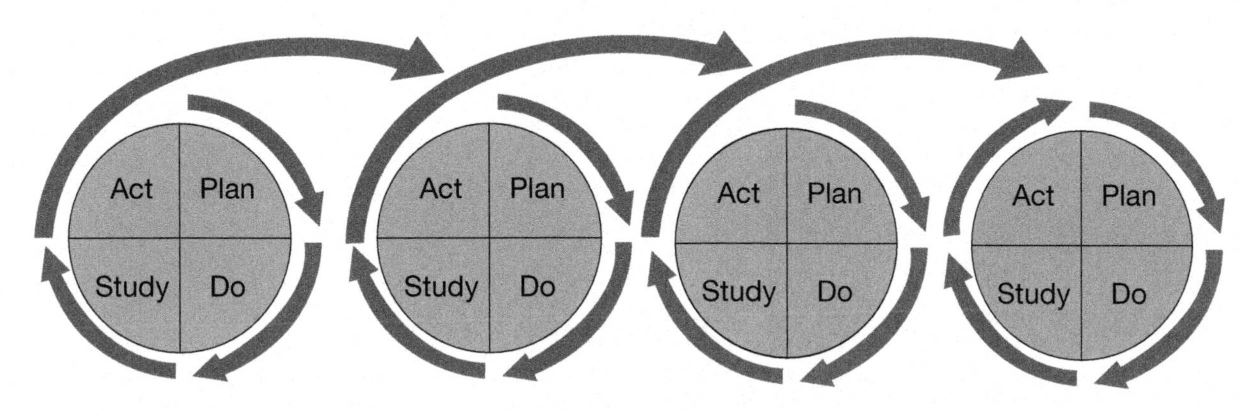

Figure 10.2 Model for Improvement.
Source: Institute for Healthcare Improvement. (2019a). How to improve. Retrieved from http://www.ihi.org/resources/Pages/HowtoImprove/default.aspx

NEXT STEPS

- Discuss your plans with your DNP team.
- Consider running multiple rapid PDSA cycles each with unique focus.
- Continue to utilize the Model for Improvement beyond DNP graduation.

REFERENCES AND RESOURCES

Institute for Healthcare Improvement. (2018, December). IHI national forum on quality improvement in health care. Retrieved from http://www.ihi.org/education/Conferences/Forum2017/Pages/2018-National-Forum.aspx

Institute for Healthcare Improvement. (2019a). How to improve. Retrieved from http://www.ihi.org/resources/Pages/HowtoImprove/default.aspx

Institute for Healthcare Improvement. (2019b, March). IHI/BMJ international forum on quality and safety in healthcare. Retrieved from http://internationalforum.bmj.com/

Institute for Healthcare Improvement. (2019c). Tools. Retrieved from www.ihi.org/resources/Pages/HowtoImprove/default.aspx

Institute for Healthcare Improvement. (2019d). Open school online courses. Retrieved from http://app.ihi.org/lmsspa/#/6cb1c614-884b-43ef-9abd-d90849f183d4

Langley, G. J., Moen, R. D., Nolan, K. M., Nolan, T. W., Norman, C. L., & Provost, L. P. (2009). *The improvement guide: A practical approach to enhancing organizational performance* (2nd ed.). San Francisco, CA: Jossey-Bass.

Western Institute of Nursing National Conference. (2019a, April). Improving diabetes care with TEAM engagement: A QI project (podium). Retrieved from https://www.winursing.org/2019-researchconference/

Western Institute of Nursing National Conference. (2019b, April). Improving diabetes care in a nurse-practitioner-led clinic: A QI project (poster). Retrieved from https://www.winursing.org/2019-researchconference/

RELATED TEXTBOOKS

Christenbery, T. (Ed.). (2018). *Evidence-based practice in nursing*. New York, NY: Springer Publishing Company.

Chapter 14: Quality Improvement Processes and Evidence-Based Practice

Hickey, J. V., & Brosnan, C. A. (Eds.). (2017). *Evaluation of health care quality for DNPs* (2nd ed.). New York, NY: Springer Publishing Company.

Chapter 8: Quality Improvement

Lesson 10.3

DNP PROJECT PROFILE: COMMUNITY-BASED PROJECTS AND POPULATION HEALTH

Contributing DNP Student: Martha De Crisce

BACKGROUND

"Population health" is classically defined as the health outcomes of a group of individuals (Kindig & Stoddart, 2003). The American Association of Colleges of Nursing (AACN, 2015) recommends that a DNP

Project has a population focus. Remember that populations exist in various places and healthcare is not always delivered in traditional clinic-based settings or hospitals. Where does your population of interest exist?

Providing healthcare to populations in a community-based setting is a feasible context for a DNP Project. The DNP Project profiled in this lesson embodies population health, evidence-based practice, engagement of community stakeholders, and collaboration with both healthcare colleagues and religious leaders. It was developed using the Centers for Disease Control and Prevention's (CDC) framework for program evaluation.

LEARNING OBJECTIVES

- Determine the importance of a "needs survey" for your DNP Project.
- Identify experts who may contribute to intervention development.
- Relate the CDC's framework for program evaluation to your current and future practice (Figure 10.3).

PROJECT PROFILE

Student: Martha De Crisce
Project title: "Addressing Pregnancy Loss Among Jewish Women" (see Supplement 10.3 available at connect.springerpub.com/content/book/978-0-8261-7433-8/ch10).

Problem: Orthodox Jewish women were lacking access to culturally appropriate resources after experiencing pregnancy loss. The current literature describes evidence for support after pregnancy loss, but it was not customized to the target population.

Purpose statement: The purpose of this DNP Project was to develop, implement, and evaluate a culturally appropriate, evidence-based support group for Orthodox Jewish women who have experienced pregnancy loss.

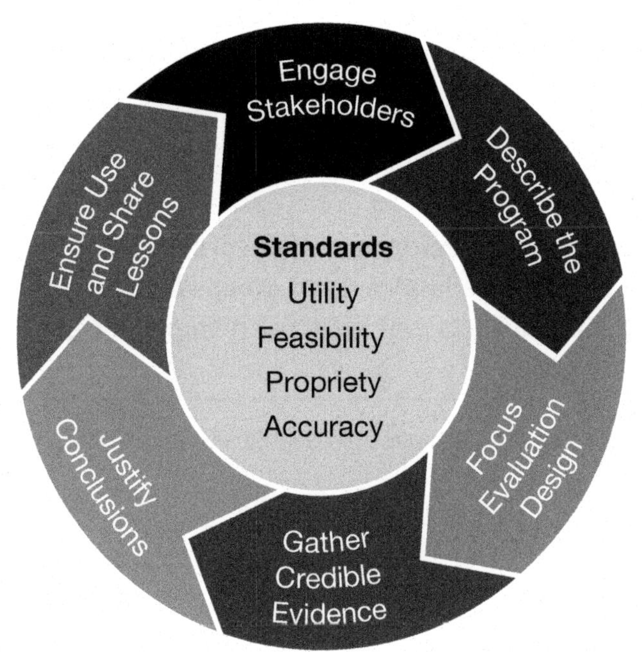

Figure 10.3 Centers for Disease Control and Prevention framework for program evaluation.
Source: Centers for Disease Control and Prevention. (1999). Framework for program evaluation in public health. *Morbidity and Mortality Weekly Report, 48*(RR-11).

"My top three challenges for this project were:

1. Lack of population-specific, evidence-based literature
2. Lack of community support
3. Fear of stigma associated with pregnancy loss among the targeted population."

"There was not much that I could do about the literature, but I could gather suggestions from the literature on pregnancy loss in other populations. There were common themes about how they perceived their loss and dealt with their emotions."

"I used this evidence to create a needs survey. It was very important for me to document the needs of my population to support the importance of my project. I used the results of the survey to design my support group. The local YM–YWHA, or Jewish Community Center, was willing to host my project. Because many Jewish women from my community were members, the center allowed me to send the survey out via its mailing list. The needs survey captured important data to present to my stakeholders." — Martha De Crisce

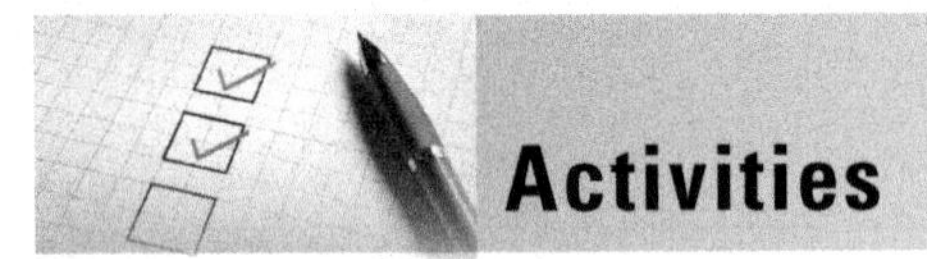

Reflecting on this DNP Project, complete these activities:

Q: Should a needs survey be conducted to assess your target population? Write your thoughts here to share with your DNP team.

- What are key findings in the literature that need to be affirmed or denied?

- Are there logical questions you need to ask?

The DNP experience hours can be critical to the development of the project intervention. "Before implementing my project, I attended several support groups for pregnancy loss. Some were for my target population and some were not, but it helped me get a sense of what worked and what didn't." Martha De Crisce

---

Q: Could you attend similar events related to your DNP Project? Explore possible events and list them here:

Community leaders, experts, and stakeholders can help operationalize the DNP Project.

"I engaged the support of the local rabbi(s). They saw a need and were open to embracing a support group. The sensitive, religious nature of this topic and this population made their input critical. I was also supported by a psychiatrist, who was instrumental in developing the content of each session for the support group. I did undergo full IRB review since my target population was a vulnerable population." —Martha De Crisce

Q: Are there leaders, experts, or stakeholders who could/should contribute to your DNP Project? Write your notes here, listing names and possible contributions.

Q: Are you involved in a community-based program (project related or otherwise) that would benefit from improved evaluation? How can you use your DNP skills to be instrumental in evaluating the program's success? Write your notes here.

NEXT STEPS

- "Focus on a problem you are passionate about. It would be difficult to put forth so much hard work and effort toward a topic/problem that has little meaning to you."
- "Find a team that supports your vision that has open-minded members. A good team is one that supports your project and makes good recommendations to improve it." —Martha De Crisce

REFERENCES AND RESOURCES

American Association of Colleges of Nursing. (2015). *The doctor of nursing practice: Current issues and clarifying recommendations* [White paper]. Retrieved from https://www.aacnnursing.org/Portals/42/News/White-Papers/DNP-Implementation-TF-Report-8-15.pdf

Centers for Disease Control and Prevention. (2019). Framework for program evaluation. Retrieved from https://www.cdc.gov/eval/framework/index.htm

Centers for Disease Control and Prevention. (1999). Framework for program evaluation in public health. *Morbidity and Mortality Weekly Report, 48*(RR-11).

De Crisce, M. (2018, May). *Addressing pregnancy loss among Jewish women.* Poster session presented at the Orthodox Jewish Nurses Association Annual Conference, New York, NY. Retrieved from https://jewishnurses.org/past-conferences/conference/

Kindig, D., & Stoddart, G. (2003). What is population health? *American Journal of Public Health, 93*(3), 380–383.

RELATED TEXTBOOK

Curley, A. L., & Vitale, P. A. (2016). *Population-based nursing.* New York, NY: Springer Publishing Company.

Chapter 2: Identifying Outcomes

Chapter 10: Challenges in Program Implementation

Lesson 10.4

DNP PROJECT PROFILE: ADVOCACY TO CREATE A BODY OF SCHOLARSHIP

Contributing DNP Student: Aleksandra Novik

BACKGROUND

The DNP Project profiled in this lesson demonstrates a practice change in a small, private primary care office that eventually made an impact at the state and national levels by engaging in advocacy. Advocacy was accomplished by a series of presentations, contact with local legislators, and publication of the project on a public website. These DNP experiences generated interest that eventually caught the attention of the governor's office and Dr. Margaret Fitzgerald.

The American Association of Colleges of Nursing (AACN, 2015) advocates for use of the DNP Project as a platform for future scholarship. We add that the DNP experience also provides an opportunity to create a body of scholarship.

PROJECT PROFILE

Student: Aleksandra Novik
Project title: "Use of Controlled Dangerous Substance Tools by Advanced Practice Nurses in the State of New Jersey" (see Supplements 10.4 and 10.5, available at connect.springerpub.com/content/book/978-0-8261-7433-8/ch10).

Problem: Nurse practitioners and other providers prescribing opioids may not fully utilize available resources or best evidence. In a small, private practice, a nurse practitioner (NP) requested development of a better form to use when signing controlled substance contracts with patients. Also, at the time, there was a new requirement to inform patients of local places to drop off unused prescription drugs, but many providers were unaware of the resource.

The purpose of this DNP Project was to close this practice gap by:

- Creating an evidence-based controlled substance agreement form meeting the requirements of the state and at the appropriate level of health literacy.
- Vetting the form through practicing NPs and implementing it into practice.
- Developing an advocacy initiative to utilize state resources, such as the controlled substance monitoring program and prescription drop-off locations.

Purpose statement: The purpose of this lesson is to demonstrate the impact of advocacy as a strategy to impact both organizational and public policy as well as build a body of scholarship.

LEARNING OBJECTIVES

- Discuss opportunities to scale DNP Projects with advocacy.
- Develop a plan to create multiple presentations and a body of DNP scholarship.

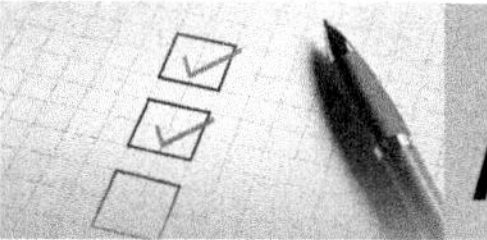

Activities

When DNP Projects occur in small settings, there is often concern that the practice change is "not enough" for doctoral work. Advocating for best practices by offering tools is a way to scale the DNP Project and impact policy. Review the components of this project, listed on the left. Next to each activity, identify and discuss opportunities related to your DNP Project.

ADVOCACY EXAMPLE	ADVOCACY OPPORTUNITY FOR YOUR DNP PROJECT
Offer evidence-based tools via a website platform. Visit this project's website at https://aleksandranovik.wixsite.com/cdsmonitoringtools	
Foster local engagement of patients by sharing information on controlled substances at a local health fair.	
Gain state wide engagement of nursing professionals by using poster presentation regarding state policy at prescription drop-off points.	
Encourage national engagement of NPs via poster presentation regarding the outcome of the project survey and the evidence-based controlled substance agreement.	
Schedule meeting with local legislators' offices to share evidence-based tools related to public policies.	

Pearls and Evidence of Advocacy Success

"Participate in conferences and presentations as much as possible at all levels. Pick different components of your work to focus on at each presentation so that the presentations are not identical. This provides an opportunity to become known as a topic expert and leads to new opportunities. For example, Dr. Margaret Fitzgerald approached me at my poster at the American Association of Nurse Practitioner's national conference and invited me to contribute to her monthly newsletter!"— Aleksandra Novik

"I was invited to speak at a conference on opioids at Drew University. A member of the governor's office was in attendance and approached me afterward to share my work with a state task force on opioid prescribing policies. Having my tool on a website platform made sharing the work easy. The fact that I vetted the form and surveyed nurse practitioners to understand their habits regarding controlled substances provided data and credibility to my work." — Aleksandra Novik

NEXT STEPS

- "Learn about what your DNP colleagues are doing and identify opportunities to work together. For example, I partnered with a DNP student to review my tool for components of health literacy. If you develop tools to use with patients, ensure they are both evidence based and health literacy appropriate." — Aleksandra Novik
- "Prior to DNP graduation, I completed three poster presentations and two podium presentations. Work with faculty who are both knowledgeable but also vested in the subject matter. I learned about the importance of sharing the changes I make in my clinical practice with others. I encourage you to do the same." — Aleksandra Novik

REFERENCES AND RESOURCES

American Association of Colleges of Nursing. (2015). *The doctor of nursing practice: Current issues and clarifying recommendations* [White paper]. Retrieved from https://www.aacnnursing.org/Portals/42/News/White-Papers/DNP-Implementation-TF-Report-8-15.pdf

Bradshaw, M., VanWyck, K., & Novik, A. (2017, April 3). *Research to reality: Taking action in primary care to address the opioid epidemic.* Podium presentation at the Symposium on Combating Opioids and the Addiction Crisis, Drew University, Madison, NJ.

Fitzgerald Health Education Associates. (2017). *Controlled dangerous substance agreement form. Newsletter,* October 2017. *Retrieved from* https://www.fhea.com/newsletter.aspx

Novik, A. (2017). CDS monitoring tools. Retrieved from https://aleksandranovik.wixsite.com/cdsmonitoringtools/results

Novik, A., Padovano, C., & Bradshaw, M. (2016a). *NJ prescription monitoring program.* Poster presented at the Morristown Medical Center, Morristown, NJ.

Novik, A., Padovano, C., & Bradshaw, M. (2016b). *Project medicine drop.* Poster Presentation, New Jersey State Nurses' Association Annual Conference, Atlantic City, NJ.

Novik, A., Padovano, C., & Bradshaw, M. (2017). *Use of CDS agreement forms by NJ NPs.* Poster presentated at the American Association of Nurse Practitioner National Conference, Philadelphia, PA.

RELATED TEXTBOOKS

Goudreau, K. A., & Smolenski, M. C. (2018). *Health policy and the advanced practice nurse.* New York, NY: Springer Publishing Company.

Grady, P. A., & Hinshaw, A. S. (2017). *Using nursing research to shape health policy.* New York, NY: Springer Publishing Company.

Zalon, M., & Patton, R. (2019). *Nursing making policy* (2nd ed.). New York, NY: Springer Publishing Company.

Lesson 10.5

DNP PROJECT PROFILE: RECOVERING AFTER YOUR TOPIC CHANGES

Student Contributor: Margaret Zoellers

BACKGROUND

The goals of the partnering agency and DNP student must be in alignment, following an agreed-upon timetable. Despite the best efforts to collaborate and/or control variables, sometimes there are complicating circumstances arise. The DNP student may need to change topics and/or change the location of the DNP Project as a result.

LEARNING OBJECTIVES

- Review the DNP Project profile.
- Remember to utilize the recovery questions if needed.

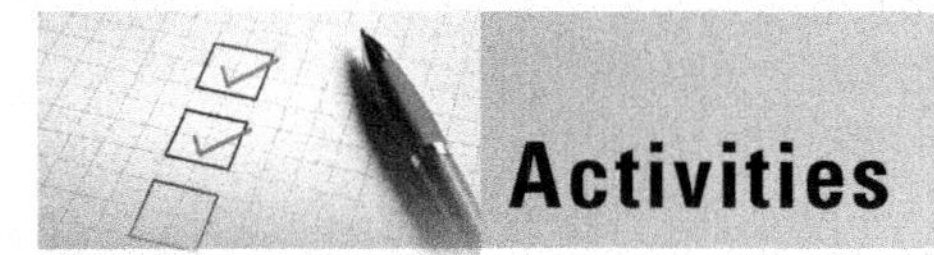

Activities

Review the following DNP Project profile.

Project Profile

Student: Margaret Zoellers

Project title: "A Process Improvement for Depression Screening and Management in a University Health Clinic" (see Supplement 10.6 available at connect.springerpub.com/content/book/978-0-8261-7433-8/ch10).

"My initial DNP Project site was awesome! An employer had established on-site primary care for employees and their dependents. I spent some time there helping them collect data on health indicators such as A1c, lipid levels, BMI, blood pressure, and so on. I was ultimately planning to implement my DNP Project there. Unfortunately, there was an unexpected health challenge for the clinic director, who had to be temporarily replaced during recovery. As a result, the employer/clinic owner felt adding a DNP Project during this period would become too difficult to manage. I had to change sites, which meant changing topics." —Margaret Zoellers

INITIAL PROJECT	FINAL PROJECT
Location: On-site, employer-sponsored health clinic	Location: University student health clinic
Target population: Employees and dependents of the agency	Target population: Students and providers involved in student health services
Problem: Identification of chronic disease indicators and improvement of population health through primary care services and lifestyle modification (Model presented to the CDC)	Problem: Improving process for depression screening and treatment

Reflect on the circumstances described here and discuss the scenario with your DNP team.

- Is it appropriate to "relocate" a project from one site to another?
- What are the challenges associated with that?

In the event of unforeseen circumstances, reflect on these recovery questions:

- Is there a different organization interested in the same problem?
- Would that organization be willing to partner with the DNP student?
- What elements of the project would change if the location changes?

"A change of agency after beginning to formulate a project plan was disheartening. I lost a semester of work and time that would have provided the groundwork for my project. There was no option except to begin again with a new agency/problem. I utilized the skills from my core DNP courses to start again. Feeling overwhelmed by the unfamiliar process, I reached out to my DNP advisor often, but also peers and other qualified people for input, guidance, and encouragement." — Margaret Zoellers

Make a list of people who you can reach out to for input, guidance, and encouragement during your DNP Project process:

1.

2.

3.

As you have noticed, there have been several steps and hurdles to overcome as you plan, develop, and implement your project. Your project has likely evolved from the time you starting thinking about what you would like to study. However, sometimes along the way, for a variety of reasons, the project changes. This is different from the project evolving. This may require a complete change in focus or topic. Although this may be extremely discouraging and outside your control, being equipped with strategies to recover will help you navigate this process.

Be proactive rather than reactive. Certainly, it is understandable that you may be upset about the circumstances surrounding why your project has changed, but be proactive and keep yourself moving forward. This too shall pass and soon enough you will be well on your way with a new topic.

Be adaptable and flexible. Recognize that although you were committed to the previous project, it is now necessary to be adaptable and flexible in considering the new project topic.

Consider uncertainties that come along with a project. You have already had to adjust to different stakeholders influencing the development of the project and what that entails. That said, you will want to consider how they may contribute to any uncertainties related to your project.

Remain confident. We could argue the point that everything happens for a reason, but that may provide little consolation while you are in the thick of it and trying to start from scratch.

NEXT STEPS

- "Identify a student peer for collaboration and moral support."
- "Realize that you are likely not going to change the world with your DNP Project—but you will make a difference." — Margaret Zoellers

REFERENCE AND RESOURCE

Zoellers, M. H. (2018). A process improvement for depression screening and management in a University Health Clinic. *Doctor of Nursing Practice Capstone Projects*, 34. Retrieved from https://encompass.eku.edu/dnpcapstones/34

RELATED TEXTBOOK

White, K. M., Dudley-Brown, S., & Terhaar, M. F. (Eds.). (2020). *Translation of evidence into nursing and healthcare* (3rd ed.). New York, NY: Springer Publishing Company.

Chapter 15: Best Practices in Translation: Challenges and Barriers in Translation

Lesson 10.6

THE APPROACH TO "NEGATIVE" OR "BAD" RESULTS

BACKGROUND

It is helpful to remember that the DNP Project is a learning experience. It is an opportunity to develop, implement, and evaluate practice improvements with the help and support of your DNP team. The list that follows contains some frequently asked questions regarding negative or bad results.

LEARNING OBJECTIVES

- Appreciate the importance of a "negative" or "bad" result.
- Articulate DNP Project limitations with transparency.

Q: *"What if my DNP Project does not show 'statistical' significance?"*
A: *Statistical significance* refers to the amount of certainty there is that the intervention (independent variable) caused the result. Its lack does not mean that the DNP Project is not meaningful.

Q: *"What if my DNP Project results are 'negative' or 'bad'?"*
A: Even evidence-based interventions can be unsuccessful. But that's okay! According to Dr. Irina Benenson, "If an intervention doesn't produce the outcome we want, we should consider abandoning the practice or trying a different approach." A negative result simply means that you have to do something different.

Q: *"Should I only report the good information and omit the bad?"*
A: No, report results and limitations with accuracy and transparency. As a student, you should try to consider what factors contributed to the negative result. Report things as they actually happened. Discuss the limitations of the DNP Project.

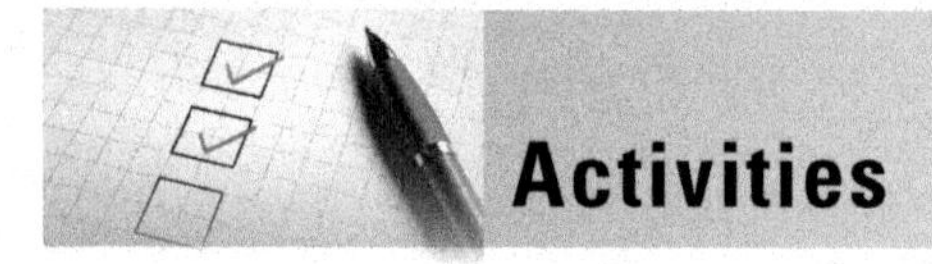

Activities

Talk to your faculty members hypothetically about what happens if the outcome of your DNP Project is not favorable. Record the key points of the discussion here.

Expert Commentary: Tracy R. Vitale, DNP, RNC-OB, C-EFM, NE-BC

When I conducted my DNP Project, I was devastated when I completed my data analysis and found negative results. As some background, I was looking to identify how participating in a structured mentorship program impacted nurse leaders' transformational leadership practices and job satisfaction. I double- and triple-checked my results because I must have done something wrong in the analysis. Maybe I had mixed up my categories? Maybe I had clicked the wrong button? But no ... I had negative results!

I felt defeated, disappointed, and as if all my work had been for nothing. After a long (ugly) cry, I reached out to my project chair and asked for help. He calmly talked me down and said, "Your data are your data. You can't change that. What you can do is to examine your results and consider possible reasons why that happened and speak to it." If you have negative results, use the information for your benefit and speak to what may have influenced the results. In my case, most of my sample of nurse leaders were in their mid-50s. It is likely that regardless of having participated in the structured mentoring, the two groups likely received mentoring in some capacity, at some point in their 20- to 30+-year nursing careers. My results could also have been different had I used a better project design. There are several factors (limitations) that may have been the reason for my results. The bottom line is your results are your results ... and that's okay!

Looking back, I wish someone would have prepared me for the possibility of negative results. Perhaps then I would not have panicked like I did or worried that I would not be able to graduate. In fact, the more I talked about my results and surprised people with them, the more confidently I was able to speak to the potential whys, how I could have improved my project, or how I can use those results for future research and scholarly work. There was a benefit in having my results be what they were; I was able to use my DNP education and speak to how the results align/do not align with existing evidence. I am able to see the importance of project design and methodology impacting the quality of the DNP Project. Also, perhaps what I am most proud of is that in a time when we encourage students to work toward publishing their DNP work, I, too, was able to publish the results of my DNP Project—negative results and all!

So, although your results may be negative, you must stay positive! Learn from the experience and use the fundamentals you studied in your doctoral classes to identify and analyze why you had those results, recommend opportunities to address those factors and limitations, and keep moving forward! Remember ... negative results do not equal failure, but rather more evidence to contribute to the greater body of knowledge. Your data matter just as much as everyone else's data, so keep your chin up and be proud of the work you have done.

NEXT STEPS

- Discuss the potential outcomes of negative results with your DNP team.
- Stay encouraged even if the results of the project are not what you expect.

RELATED TEXTBOOK

Sylvia, M. L., & Terhaar, M. F. (2019). *Clinical analytics and data management for the DNP*. New York, NY: Springer Publishing Company.

Lesson 10.7

FINISHING ON A NOTE OF EMPOWERMENT

BACKGROUND

The DNP Project and the DNP degree are instruments of nursing empowerment. "Empowerment" essentially means being equipped or having the ability to get things done (Christenbery, 2018). You are now equipped with essential skills to solve complex healthcare problems and lead interprofessional teams. You can develop, implement, and evaluate the impact of evidence-based solutions on patient outcomes.

LEARNING OBJECTIVES

- Describe the contribution your doctoral work has made.
- Relate the meaning of the work to elements of an empowered organization.

What do you think of when you think of empowerment? How do you empower yourself? How do you empower others?

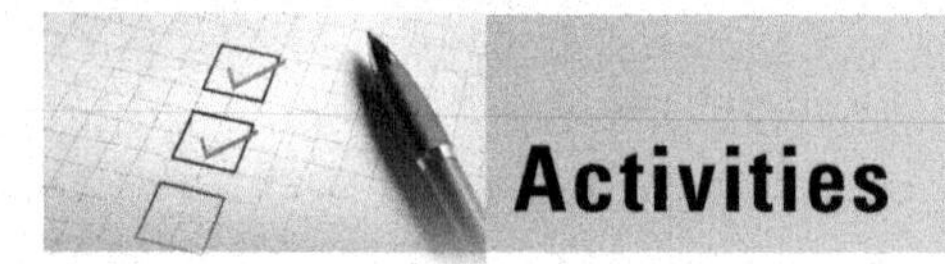

Activities

Consider the empowering behaviors listed in Box 10.1. Highlight the three that are most important to you.

BOX 10.1 Example of Empowering Behaviors

Organizations that encourage empowerment provide the following:

- Opportunities for professional growth and development
- Stimulating and challenging work
- Opportunities to gain new work-related knowledge and skills
- Access to resources to accomplish work
- Time allotted to complete work
- Encouragement to find meaning in work
- Information needed to accomplish work
- Support from management to meet responsibilities and work activities
- Opportunities to work collaboratively with other departments and interprofessional teams
- Recognition for work well done
- Tangible recognition from organizational leadership for the work done

Source: From Christenbery, T. (Ed.). (2018). *Evidence-based practice in nursing.* New York, NY: Springer Publishing Company.

Based on your selections, list two ways that you will continue to foster these behaviors after graduation:

1.

2.

Briefly describe the meaning and contribution your doctoral work has made.

Contribution to your personal/professional growth:

Contribution to your partnering organization:

Contribution to the nursing profession:

NEXT STEP

- Empower self and others in your future endeavors.

REFERENCE AND RESOURCE

Christenbery, T. (Ed.). (2018). *Evidence-based practice in nursing.* New York, NY: Springer Publishing Company.

RELATED TEXTBOOKS

Christenbery, T. (Ed.). (2018). *Evidence-based practice in nursing.* New York, NY: Springer Publishing Company.

Chapter 15: Evidence-Based Practice: A Culture of Organizational Empowerment

Chapter 20: Evidence-Based Practice: Empowering Nurses

CHAPTER SUMMARY

Consider how far you have come since you started this journey toward the DNP. You will soon be a doctorally prepared nurse leader. You will be qualified at the highest level of nursing practice. Take a minute to look back at where you started just a short time ago. It is likely that somewhere along the way you were inspired by another nurse leader, a colleague, a faculty member, or even another student. Remember to be that source of inspiration for others in the future. It is now your moment to carry that forward and, as Mahatma Gandhi said, "be the change you wish to see in the world." We are confident that you will finish strong!

NOTES

Appendix
Project Management Resources

COMMUNICATION FORM

DNP student:

Other attendees:

Date:

Purpose of the meeting/communication:

Notes:

Action items:

Timeline for completion:

Next scheduled meeting:

Other plans for follow-up:

GROUP PROJECT PLANNING FORM

The American Association of Colleges of Nursing (AACN, 2015) specifies that although group projects can be valuable, they do present some challenges, especially when it comes to evaluation/grading them. AACN (2015) also indicates that each member of a project team must successfully meet all expectations of planning, implementation, and evaluation and the work of each must be evaluated separately. Students who are completing a group DNP project should submit this form to the DNP chair for approval at the beginning of the DNP planning process.

REQUIREMENTS	STUDENT A ________	STUDENT B ________
Describe the contributions to overall DNP project planning		
Describe the aim/objectives for which student is taking a leadership role		
Describe contributions to: • Writing the DNP project proposal • Proposal presentation • IRB Submission • Developing Plan for Experience • Hours		
Describe the contributions to: • Project Planning • Project implementation • Project evaluation/data analysis and synthesis		
Describe the contributions to methods of dissemination: • Final project paper • Final project poster • Final project presentation		
Other project-related contributions:		
Student signatures:		

Approved by DNP chair:

Name: **Date:**

EXPERIENCE LOG

DATE	COURSE	DESCRIPTION OF EXPERIENCE ACTIVITY	DNP ESSENTIAL	# OF HOURS ANTICIPATED	# OF HOURS COMPLETED	CUMULATIVE HOURS

DATE	COURSE	DESCRIPTION OF EXPERIENCE ACTIVITY	DNP ESSENTIAL	# OF HOURS ANTICIPATED	# OF HOURS COMPLETED	CUMULATIVE HOURS

DATE	COURSE	DESCRIPTION OF EXPERIENCE ACTIVITY	DNP ESSENTIAL	# OF HOURS ANTICIPATED	# OF HOURS COMPLETED	CUMULATIVE HOURS

DNP ESSENTIALS	
1 - Scientific Underpinnings for Practice	1
2 - Organizational and Systems Leadership for Quality Improvement and Systems Thinking	2
3 - Clinical Scholarship and Analytical Methods for Evidence-Based Practice	3
4 - Information Systems/Technology and Patient Care Technology for the Improvement and Transformation of Healthcare	4
5 - Healthcare Policy for Advocacy in Healthcare	5
6 - Interprofessional Collaboration for Improving Patient and Population Health Outcomes	6
7 - Clinical Prevention and Population Health for Improving the Nation's Health	7
8 - Advanced Nursing Practice	8

REFERENCE

American Association of Colleges of Nursing. (2015). *The doctor of nursing practice: Current issues and clarifying recommendations* [White paper]. Retrieved from https:// www.aacnnursing.org/ Portals/42/News/White- Papers/ DNP- Implementation-TF- Report-8-15.pdf

Index